Advances in the Diagnosis and Treatment of Genitourinary Cancers

Advances in the Diagnosis and Treatment of Genitourinary Cancers

Guest Editors

Piotr Radziszewski
Łukasz Zapała

MDPI

Basel • Beijing • Wuhan • Barcelona • Belgrade • Novi Sad • Cluj • Manchester

Guest Editors
Piotr Radziszewski
Clinic of General, Oncological
and Functional Urology
Medical University of Warsaw
Warsaw
Poland

Łukasz Zapała
Clinic of General, Oncological
and Functional Urology
Medical University of Warsaw
Warsaw
Poland

Editorial Office
MDPI AG
Grosspeteranlage 5
4052 Basel, Switzerland

This is a reprint of the Special Issue, published open access by the journal *Cancers* (ISSN 2072-6694), freely accessible at: https://www.mdpi.com/journal/cancers/special_issues/303JT7BB09.

For citation purposes, cite each article independently as indicated on the article page online and as indicated below:

Lastname, A.A.; Lastname, B.B. Article Title. *Journal Name* **Year**, *Volume Number*, Page Range.

ISBN 978-3-7258-6776-9 (Hbk)
ISBN 978-3-7258-6777-6 (PDF)
https://doi.org/10.3390/books978-3-7258-6777-6

Contents

cancers

MDPI

Article

Does the Administration of Intravenous Fluid Matter in the Context of the Incidence of Postoperative Complications After Radical Cystectomy?

Paweł Lipowski [1,*], Adam Ostrowski [1], Jan Adamowicz [1,2], Przemysław Jasiewicz [3], Filip Kowalski [1], Tomasz Drewa [1] and Kajetan Juszczak [1,*]

1 Department of Urology and Andrology, Collegium Medicum, Nicolaus Copernicus University, M. Curie Skłodowskiej 9, 85-094 Bydgoszcz, Poland; adostro@gmail.com (A.O.); adamowicz.jz@gmail.com (J.A.); urologpolska@gmail.com (F.K.); t.drewa@wp.pl (T.D.)

2 Department of Regenerative Medicine, Collegium Medicum, Nicolaus Copernicus University, M. Curie Skłodowskiej 9, 85-094 Bydgoszcz, Poland

3 Department of Anesthesiology and Intensive Care, Collegium Medicum, Nicolaus Copernicus University, 85-094 Bydgoszcz, Poland; pjasiewicz@cm.umk.pl

* Correspondence: pavelipovsky@gmail.com (P.L.); kaj.juszczak@gmail.com (K.J.); Tel.: +48-52-585-60-80 (P.L. & K.J.)

Simple Summary: Intravenous fluid management plays a key role in perioperative care, particularly in patients undergoing radical cystectomy (RC) within enhanced recovery after surgery (ERAS) protocols. This study analyzed 288 patients who underwent laparoscopic RC with urinary diversion to evaluate the impact of fluid administration on postoperative complications assessed 30 days after surgery. Patients were categorized based on the type of urinary diversion (ureterocutaneostomy or ileal conduit) and the volume of intraoperative fluids administered (less than or more than 1000 mL). The results showed that administering more than 1000 mL of fluids was initially associated with an increased risk of complications, but this association lost statistical significance after adjusting for surgery duration and BMI. Indices such as the absolute Vascular Bed Filling Index (aVBFI) and the adjusted Vascular Bed Filling Index (adjVFBI) revealed differences in complication severity 30 days after surgery depending on the type of urinary diversion and fluid management strategy.

Abstract: Introduction: Intravenous fluid management is integral to perioperative care, particularly under enhanced recovery after surgery (ERAS) protocols. In radical cystectomy (RC), which carries high risks of complications and mortality, optimizing fluid management poses a significant challenge due to the absence of definitive guidelines. **Aim:** the purpose of this study was to investigate the effects of intravenous fluid administration on postoperative complications in patients undergoing RC. **Material and methods:** This study involved 288 patients who underwent laparoscopic RC and urinary diversion from 2018 to 2022. ERAS protocols were implemented for all patients. Participants were divided into four groups based on the type of urinary diversion (ureterocutaneostomy vs. ileal conduit) and the intraoperative fluid volume input (less than 1000 mL vs. more than 1000 mL). Postoperative complications were evaluated at 30 and 90 days post-surgery using the Clavien-Dindo scale. The fluid management effectiveness was measured using the absolute Vascular Bed Filling Index (aVBFI) and the adjusted Vascular Bed Filling Index (adjVFBI). **Results:** The UCS is associated with a lower risk of increased severity of postoperative complications. The administration of more than 1000 mL of fluids was associated with a higher risk of complications ($p = 0.035$). However, after adjusting for the duration of the surgery and BMI, this association did not hold statistical significance, indicating that fluid volume alone is not a direct predictor of postoperative complications. At aVBFI values between zero and eight, urinary diversion using the UCS method is associated with a lower risk of complications compared to the IC. When aVBFI equals eight, the differences in the severity of complications between the UCS and the IC are minimal. However, when aVBFI exceeds eight, the IC is associated with fewer complications during the 30 days post-operation compared to the UCS. The correlation between the adjVFBI (B = −0.27; 95% CI: −0.45 to −0.08; p = 0.005) and the severity of complications up to 30 days postoperatively is similar to that seen with the aVBFI. Similarly, the correlation of the adjVFBI with the method of urinary diversion (B = 0.24; 95% CI: 0.06 to 0.43; p = 0.011) resembles that of the aVBFI. The volume of fluids administered and the indices aVBFI and adjVFBI did not influence the occurrence of complications 90 days postoperatively. **Conclusions:** The volume of fluids administered is not a factor directly affecting the occurrence of complications following RC when the ERAS protocol is used. The amount of intraoperative fluid administration should be adjusted according to the intraoperative blood loss. Our findings endorse the utility of aVBFI and adjVFBI as valuable tools in guiding fluid therapy within the framework of ERAS protocols. However, further multicenter randomized trials are needed to definitively determine the best fluid therapy regimen for patients undergoing RC.

Keywords: radical cystectomy; bladder cancer; ERAS protocol; fluid therapy

1. Introduction

Intravenous fluid restoration is an essential part of perioperative and postoperative care. Adequate intravenous fluid administration maintains proper water and electrolyte balance. The optimal amount of intravenous fluids during and after general surgery still remains undefined [1]. Previous studies have revealed that personalized perioperative fluid management has improved the duration of postoperative ileus (with a lower complication rate) [1,2]. According to some surgical guidelines, fluid intake should be restricted to a maximum of 3 L on the day of surgery [3].

It is worth noting that a restricted postoperative fluid regime reduces complications and postoperative hospital stay after surgery, especially when using the ERAS (Enhanced Recovery After Surgery) protocol [4,5]. Upon achieving promising results in general surgery, the ERAS protocol also began to be implemented in patients undergoing urological procedures. Radical cystectomy (RC) remains the gold standard for treating muscle-invasive urinary bladder cancer, but it is associated with a significant risk of complications and mortality [6–8]. It is worth noting that LND is associated with higher perioperative morbidity and mortality in patients with muscle-invasive bladder cancer undergoing radical cystectomy. Moreover, extended LND did not result in improved disease-free or overall survival in comparison with standard LND [9]. Moreover, Pfail et al. [10] showed that patients with muscle-invasive bladder cancer and with clinically positive lymph nodes, especially in N2-N3 disease, require a tailored approach. While neoadjuvant chemotherapy followed by radical cystectomy is standard for N1 disease, the role of surgery in advanced nodal stages is growing because of better patient selection and treatment strategies [10]. Neoadjuvant chemotherapy improves cancer-specific mortality (CSM) compared to RC alone, both in organ- and non-organ-confined urinary bladder cancer [11]. Additionally, de Angelis et al.'s [12] study showed that neoadjuvant chemotherapy before RC does not result in a statistically significant CSM benefit relative to RC followed by adjuvant chemotherapy.

The implementation of the ERAS protocol for patients undergoing RC can reduce the hospitalization time and may improve the cancer-specific survival (CCS) and the 5-year overall survival (OS) [13–16]. Moreover, meta-analyses demonstrate that applying the ERAS protocol in patients undergoing RC reduces the complication rate and accelerates the return of bowel function [17]. The introduction of less invasive modern surgical techniques allows for a reduction in hospitalization time and a decrease in the number of complications [18].

While working on the study, we hypothesized that excessive fluid administration during cystectomy could lead to edema of the intestinal-to-intestinal or uretero-intestinal anastomoses, particularly in patients from the ileal conduit group. Additionally, the ERAS protocol and its components are implemented differently across various centers. With this study, we aimed to emphasize the importance of restrictive fluid management and the necessity of considering vascular bed filling.

From a pathophysiological point of view, proper water, electrolyte, protein and acid–base balance is crucial for the quick recovery of patients undergoing major surgery. Thus, restrictive fluid therapy remains an important component of the ERAS protocol.

Currently, knowledge regarding the influence of fluid supply during RC is scarce. Several studies on the optimal method of fluid therapy in patients undergoing RC have been conducted by both anesthesiologists and urologists. Previous randomized clinical trials evaluating various fluid therapy regimens did not conclusively determine the management of fluid therapy in patients undergoing RC for urinary bladder cancer [19–22].

Previous knowledge regarding the effect of fluid therapy during and after RC is still inconclusive.

Therefore, the main purpose of this study was to investigate the effects of intravenous fluid administration on postoperative complications in patients undergoing RC.

2. Materials and Methods

2.1. Study Protocol

Two hundred eighty-eight consecutive patients with muscle-invasive urinary bladder cancer who underwent laparoscopic RC with lymphadenectomy and urinary diversion (ureterocutaneostomy or ileal conduit) from 2018 to 2022 were enrolled in a retrospective cohort study. The same surgeon performed all RCs. In each patient of our cohort who underwent radical cystectomy, lymph node dissection (LND) was performed. The standard LND in muscle-invasive bladder cancer involves the removal of nodal tissue cranially up to the common iliac bifurcation, with the ureter being the medial border, and includes the internal iliac, presacral, obturator fossa and external iliac nodes. The lateral borders are the genitofemoral nerves, caudally the circumflex iliac vein, the lacunar ligament and the lymph node of Cloquet [11]. The cohort included patients of various cancer stages, ages and comorbidities.

Patients after RC were divided into four groups based on the urinary diversion technique [ureterocutaneostomy (UCS) and ileal conduit (IC)] and the amount of intravenous fluid (crystalloids) administration [< or >1000 mL], as follows: (1) group 1 [UCS + fluid intake < 1000 mL], (2) group 2 [UCS + fluid intake > 1000 mL], (3) group 3 [IC + fluid intake < 1000 mL] and (4) group 4 [IC + fluid intake > 1000 mL].

ERAS protocols were implemented in each patient who underwent RC, incorporating both preoperative and postoperative measures.

Preoperative measures included promoting increased physical activity and a high-protein diet approximately four weeks prior to RC. No bowel preparation or enemas were used. Carbohydrate- and electrolyte-rich fluids were administered the day before and the morning of the surgery to mitigate insulin resistance. Perioperatively, gabapentin was employed as a co-analgesic. Postoperative management allowed fluid intake on the day of surgery, with oral nutrition initiated on the first postoperative day. Gastric tubes were not used postoperatively, and the route of drug administration was switched to the oral route as tolerated. Low-molecular-weight heparin was administered for thromboprophylaxis.

The collected data included gender, age, body mass index (BMI), Charlson comorbidity index (CCI), nutrition scale (nutrition risk screening, NRS), anesthesiological risk using the ASA (American Society of Anesthesiologists) score, baseline hemoglobin levels and the presence of comorbidities such as hypertension, type 2 diabetes, heart failure, where patients with heart failure were classified as those diagnosed with a reduced left ventricular ejection fraction (LVEF) of <50% during cardiological evaluation, and chronic kidney disease.

Several parameters closely related to the surgical procedure, such as the operation time, blood loss and the method of urinary diversion (UCS or IC) were also taken into account.

These groups were compared in terms of complications at 30 and 90 days post-surgery, and 30- and 90-day post-surgery complications and their relationships were assessed in all experimental groups. Complications were assessed using the Clavien-Dindo scale.

In assessing complications, the ratio of the volume of fluids administered relative to body weight (mL/kg), BMI (mL/kg/m^2), duration of the procedure and combined ratio, taking into account procedure time and body weight (mL/hour/kg), were used. Additionally, two novel clinical parameters were introduced (see Section 2.2).

Propensity score matching (PSM) was conducted to balance baseline characteristics between the UCS group (n = 240) and the ileal conduit diversion group (n = 48). To achieve covariate balance between the groups, the validity of subsequent comparisons was enhanced. PSM was implemented using a nearest-neighbor matching algorithm with a 1:1 matching ratio, ensuring that each patient in the IC group was matched with one patient from the UCS group based on similar propensity scores. The propensity scores were estimated using a logistic regression model, with patient age, CCI (Charlson Comorbidity Index) and clinical tumor stage as predictors.

2.2. Novel Clinical Parameters

Due to the high heterogeneity of patients undergoing RC related to different patient weights and operation time (which is influenced, among others, by the type of urinary diversion), we have defined two novel clinical parameters (aVBFI and adjVFBI), which allow for the unification of experimental groups, allowing for a reliable comparison between groups.

The absolute Vascular Bed Filling Index (aVBFI) assesses vascular bed filling during the procedure. The aVBFI is calculated as the ratio of fluids administered during the procedure due to blood loss.

The adjusted Vascular Bed Filling Index (adjVFBI) is a more accurate parameter than aVBFI because it also considers the procedure's duration. The adjVFBI is calculated as the ratio of the aVBFI to the duration of the procedure in minutes.

Moreover, in further analysis, we assumed that fluid loss through evaporation, respiration and convection remains constant, and that in laparoscopic interventions, it is not as significant as in open surgeries.

2.3. Statistical Analysis

Data analysis was conducted, adhering to rigorous methodological and statistical standards, with a significance level set at $\alpha = 0.05$, which is standard in biomedical sciences, minimizing the risk of Type I error. Descriptive statistics tailored to the type of data were utilized. For quantitative variables, the median was used as it is less sensitive to outliers than the arithmetic mean, and the first and third quartiles were presented, allowing for a fuller understanding of the data distribution.

For categorical variables, the number of observations and percentages were used, facilitating the interpretation of the distribution. To assess the significance of differences between groups, the Wilcoxon rank-sum test was used for quantitative variables and the Pearson Chi-square test, Fisher's exact test or a proportions test for categorical variables, depending on the sample size and data characteristics.

A multivariate analysis was conducted using a multiple regression model to identify factors affecting the severity of postoperative complications, enabling the assessment of relationships between multiple independent and dependent variables. A robust estimator (M-Huber) that is less sensitive to outliers was used in the analysis, ensuring greater reliability of the results.

The analysis provides information on the risk profile and enables the identification of high-risk groups as well as risk factors that can be targeted for intervention to improve treatment outcomes. The statistical analysis results are presented with 95% confidence intervals and p-values, allowing for the precise interpretation of the strength and direction of the statistical relationships.

Propensity score matching analyses were conducted using the R Statistical language (version 4.3.3; R Core Team, 2024) on Windows 11 pro 64 bit (build 22631), using the packages cobalt (version 4.5.5; Greifer N, 2024), MatchIt (version 4.5.5) [23].

3. Results

3.1. Characteristics of Experimental Groups

The median age of the patients was 68.5 years (63 to 74 years). The gender distribution in the study group showed a significant predominance of males, who comprised 78.1% (225 patients), compared to females, who accounted for 21.9% (63 patients). The median body weight of the patients was 80 kg (70 to 89 kg). The median BMI was 26.95 kg/m^2 (24.30 to 30.05 kg/m^2). Ureterocutaneostomy and ileal conduit were conducted in 240 and 48 patients, respectively.

The hospitalization stay was 10 days (8 to 13 days). The duration of hospitalization did not differ significantly between all experimental groups ($p = 0.153$).

Hypertension (HT) was the most common comorbidity, which affected 65.3% of all patients. In patients with IC, the incidence of HT was lower at 54.1% compared to the group with UCS, which had a prevalence of 67.5%. However, this difference did not reach statistical significance ($p = 0.077$). Diabetes mellitus (DM) was present in 24.7% of the participants, with a slightly higher frequency in the patients with IC (29.2%) compared to the patients with UCS (23.8%), although this difference was also not statistically significant ($p = 0.427$). Similarly, the incidence of heart failure (HF) did not differ significantly between groups, with 14.6% in the IC and 19.1% in the UCS patients ($p = 0.454$). In our cohort, a statistically significant difference was observed in the case of chronic kidney disease (CKD). In the group of patients after IC, the percentage of patients with CKD was significantly lower (8.3%) compared to the patients with UCS (30%), with a p-value of 0.002. (Table 1)

Patients in the IC group were statistically younger than those in the USC group. The median age for the IC group was 64 years, compared to 69 years for the USC group ($p < 0.001$).

According to the Charlson comorbidity index (CCI) results, the majority of patients (59.7%) had a score greater than four, suggesting the presence of comorbid conditions that worsen the prognosis. A statistically significant difference ($p < 0.001$) between urinary diversion techniques indicates that a higher percentage of patients with ileal conduit had a better CCI outcome (<4) (64.6%) compared to the patients with UCS (35.4%).

For older and comorbid patients, the uretero-ureterocutaneous fistula (UCN) without the use of intestinal interposition devices is an alternative and safe procedure [24]. In our population of 417 patients, the operation time (incision–suture time: median 82 min; range 63–121 min) and mortality (2.1%) are low despite a pronounced negative selection of comorbid in elderly patients (mean age 79 years). A potential disadvantage compared to the ileum conduit is the obligatory ureteral splinting.

Table 1. Characteristics of the study group.

Characteristic	N = 288	Overall in Sample [a]	Urinary Diversion		p^b
			IC [a], $n = 48$	UCS [a], $n = 240$	
Hypertension		188 (65.28%)	26 (54.2%)	162 (67.5%)	0.077
Diabetes mellitus		71(24.65%)	14(29.2%)	57 (23.8%)	0.427
Heart failure		53(18.40%)	7 (14.6%)	46 (19.2%)	0.454
Chronic kidney disease		76(26.39%)	4 (8.3%)	72 (30.0%)	0.002
Neoadjuvant chemotherapy		44 (15.3%)	5 (10.4%)	39 (16.3%)	0.305 [b]
cTNM:					
cT2		101 (35.1%)	25 (52.1%)	76 (31.7%)	0.007 [d]
cT3		118 (41.0%)	20 (41.7%)	98 (40.8%)	0.915 [d]
cT4		68 (23.6%)	2 (4.2%)	66 (27.5%)	0.001 [c]
N1		33 (11.5%)	1 (2.1%)	32 (13.3%)	0.025 [c]

[a] n (%); [b] Pearson Chi-square test; [c] Fisher's exact test; [d] proportions test.

The assessment of the ASA scale score revealed significant differences between the groups ($p = 0.004$). In the patients with IC, a larger percentage of patients had a lower risk class, ASA2 (41.7%), compared to the UCS patients (19.2%), while the higher risk class, ASA3, was more common in the UCS patients (79.2%) than in the IC patients (58.3%). The NRS (nutritional risk score) also showed a statistically significant difference ($p = 0.022$), with the median score in the IC patients being lower than that in the UCS patients.

The study observed a statistically significant difference in preoperative hemoglobin (HGB) levels between the groups, where patients with IC creation had a higher median HGB (13.80 g/dL) compared to the patients with UCS (12.30 g/dL). The differences remained significant postoperatively, with higher HGB in the IC patients (11.95 g/dL) compared to the UCS patients (10.65 g/dL). The loss of hemoglobin did not differ significantly between the groups.

The use of neoadjuvant chemotherapy (CHTx) in this cohort was relatively low, at 15.3% (44 individuals)—5 patients from the IC group (10.4%) and 39 patients from the UCS group (16.3%). The neoadjuvant CHTx used for our patients was based on cisplatin agents.

The low percentage of patients receiving neoadjuvant chemotherapy results from the significant comorbidity of the Polish population compared to other European populations [25]. Scientific reports indicate that the risk of malnutrition in the Polish population over 65 years old can reach 44.2% [26] and 39.2% in the oncological patient group [27]. The prevalence of overweight is 63% in men and 43% in women [28]. This also explains why the simplest form of urinary diversion is often chosen after cystectomy (CR).

The results indicate statistically significant differences ($p < 0.05$) in terms of clinical tumor stage (cT). In the UCS group, individuals with advanced cT4 tumors constituted

27.5%, while the patients with IC constituted only 4.17% (p = 0.001). (Table 1) A higher proportion of patients in the UCS group was suspected of having lymph node metastases compared to the IC group (13.3% vs. 2.1%, p = 0.025). Patients in the IC group more frequently had organ-confined disease (cT2)—52.1%, compared to 31.7% in the UCS group (p = 0.007). The percentage of patients with cT3 advancement did not differ significantly between the groups, with 41.6% in the IC group and 40.1% in the UCS group (p = 0.915). However, the presence of hydronephrosis was significantly less common in the IC group (10.4%) compared to the UCS group (34.2%) [p = 0.001].

Preventing infections, including wound infections, appears to play a crucial role during radical cystectomy and in the perioperative period. Infectious complications can account for up to 25% of complications following radical cystectomy procedures during RARC [29]. If open access is used during radical cystectomy (ORC), the use of Alexis wound protectors has been shown to effectively reduce the rate of postoperative wound infections [30]. In our study, all procedures were performed laparoscopically, and we used standard extraction bags. We observed only incidental cases of wound infections or pneumonia after laparoscopy.

The median operation time was 200 min (from 175 to 241 min.). The duration of the procedure was significantly longer in the group of patients using the IC creation (average 260 min.) compared to the UCS creation (average 190 min.; p < 0.001). The median blood loss was 250 mL (ranging from 150 to 350 mL). Concurrently, there was no significant difference in blood loss between the UCS and IC groups (p = 0.962). (Table 2).

Table 2. Parameters of perioperative factors in the sample, stratified by urinary diversion technique after cystectomy.

Characteristic	N = 288	Overall in Sample [a]	Urinary Diversion		p [c]
			IC [a], n = 48	UCS [a], n = 240	
Surgery time min		200 (175–241)	260 (242–285)	190 (165–220)	<0.001
Blood loss mL		250 (150–350)	250 (200–350)	250 (150–350)	0.962
Fluids administrated during surgery mL		1000 (500–1900)	1350 (800–1900)	1000 (500–1900)	0.011
Fluids administrated/Surgery time/Weight mL/hr/kg		4.28 (3.34–5.41)	3.69 (2.55–4.60)	4.41 (3.58–5.79)	<0.001
Fluids/BMI ml/kg/m^2		140.5 (124.0–158.0)	143.0 (124.0–152.25)	140.0 (124.0–159.25)	0.998
aVBFI (1)		4.80 (3.18–7.04)	5.00 (3.63–8.08)	4.33 (3.0–7.0)	0.107

[a] Mdn (Q1, Q3); [c] Wilcoxon rank-sum test.

The ratio of fluids administered per hour of surgery per kilogram of body weight (mL/hour/kg) was significantly lower in the IC group (3.69) compared to the UCS group (4.41; p < 0.001).

This may be due to the fact that patients in the IC group statistically weighed more than those in the USC group—84 kg vs. 79 kg (p = 0.011). However, no differences between the groups were noted after calculating the BMI.

The rate of blood product transfusions was higher in the UCS group (34.2%) than in the IC group (14.6%; p = 0.007). No statistically significant differences were observed in the percentage of patients requiring intensive care unit support (p = 0.228).

There was a statistically significant difference in the incidence of ileus (p = 0.001), with a higher frequency of cases in the IC group (27.1%) compared to the UCS group (9.6%).

3.2. Postoperative Complications According to the Clavien-Dindo Classification Within 30 Days

The frequency of complications, as measured by the Clavien-Dindo scale, did not differ significantly, regardless of the method of urinary diversion or the amount of fluids administered. The distribution of complications in each group is attached in Table 3.

Table 3. Complications depending on the type of urinary diversion type.

Characteristic	N	Overall in Sample [a]	Urinary Diversion		p [b]
			IC [a], $n = 48$	UCS [a], $n = 240$	
Clavien-Dindo 30 days	288				0.354
1		126 (43.8%)	19 (39.6%)	107 (44.6%)	
2		70 (24.3%)	19 (20.8%)	60 (25.0%)	
3a		37 (12.9%)	8 (16.7%)	29 (12.1%)	
3b		32 (11.1%)	9 (18.8%)	23 (9.6%)	
4		6 (2.1%)	0 (0.0%)	6 (2.5%)	
5		8 (2.8%)	0 (0.0%)	8 (3.3%)	
Clavien-Dindo 90 days	280				0.176
1		46 (16.4%)	4 (8.3%)	42 (18.1%)	
2		71 (25.4%)	11 (22.9%)	60 (25.9%)	
3a		29 (10.4%)	8 (16.7%)	21 (9.0%)	
3b		4 (1.4%)	1 (2.1%)	3 (1.3%)	
4		1 (0.4%)	0 (0.0%)	1 (0.4%)	
5		11 (3.9%)	0 (0.0%)	11 (4.7%)	

[a] n (%); [b] Fisher's exact test.

However, several factors that influence the severity of complications were identified (Table 4).

Table 4. Factors determining the complications 30 days after RC.

Explanatory Variables	Severity of Complications (Clavien-Dindo) B	CI 95%	p
Age years	0.01	−0.01–0.03	0.283
BMI kg/m^2	−0.03	−0.06–−0.00	0.045
Fluids administrated (>1000 mL)	0.28	0.02–0.54	0.035
Fluids to surgery time to patient weight ratio ml/hr/kg	−0.04	−0.11–0.04	0.337
Neoadjuvant CHTx	−0.00	−0.30–0.30	0.999
Hypertension	0.11	−0.14–0.36	0.396
Diabetes mellitus	0.08	−0.19–0.35	0.572
Heart failure	−0.07	−0.37–0.24	0.669
Chronic kidney disease	0.11	−0.19–0.41	0.467
Hydronephrosis	0.09	−0.17–0.36	0.476
Acute kidney injury	0.11	−0.13–0.36	0.358
Urinary diversion (IC) *	-	-	-
Urinary diversion (UCS)	−0.53	−0.99–−0.07	0.024
aVBFI	−0.07	−0.12–−0.03	0.002
adjVBFI	−0.27	−0.45–−0.08	0.005
Transfusion	0.24	−0.04–0.51	0.092
Hospitalization days	0.02	0.00–0.03	0.011
Reoperation	2.11	1.78–2.44	<0.001
aVBFI × Urinary diversion (UCS)	0.07	0.02–0.12	0.011
adjVBFI × Urinary diversion (UCS)	0.24	0.06–0.43	0.011

Annotations: B—regression model coefficient; CI 95%—confidence interval 95%; p—p-value of the statistical test. *—No value is given for the urinary diversion (IC) variable because urinary diversions were compared to each other.

The administration of fluid volumes above 1000 mL is associated with a higher severity of complications ($p = 0.035$) within 30 days post-surgery when not accounting for additional factors such as the duration of the operation and patient weight. However, the lack of statistical significance in this area after adjusting the volume of administered fluids for the duration of the operation and patient BMI indicates that fluid volume alone is not a reliable predictor of the severity of complications after RC. Using the UCS after RC is associated with less severe complications according to the Clavien-Dindo scale, suggesting its potential benefits in a postoperative context (B = −0.53, p = 0.024). However, the significance of this variable becomes more complex when considering its interaction with the absolute Vascular Bed Filling Index (aVBFI). A direct comparison of the four experimental groups, based solely on the number of fluids administered (< or >1000 mL), showed no differences.

However, after applying the aVBFI, it was found that there was a significant interaction between aVBFI and the type of urinary diversion (UCS/IC) (B = 0.07, p = 0.011).

At aVBFI values between zero and eight, urinary diversion using the UCS is associated with a lower risk of complications compared to the IC. When aVBFI equals eight, the differences in the severity of complications between the UCS and the IC are minimal. However, when aVBFI exceeds eight, the IC creation is associated with fewer complications within 30 days postoperatively compared to UCS (Figure 1) .

The correlation between the adjusted Vascular Bed Filling Index (adjVFBI) (B = −0.27; 95% CI: −0.45 to −0.08; p = 0.005) and the severity of complications up to 30 days postoperatively is similar to that seen with aVBFI. Similarly, the correlation of adjVFBI with the method of urinary diversion (B = 0.24; 95% CI: 0.06 to 0.43; p = 0.011) resembles that of aVBFI.

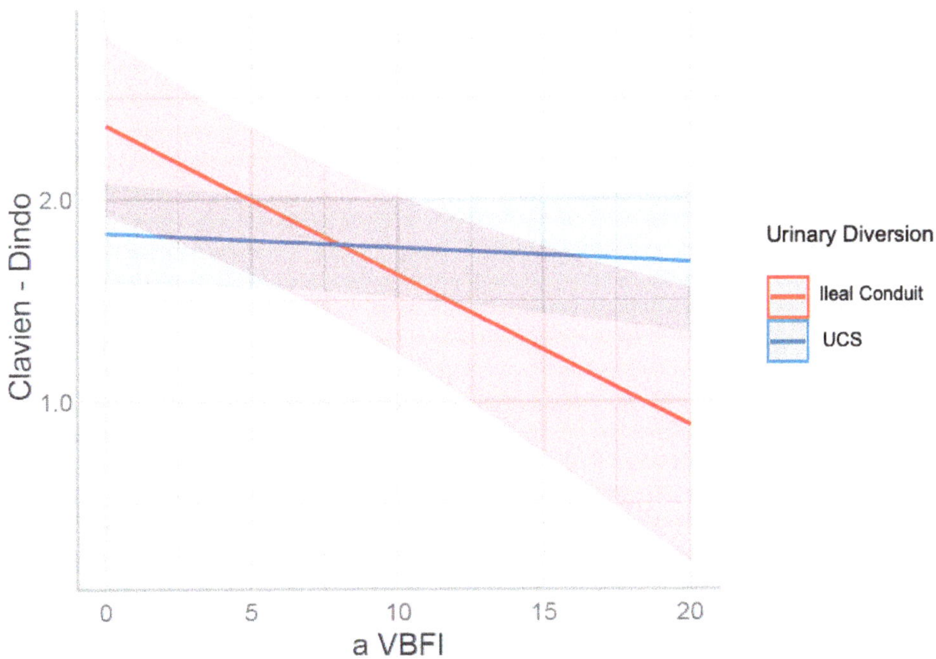

Figure 1. The interaction effect between aVBFI and the urinary diversion on the severity of complications using the Clavien-Dindo scale one month after RC.

3.3. *Complications According to the Clavien-Dindo Classification After 90 Days*

The different amounts of intravenous fluid administration did not influence the severity of complications in 90 days postoperatively.

The statistical analysis based on two hundred and eighty observations (eight patients died before reaching 90 days post-surgery) indicated that the occurrence of acute kidney injury in the postoperative period was associated with a higher degree of complication severity (B = 0.40; 95% CI: 0.04–0.75; p = 0.028). A longer hospitalization time was also significantly associated with a higher degree of complication severity (B = 0.04; 95% CI: 0.02–0.06; p < 0.001). No significant associations were observed between other factors and complications after 90 days from the procedure.

3.4. Propensity Score Matching

The propensity score matching procedure was successful in balancing covariates between the UCS group and the ileal conduit diversion group. Prior to matching, significant imbalances were observed across several covariates. For instance, the standardized mean differences (SMD) indicated substantial differences in age (SMD = −0.80), CCI scale ("good" vs. "burdened" SMD = 0.61 and −0.61, respectively) and tumor stage, particularly for cT4 (SMD = −1.17). These imbalances suggest that patients in the UCS group were older, had a higher burden of comorbidities and were more likely to present with advanced tumor stages compared to the ileal conduit group.

After matching, covariate balance improved considerably. The standardized mean differences for all covariates were reduced to within acceptable thresholds, with SMD values for age (−0.08), CCI categories (0.00 for both ("good" vs. "burdened") and tumor stages (e.g., cT1-cT2: SMD = 0.13, cT3: SMD = −0.17, cT4: SMD = 0.10) indicating minimal residual imbalance. The mean difference in propensity scores between the groups was also reduced (SMD = 0.05), reflecting the successful alignment of treatment probabilities between the matched groups. The variance ratios for continuous variables, such as age (0.72), and eCDF differences for categorical variables (all ≤0.13) further confirm improved balance post-matching (see Figure 2 for visualized covariate balance).

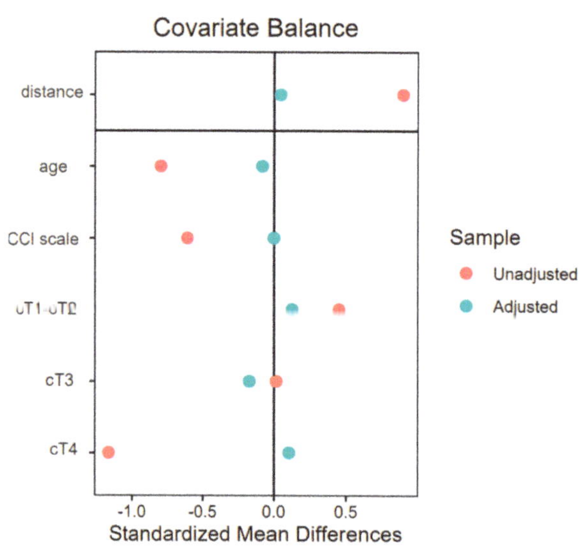

Figure 2. Standardized mean differences for covariate balance before and after propensity score matching.

The matching process retained all 48 patients in the ileal conduit group and matched them to 48 patients in the UCS group, reducing the control group from 240 to 48 for direct comparisons. This ratio ensured equal representation of both groups in the matched dataset, minimizing bias in subsequent analyses. Importantly, no patients were discarded or excluded due to extreme propensity scores, indicating that overlap in treatment probabilities was sufficient for reliable matching.

These results imply that the matched dataset provides a robust basis for comparing outcomes between the UCS and IC groups, free from the confounding influences of age, comorbidities and tumor stage. The improved balance after matching allows for more accurate estimation of the effect of urinary diversion type on patient outcomes, without the bias introduced by baseline differences between the groups.

The assessment of the impact of the urinary diversion method using the covariate balance sample (N = 96, n IC = n UCS = 48) reproduced the results of the previously reported regression models. The UCS diversion was associated with a significantly lower severity of complications one month after surgery (B = −0.51, 95% CI: −0.99–−0.03, $p = 0.036$) compared to the IC diversion. However, the urinary diversion method did not have a significant effect on the Clavien-Dindo parameter at three months post-surgery ($p = 0.415$).

4. Discussion

The results of this study indicate that the amount of intravenous fluids administration as an isolated parameter does not correlate with the severity of early and late postoperative complications after RC. The significant effects observed with newly defined clinical parameters such as absolute and adjusted Vascular Bet Filling Index (aVBFI and adjVBFI) suggest that the appropriate ratios of fluid resuscitation relative to blood loss are crucial for improving postoperative outcomes and can effectively reduce the severity of complications. Our findings also suggest that simpler methods of urinary diversion should be considered during procedures associated with significant blood loss.

In various single-center studies of radical cystectomy, the incidence of complications remains high even when tumors are slightly less advanced. Additionally, the rate of blood transfusions has been reported to be as high as 54.8%, as detailed in the study by Anil Erdik et al. [31].

Bazargani et al. [19] found no correlation between the amount of perioperative fluids input (including crystalloids, colloids, and blood products) and complications at 30 and 90 days post-surgery in 180 patients after open RC. Additionally, fluid administration did not affect the length of hospital stay.

On the other hand, Wuetrich et al. [32] randomized 166 patients into two groups and demonstrated that reduced fluid administration at a rate of 3 mL/kg/hour during surgery, combined with intraoperative noradrenaline infusion, reduced complications by 21% (52% vs. 73%) compared to administering 6 mL/kg/hour without noradrenaline. This approach also decreased the risk of death within 90 days after RC by 4.8% (0% vs. 4.8%). However, their study did not utilize the ERAS protocol, whose components may positively influence the frequency of complications and postoperative stress. This might be the reason for conflicting results regarding fluid therapy alone in these patients.

Similarly, Furrer et al.'s [33] study, in a group of 775 patients undergoing RC without the ERAS protocol, demonstrated that a reduced crystalloid administration of 3.5 vs. 4.2 mL/kg body weight during the procedure may contribute to developing postoperative renal failure. However, no effect of colloids on postoperative renal failure was demonstrated.

Studies emphasize that fluid administration should be individualized and based on objective measurements of flow rates to achieve optimal preload values. This involves adjusting fluid delivery according to the filling of the vascular bed, which can be monitored using tools like an esophageal Doppler probe placed in the patient. Goal-directed fluid therapy (GDFT) has been particularly studied in terms of the recovery of gastrointestinal

(GI) function after surgical procedures, and several meta-analyses have been conducted on this topic.

Giglio and colleagues analyzed 16 studies and demonstrated that GDFT reduces the frequency of severe GI complications compared to the control groups [34]. Additionally, Gomez-Isquierdo et al. [1] concluded that GDFT decreases the incidence of postoperative nausea and vomiting, allows patients to tolerate a diet sooner and shortens the time to the first bowel movement. These benefits did not extend to patients who were managed under the ERAS protocol. Also, Srinivasa et al. [35] analyzed 691 patients where GDFT was combined with the ERAS protocol in colorectal surgery and found no differences in complications or length of hospital stay among the patients.

The impact of GDFT has also been studied in patients with urinary bladder cancer undergoing RC. After analyzing two fairly large groups of patients who underwent open RC, where GDFT was applied in the experimental group without the ERAS protocol, Arslan-Carlon et al. [22] did not demonstrate a positive impact of this fluid therapy approach on either intestinal function or the number of high-grade postoperative complications. They observed a higher risk of acute kidney injury (AKI) in patients from the GDFT group. On the other hand, Pillai and colleagues demonstrated that using GDFT in patients undergoing RC reduces GI complications and improves wound healing [2]. However, the experimental and control groups were small; the procedure duration significantly differed between groups, and the ERAS protocol was not implemented in this study.

Ghoreifi et al. [20] studied the application of GDFT in patients undergoing RC and the ERAS protocol implementation. They evaluated kidney function, the length of stay, complications and rehospitalization 90 days post-surgery. No significant differences were found between the experimental and control groups. Additionally, stroke volume variation (SVV) was studied by Kong et al. [21] in patients undergoing RC. SVV is gaining increasing attention as a reliable index for protocolized fluid management (specifically maintaining SVV within the 10–20% range) to minimize vascular congestion in surgical areas and intraoperative blood loss during procedures such as living-donor hepatectomy. However, this study did not show the impact of this method of fluid transfusion on postoperative outcomes. Nevertheless, it did help to reduce blood loss and the number of transfusions of blood products.

The results of the studies presented above are conflicting, yet they suggest that intraoperative fluid administration based on the filling of the vascular bed or blood loss may influence the complications following RC.

We would also like to mention that a limitation of our study is the retrospective nature of the data analysis. We also did not exclude patients with advanced cancer or those undergoing palliative cystectomy from the analysis. The group of patients in whom urinary diversion was performed using the IC is significantly smaller, and these patients had lower CCI scores and initial cancer staging. Patients in the UCS group also had a higher risk of malnutrition, which is an independent risk factor for the occurrence of complications 30 days after the procedure [36]. However, comparing the results of our study with those of other researchers suggests that optimizing fluid administration based on the filling of the vascular bed could have a positive impact on complications in patients undergoing RC together with the application of the ERAS protocol.

Additionally, it seems that newly defined clinical parameters, such as absolute and adjusted Vascular Bed Filling Index (aVBFI and adjVBFI), seem useful in everyday urological practice in assessing the risk of postoperative complications after RC.

5. Conclusions

The volume of fluids administered does not directly affect the severity of complications following RC when the ERAS protocol is used. The amount of intraoperative fluid administration should be adjusted according to the intraoperative blood loss. In procedures with significant blood loss, simpler methods of urinary diversion should be considered.

The findings endorse the utility of novel clinical parameters such as aVBFI and adjVBFI as valuable clinical tools in guiding fluid therapy within the framework of ERAS protocols. However, further multicenter randomized trials are needed to definitively determine the best fluid therapy regimen for patients undergoing RC.

Author Contributions: Conceptualization, P.L. and T.D.; methodology, P.L. and K.J. and A.O.; software, A.O. and F.K.; validation, T.D., K.J. and J.A.; formal analysis, P.L. and A.O.; investigation, P.L.; resources, P.J.; data curation, P.L.; writing—original draft preparation, P.L.; writing—review and editing, K.J, T.D., A.O. and J.A.; visualization, A.O., F.K., P.J.; supervision, K.J., T.D.; project administration, P.L. and K.J. All authors have read and agreed to the published version of the manuscript.

Funding: This research received no external funding.

Institutional Review Board Statement: The study was conducted in accordance with the Declaration of Helsinki, and approved by the Ethics Committee.

Informed Consent Statement: Patient consent was waived due to inability to identify the patient in this study and retrospective nature of the study.

Data Availability Statement: Data is contained within the article.

Conflicts of Interest: The authors declare no competing interests.

References

1. Gõmez-Izquierdo, J.C.; Feldman, L.S.; Carli, F.; Baldini, G. Meta-analysis of the effect of goal-directed therapy on bowel function after abdominal surgery. *Br. J. Surg.* **2015**, *102*, 577–589. [CrossRef]
2. Pillai, P.; McEleavy, I.; Gaughan, M.; Snowden, C.; Nesbitt, I.; Durkan, G.; Johnson, M.; Cosgrove, J.; Thorpe, A. A double-blind randomized controlled clinical trial to assess the effect of doppler optimized intraoperative fluid management on outcome following radical cystectomy. *J. Urol.* **2011**, *186*, 2201–2206. [CrossRef]
3. Schwenk, W.; Flemming, S.; Girona-Johannkämper, M.; Wendt, W.; Darwich, I.; Strey, C. Structured implementation of fast-track pathways to enhance recovery after elective colorectal resection: First results from five German hospitals. *Chirurgie* **2024**, *95*, 148–156. [CrossRef] [PubMed]
4. Gustafsson, U.O.; Hausel, J.; Thorell, A.; Ljungqvist, O.; Soop, M.; Nygren, J. Adherence to the enhanced recovery after surgery protocol and outcomes after colorectal cancer surgery. *Arch. Surg.* **2011**, *146*, 571–577. [CrossRef] [PubMed]
5. Brandstrup, B.; Tønnesen, H.; Beier-Holgersen, R.; Hjortsø, E.; Ørding, H.; Lindorff-Larsen, K.; Rasmussen, M.S.; Lanng, C.; Wallin, L.; Iversen, L.H.; et al. Effects of Intravenous Fluid Restriction on Postoperative Complications: Comparison of Two Perioperative Fluid Regimens—A Randomized Assessor-Blinded Multicenter Trial. *Ann. Surg.* **2003**, *238*, 641–648. [CrossRef] [PubMed]
6. Nielsen, M.E.; Mallin, K.; Weaver, M.A.; Palis, B.; Stewart, A.; Winchester, D.P.; Milowsky, M.I. Association of hospital volume with conditional 90-day mortality after cystectomy: An analysis of the National Cancer Data Base. *BJU Int.* **2014**, *114*, 46–55. [CrossRef] [PubMed]
7. Hautmann, R.E.; De Petriconi, R.C.; Volkmer, B.G. Lessons learned from 1,000 neobladders: The 90-day complication rate. *J. Urol.* **2010**, *184*, 990–994. [CrossRef]
8. Stein, J.P.; Skinner, D.G. Radical cystectomy for invasive bladder cancer: Long-term results of a standard procedure. *World J. Urol.* **2006**, *24*, 296–304. [CrossRef] [PubMed]
9. Lerner, S.P.; Tangen, C.; Svatek, R.S.; Daneshmand, S.; Pohar, K.S.; Skinner, E.; Schuckman, A.; Sagalowsky, A.I.; Smith, N.D.; Kamat, A.M.; et al. Standard or Extended Lymphadenectomy for Muscle-Invasive Bladder Cancer. *N. Engl. J. Med.* **2024**, *391*, 1206–1216. [CrossRef] [PubMed]

10. Pfail, J.; Lichtbroun, B.; Golombos, D.M.; Jang, T.L.; Packiam, V.T.; Ghodoussipour, S. The role of radical cystectomy and lymphadenectomy in the management of bladder cancer with clinically positive lymph node involvement. *Curr. Opin. Urol.* **2025**, *35*, 115–122. [CrossRef]
11. de Angelis, M.; Jannello, L.M.I.; Siech, C.; Baudo, A.; Di Bello, F.; Goyal, J.A.; Tian, Z.; Longo, N.; de Cobelli, O.; Chun, F.K.; et al. Neoadjuvant chemotherapy before radical cystectomy in patients with organ-confined and non-organ-confined urothelial carcinoma. *Urol. Oncol. Semin. Orig. Investig.* **2025**, *43*, 62.e1–62.e6. [CrossRef]
12. de Angelis, M.; Siech, C.; Jannello, L.M.I.; Di Bello, F.; Peñaranda, N.R.; Goyal, J.A.; Touma, N.; Tian, Z.; Longo, N.; de Cobelli, O.; et al. Neoadjuvant Versus Adjuvant Chemotherapy in Non-Metastatic Locally-Advanced Stage Radical Cystectomy Candidates. *Clin. Genitourin. Cancer* **2024**, *22*, 102132. [CrossRef] [PubMed]
13. Daneshmand, S.; Ahmadi, H.; Schuckman, A.K.; Mitra, A.P.; Cai, J.; Miranda, G.; Djaladat, H. Enhanced recovery protocol after radical cystectomy for bladder cancer. *J. Urol.* **2014**, *192*, 50–56. [CrossRef] [PubMed]
14. Frees, S.K.; Aning, J.; Black, P.; Struss, W.; Bell, R.; Chavez-Munoz, C.; Gleave, M.; So, A.I. A prospective randomized pilot study evaluating an ERAS protocol versus a standard protocol for patients treated with radical cystectomy and urinary diversion for bladder cancer. *World J. Urol.* **2018**, *36*, 215–220. [CrossRef] [PubMed]
15. Persson, B.; Carringer, M.; Andrén, O.; Andersson, S.O.; Carlsson, J.; Ljungqvist, O. Initial experiences with the enhanced recovery after surgery (ERAS®) protocol in open radical cystectomy. *Scand. J. Urol.* **2015**, *49*, 302–307. [CrossRef] [PubMed]
16. Crettenand, F.; M'baya, O.; Grilo, N.; Valerio, M.; Dartiguenave, F.B.; Cerantola, Y.; Roth, B.; Rouvé, J.-D.; Blanc, C.; Lucca, I. ERAS® protocol improves survival after radical cystectomy: A single-center cohort study. *Medicine* **2022**, *101*, e30258. [CrossRef]
17. Tyson, M.D.; Chang, S.S. *Enhanced Recovery Pathways Versus Standard Care After Cystectomy: A Meta-Analysis of the Effect on Perioperative Outcomes*; Elsevier: Amsterdam, The Netherlands, 2016. [CrossRef]
18. Rahota, R.G.; Beauval, J.-B.; Gautier, J.-R.; Almeras, C.; Garnault, V.; Loison, G.; Salin, A.; Tollon, C.; Ploussard, G. Impact of outcomes and costs for implementation of robotic radical cystectomy with full intracorporeal urinary diversion. *Central Eur. J. Urol.* **2023**, *76*, 305–310. [CrossRef]
19. Bazargani, S.T.; Ghodoussipour, S.; Tse, B.; Miranda, G.; Cai, J.; Schuckman, A.; Daneshmand, S.; Djaladat, H. The association between intraoperative fluid intake and postoperative complications in patients undergoing radical cystectomy with an enhanced recovery protocol. *World J. Urol.* **2018**, *36*, 401–407. [CrossRef] [PubMed]
20. Ghoreifi, A.; Basin, M.F.; Ghodoussipour, S.; Bazargani, S.T.; Amini, E.; Aslzare, M.; Cai, J.; Miranda, G.; Sugeir, S.; Bhanvadia, S.; et al. Perioperative outcomes of goal-directed versus conventional fluid therapy in radical cystectomy with enhanced recovery protocol. *Int. Urol. Nephrol.* **2021**, *53*, 1827–1833. [CrossRef] [PubMed]
21. Kong, Y.G.; Kim, J.Y.; Yu, J.; Lim, J.; Hwang, J.H.; Kim, Y.K. Efficacy and safety of stroke volume variation-guided fluid therapy for reducing blood loss and transfusion requirements during radical cystectomy: A randomized clinical trial. *Medicine* **2016**, *95*, e3685. [CrossRef]
22. Arslan-Carlon, V.; Tan, K.S.; Dalbagni, G.; Pedoto, A.C.; Herr, H.W.; Bochner, B.H.; Cha, E.K.; Donahue, T.F.; Fischer, M.; Donat, S.M. Goal-directed versus standard fluid therapy to decrease ileus after open radical cystectomy: A prospective randomized controlled trial. *Anesthesiology* **2020**, *133*, 293–303. [CrossRef] [PubMed]
23. Ho, D.; Imai, K.; King, G.; Stuart, E.A. MatchIt: Nonparametric Preprocessing for Parametric Causal Inference. *J. Stat. Softw.* **2011**, *42*, 1–28. [CrossRef]
24. Otto, T.; Barski, D.; Karig, R.T. Additions. *Dtsch. Arztebl. Int.* **2021**, *118*, 31–32. [CrossRef] [PubMed]
25. Souza, D.L.B.; Oliveras-Fabregas, A.; Minobes-Molina, E.; de Camargo Cancela, M.; Galbany-Estragués, P.; Jerez-Roig, J. Trends of multimorbidity in 15 European countries: A population-based study in community-dwelling adults aged 50 and over. *BMC Public Health* **2021**, *21*, 76. [CrossRef] [PubMed]
26. Krzyminska-Siemaszko, R.; Chudek, J.; Suwalska, A.; Lewandowicz, M.; Mossakowska, M.; Kroll-Balcerzak, R.; Wizner, B.; Tobis, S.; Mehr, K.; Wieczorowska-Tobis, K. Health status correlates of malnutrition in the polish elderly population—Results of the Polsenior Study. *Eur. Rev. Med. Pharmacol. Sci.* **2016**, *20*, 4565–4573.
27. Grabowska, I.; Ścisło, L.; Pietruszka, S.; Walewska, E.; Paszko, A.; Siarkiewicz, B.; Richter, P.; Budzyński, A.; Szczepanik, A.M. The model of perioperative risk assessment in elderly patients—Interim analysis. *Pol. Merkur. Lekarski.* **2017**, *42*, 151–157. [PubMed]
28. Gajewska, D.; Harton, A. Current nutritional status of the Polish population—Focus on body weight status. *J. Health Inequalities* **2023**, *9*, 154–160. [CrossRef]
29. Lama, D.J.; Okunowo, O.; Yamzon, J.; Zhumkhawala, A.-A.; Wilson, T.G.; Lau, C.S.; Yuh, B.E.; Chan, K.G. Long-term oncologic outcomes and complications of robot-assisted radical cystectomy for the treatment of urothelial carcinoma of the bladder. In *Urologic Oncology: Seminars and Original Investigations*; Elsevier: Amsterdam, The Netherlands, 2024. [CrossRef]

30. Galosi, A.B.; Fave, R.F.D.; Perpepaj, L.; Milanese, G.; Polisini, G.; Mantovan, M.; Brocca, C.; Palantrani, V.; Tramanzoli, P.; Antezza, A.; et al. Does Alexis Wound Protector/Retractor Reduce the Risk of Surgical Site Infections After Open Radical Cystectomy for Bladder Cancer? Results From a Single Center, Comparative Study. *Urology* **2024**, *184*, 162–168. [CrossRef]
31. Erdik, A.; Cimen, H.I.; Atik, Y.T.; Gul, D.; Kose, O.; Halis, F.; Saglam, H.S.; Ates, O.F. Sarcopenia is an independent predictor of survival in patients undergoing radical cystectomy for bladder cancer: A single-centre, retrospective study. *Central Eur. J. Urol.* **2023**, *76*, 81–89. [CrossRef]
32. Wüthrich, P.Y.; Burkhard, F.C.; Thalmann, G.; Stueber, F.; Studer, U. Restrictive Deferred Hydration Combined with Preemptive Norepinephrine Infusion during Radical Cystectomy Reduces Postoperative Complications and Hospitalization Time A Randomized Clinical Trial. *Anesthesiology* **2014**, *120*, 365–377. [CrossRef]
33. Furrer, M.A.; Schneider, M.P.; Loffel, L.M.; Burkhard, F.C.; Wuethrich, P.Y. Impact of intra-operative fluid and noradrenaline administration on early postoperative renal function after cystectomy and urinary diversion. *Eur. J. Anaesthesiol.* **2018**, *35*, 641–649. [CrossRef] [PubMed]
34. Giglio, M.T.; Marucci, M.; Testini, M.; Brienza, N. *Goal-Directed Haemodynamic Therapy and Gastrointestinal Complications in Major Surgery: A Meta-Analysis of Randomized Controlled Trials*; Oxford University Press: Oxford, UK, 2009. [CrossRef]
35. Srinivasa, S.; Lemanu, D.P.; Singh, P.P.; Taylor, M.H.G.; Hill, A.G. Systematic review and meta-analysis of oesophageal Doppler-guided fluid management in colorectal surgery. *Br. J. Surg.* **2013**, *100*, 1701–1708. [CrossRef] [PubMed]
36. Riveros, C.; Jazayeri, S.B.; Chalfant, V.; Ahmed, F.; Bandyk, M.; Balaji, K.C. The Geriatric Nutritional Risk Index Predicts Postoperative Outcomes in Bladder Cancer: A Propensity Score-Matched Analysis. *J. Urol.* **2022**, *207*, 797–804. [CrossRef]

cancers

Article

Urinary Microbiome Dysbiosis and Immune Dysregulations as Potential Diagnostic Indicators of Bladder Cancer

Matthew Uzelac [1,2], Ruomin Xin [1,2], Tianyi Chen [1,2], Daniel John [1,2], Wei Tse Li [1,2,3], Mahadevan Rajasekaran [2,4,*] and Weg M. Ongkeko [1,2,*]

1 Department of Surgery, Division of Otolaryngology-Head and Neck Surgery, University of California San Diego, La Jolla, CA 92093, USA; muzelac@ucsd.edu (M.U.); rxin@ucsd.edu (R.X.); cathytianyichen04@gmail.com (T.C.); d1john@ucsd.edu (D.J.); wtl008@ucsd.edu (W.T.L.)
2 Research Service, VA San Diego Healthcare System, San Diego, CA 92161, USA
3 School of Medicine, University of California San Francisco, San Francisco, CA 94143, USA
4 Department of Urology, San Diego VA Healthcare System, University of California, San Diego, CA 92161, USA
* Correspondence: mrajasekaran@health.ucsd.edu (M.R.); rongkeko@health.ucsd.edu (W.M.O.)

Simple Summary: Current means of bladder cancer diagnosis are invasive or lack sensitivity. Dysbiosis of the urinary microbiome has been implicated in the development of bladder cancer, though its potential as a diagnostic tool is unknown. This study attempts to characterize bladder cancer-specific dysbiosis of the urinary microbiome to explore its diagnostic potential. Numerous species were observed to be differentially abundant between the urine samples of patients with bladder cancer and healthy individuals. Specific immune modulations were observed with respect to these species, as was the enrichment of select pathways known to be implicated in the progression of bladder cancer. The study suggests that the urinary microbiome may reflect dysregulations of the tumor microenvironment. Further investigation may reveal the potential of the identified species as urinary biomarkers of this disease. In this way, the urinary microbiome may allow for the noninvasive and earlier detection of bladder cancer, regardless of stage or subtype.

Abstract: There are a total of 82,290 new cases and 16,710 deaths estimated for bladder cancer in the United States in 2023. Currently, urine cytology tests are widely used for bladder cancer diagnosis, though they suffer from variable sensitivity, ranging from 45 to 97%. More recently, the microbiome has become increasingly recognized for its role in human diseases, including cancers. This study attempts to characterize urinary microbiome bladder cancer-specific dysbiosis to explore its diagnostic potential. RNA-sequencing data of urine samples from patients with bladder cancer (n = 18) and matched controls (n = 12) were mapped to bacterial sequences to yield species-level abundance approximations. Urine samples were analyzed at both the population and species level to reveal dysbiosis associated with bladder cancer. A panel of 35 differentially abundant species was discovered, which may be useful as urinary biomarkers for this disease. We further assessed whether these species were of similar significance in a validation dataset (n = 81), revealing that the genera *Escherichia*, *Acinetobacter*, and *Enterobacter* were consistently differentially abundant. We discovered distinct patterns of microbial-associated immune modulation in these samples. Several immune pathways were found to be significantly enriched with respect to the abundance of these species, including antigen processing and presentation, cytosolic DNA sensing, and leukocyte transendothelial migration. Differential cytokine activity was similarly observed, suggesting the urinary microbiome's correlation to immune modulation. The adherens junction and WNT signaling pathways, both implicated in the development and progression of bladder cancer, were also enriched with these species. Our findings indicate that the urinary microbiome may reflect both microbial and immune dysregulations of the tumor microenvironment in bladder cancer. Given the potential biomarker species identified, the urinary microbiome may provide a non-invasive, more sensitive, and more specific diagnostic tool, allowing for the earlier diagnosis of patients with bladder cancer.

Keywords: bladder cancer; urinary microbiome; biomarker; cancer diagnosis; immune modulation

1. Introduction

In the U.S., 82,290 new cases and 16,710 deaths were reported for bladder cancer in 2023, with a 5-year survival rate of 77.9% [1]. These cancers are known to disproportionately affect older, male populations, with the median age at diagnosis being 73 [1]. Veterans are particularly susceptible to developing these diseases due to an increased risk of exposure to chemicals implicated in their pathogenesis, largely Agent Orange [2,3]. Increased usage of tobacco products, as observed in these populations, is also known to increase these individuals' risk of developing bladder cancer [4,5].

Bladder cancers are classified as either muscle-invasive or non-muscle-invasive, with treatment options varying considerably between these two groups [6,7]. In the treatment of these patients, clinicians will often select a combination of transurethral resection, adjuvant intravesical therapy, radical cystectomy, and neoadjuvant chemotherapy depending on the subtype [6,7]. However, a delayed diagnosis will result in worse prognoses irrespective of interventions [8]. As such, the early detection of bladder cancer is crucial toward improving the outcome of patients with this disease. Of the current means of diagnosis, cystoscopies are often performed when patients become symptomatic, typically presenting with urinary bleeding [9,10]. In these cases, however, the cancers have likely already reached more advanced stages, making treatment more difficult [8]. Moreover, smaller lesions may be overlooked [11,12]. For the early detection of bladder cancer, numerous biomarker screening tests have been developed and implemented [13]. Urine cytology tests, the BTA stat test, and the NMP22 test are commonly used, though they suffer from poor sensitivities in less advanced cancers [13–16]. Hence, the development of a means to diagnose bladder cancers regardless of their stages or subtypes would provide significant clinical benefit.

The progression from non-muscle-invasive to muscle-invasive bladder cancer has been heavily associated with epithelial–mesenchymal transition (EMT) [17–19]. This transition is characterized by a decrease in cell adhesion, by which epithelial cells gain mesenchymal traits [20]. The disruption of this pathway has been associated with increased cell motility and proliferation rates, ultimately promoting the acquisition of muscle-invasive bladder cancer [17–19]. The WNT/β-catenin signaling pathway has also been implicated in this transition [21,22]. Mutations in this pathway have been linked to tumorigenesis and the development of drug resistance by inducing a cancer stem cell phenotype [21]. Numerous genetic factors have been identified for their importance in EMT and WNT/β-catenin signaling, including the dysregulation of select transcriptional factors and the differential activation of associated receptors [22,23]. Epigenetic factors are less explored, though the human microbiome has been shown to indirectly regulate both EMT and WNT/β-catenin signaling [24,25].

The human microbiome is a collection of microorganisms that populate the gastrointestinal system [26]. The microbiome has become increasingly implicated in human diseases, including inflammatory bowel disease, psoriasis, and diabetes, among others [27,28]. The microbiome is thought to influence an array of biological pathways, largely through metabolite-mediated immune modulation [29,30]. As such, studies have also characterized the microbiome for its implication in various cancers, particularly colorectal cancers [31–34]. Less is known regarding the microbiome's influence beyond the gastrointestinal system, though microbial species are known to exist outside of the gut. Although previously considered sterile, the bladder has been shown to harbor a diverse population of microbiota, creating potential for the urinary microbiome to influence urological diseases [35]. In fact, studies have shown select genera to be enriched in the urine samples of patients with bladder cancer [36,37]. Urinary tract infections, too, have been shown to increase the risk of bladder cancer mortality [38]. Nonetheless, the exact mechanisms by which the urinary microbiome may mediate bladder cancer remain unknown. We have previously demonstrated the importance of the intratumoral microbiome to EMT in bladder cancer [39]. We hypothesize that by investigating the urinary microbiome for similar dysbiosis, we may identify additional microbial influences of this disease. Further, by exploring this dysbiosis for its implications in immune modulation, EMT, and WNT/β-catenin signaling, we may better understand the human microbiome's relevance to the transition between bladder cancer subtypes. With the discovery of microbial biomarkers, we may be more equipped for the early diagnosis of bladder cancers, regardless of stage or subtype.

To test our hypothesis, RNA-sequencing data of bladder cancer ($n = 18$) and normal ($n = 12$) urine samples were first downloaded from the NCBI BioProject Database. Sequences were mapped to bacterial sequences to yield species-level abundance approximations. Both population-level and species-level variations were explored, as were microbial-associated immune dysregulations and the microbial-associated enrichment of EMT and WNT/β-catenin signaling. Several species that were differentially abundant between the bladder cancer and normal samples were found to be of similar significance in a validation dataset. By assessing the urinary microbiome for its relation to these factors, we hope to demonstrate the importance of biomarker microbiota in the early diagnosis of bladder cancer.

2. Materials and Methods

2.1. Data Acquisition

RNA-Seq data were downloaded from the NCBI BioProject Database (https://www.ncbi.nlm.nih.gov/gds (accessed on 25 July 2023)) of bladder cancer ($n = 18$) and normal ($n = 12$) urine samples from three studies (PRJNA657414, PRJNA872870, and PRJNA723026). For validation, RNA-Seq data were similarly downloaded from the Genome Sequencing Archive (https://ngdc.cncb.ac.cn/gsa/ (accessed on 3 January 2024)) of bladder cancer ($n = 62$) and normal ($n = 19$) urine samples (PRJCA003781).

2.2. Bacterial Read Mapping

Sequences were mapped to bacterial species using the Pathoscope 2.0 software [40], with reference sequences sourced from the NCBI Nucleotide Database (https://www.ncbi.nlm.nih.gov/nucleotide/ (accessed on 28 July 2022)). Bacterial reads were targeted for quantification, and human reads were filtered. Standard parameters were chosen.

2.3. Gene Read Mapping

Sequences were mapped to the hg38 reference genome using the STAR 2.7.10a software [41], with reference sequences sourced from the NCBI Nucleotide Database (https://www.ncbi.nlm.nih.gov/nucleotide/ (accessed on 28 July 2022)). Standard parameters were chosen.

2.4. Cross Study Normalization

Median Absolute Deviation (MAD) normalization was performed to increase the validity of cross-study comparisons. In this technique, the median expression value of a gene is subtracted from each individual sample's expression of that gene. The resultant values are then divided by the MAD of that gene to yield relative expression values in each sample. This technique was similarly performed on species abundance values. MAD normalization assumes an equal median and distribution across samples and is resilient to outliers. MAD normalization has been shown to be robust in gene expression experiments compared to other standard normalization tools [42]. Principle coordinate analysis (PCoA) was conducted to confirm the effectiveness of this technique using Euclidean distance.

2.5. Microbial Contamination Correction

There is potential for contaminant species to be introduced upon sample collection and sequencing [43]. Across all samples, noncontaminant species are expected to be of greater abundance in samples of a greater total abundance of taxa. Contaminant species are likely introduced in a fixed amount and will not display this behavior. Spearman's correlations were computed between each species and the total abundance of all species in a sample. Species that did not show a significant correlation to the total abundance of taxa were deemed contaminants and excluded from subsequent analyses.

2.6. Global Indicator Analyses

The microbiome R package was used to perform PCoA using Euclidean distance. This package was also used to calculate alpha and beta diversity values.

2.7. Differential Abundance Analyses

The Kruskal–Wallis test was used to identify species differentially abundant between bladder cancer and normal samples ($p < 0.05$). A hypergeometric test was used to determine whether a significant number of genera were common to both the original and validation datasets.

2.8. Gene Set Enrichment Analyses

The clusterProfile R package was used to assess immune, adherens junction, and WNT signaling pathway enrichment [44]. Twenty-two immune-associated gene sets were sourced from the KEGG PATHWAY Database (https://www.genome.jp/kegg/pathway.html (accessed on 3 August 2023)). The enrichplot R package was used to visualize enrichment results.

2.9. Expression Correlation Analyses

Spearman's correlations were calculated relating species' abundances to cytokine expression. This analysis was similarly performed to relate species' abundances to the expression of the genes of the adherens junction and WNT signaling pathways. Only differentially abundant species were analyzed.

3. Results

3.1. Cross-Study Normalization and Contamination Correction

Bacterial abundance and gene expression counts were extracted from bladder cancer (n = 18) and normal (n = 12) urine samples spanning three studies (Figure 1A). MAD normalization was performed to increase the comparability of samples for subsequent analyses (see Section 2). PCoA was conducted to visualize the samples' bacterial abundance and gene expression profiles by study both before (Figure 1B) and after (Figure 1C) MAD normalization. After normalization, the samples showed closer proximity, and thus greater similarity in their expression and abundance profiles, confirming the effectiveness of the chosen normalization technique and demonstrating the comparability of the samples' abundance and expression profiles for subsequent analyses.

To identify and exclude potential contaminant species, Spearman's correlations were computed between each species and the total abundance of all species in a sample (see Section 2). Species that did not show a significant correlation to the total abundance of taxa were deemed contaminants and excluded from subsequent analyses. This procedure was performed on bladder cancer and normal samples collectively. A phylogenic tree was created to visualize the distribution of contaminant species by class or phylum (Figure 1D).

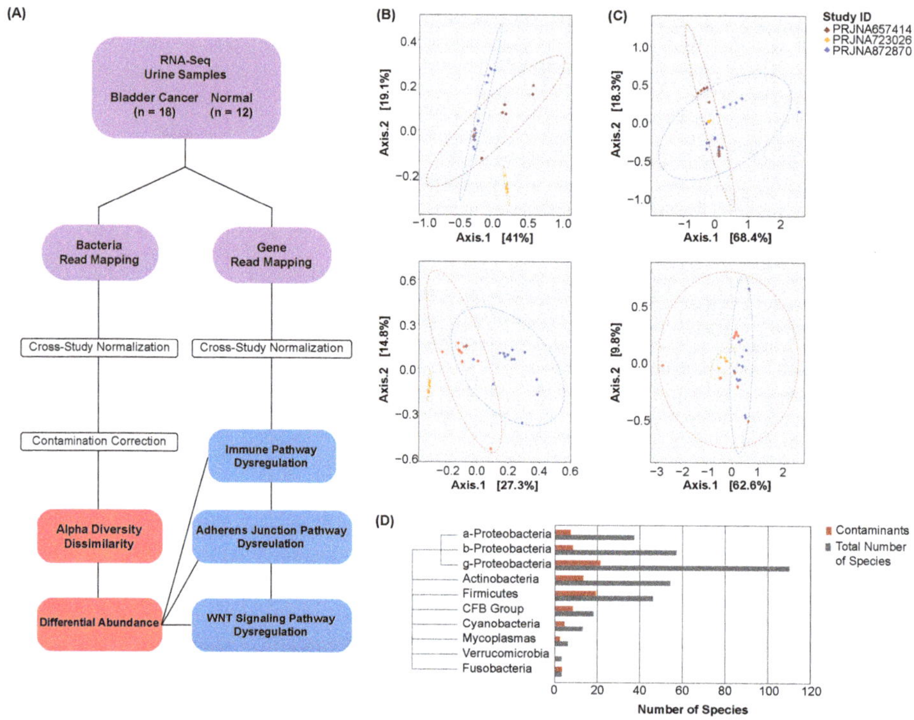

Figure 1. Analysis overview. (**A**) Overview schematic. (**B**) PCoA plots of unnormalized bacterial abundance (top) and gene expression (bottom) profiles by study. Points represent samples, with a closer proximity indicating greater similarity in the samples' bacterial abundance or gene expression profiles. (**C**) PCoA plots of normalized bacterial abundance (top) and gene expression (bottom) profiles by study. MAD normalization was performed. Points represent samples, with a closer proximity indicating greater similarity in the samples' bacterial abundance or gene expression profiles. Samples show greater comparability after normalization. (**D**) Phylogenic tree and bar chart of contaminant species by class or phylum.

3.2. Global Urinary Microbiome Dysbiosis

PCoA was conducted to characterize the samples' bacterial abundance profiles by their disease states (Figure 2A). This analysis attempts to simplify the abundance values of all microbial features in each sample into several arbitrary dimensions. In these dimensions, the proximity of one sample to another describes wholistically the samples' similarities in microbiome composition. Bladder cancer samples occupy a distinct region of the plot from normal samples, suggesting the presence of a wholistic variation in urinary microbiome composition between these disease states.

Measures of alpha and beta diversity were further computed in each sample (Figure 2B). Absolute and relative diversity were found to be significantly lesser in bladder cancer samples, while Shannon diversity was significantly greater (Figure 2C). It is unclear what factors may have influenced the observed difference in direction. Nonetheless, these metrics suggest the presence of global dysbiosis in the urinary microbiome of bladder cancer patients.

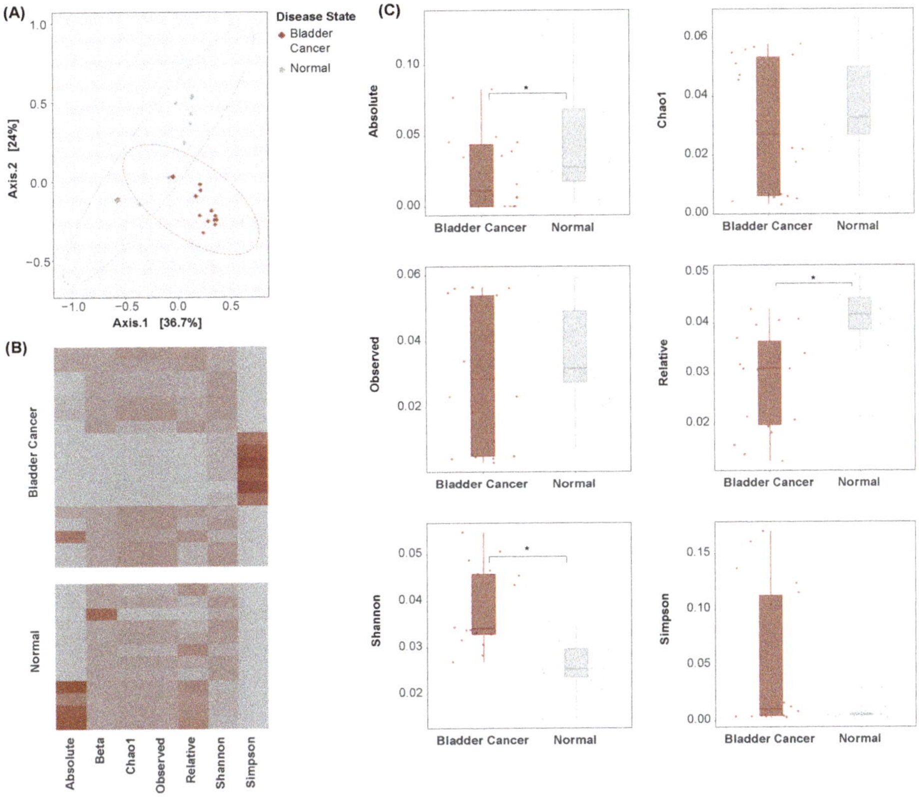

Figure 2. Global indicator dissimilarity. (**A**) PCoA plots of bacterial abundance by disease state. Points represent samples, with a closer proximity indicating greater similarity in the samples' bacterial abundance profiles. Bladder cancer samples occupy a distinct region of the plot as compared to normal samples, suggesting global dissimilarity in their urinary microbiome compositions. (**B**) Heatmap of alpha and beta diversity measures across samples. Rows represent samples. Cell values are relative, and units are arbitrary. (**C**) Boxplots of alpha diversity measures by disease state. Absolute, relative, and Shannon diversity indicators are significantly altered between bladder cancer and normal samples. * $p < 0.05$.

3.3. *Differentially Abundant Species*

The Kruskal–Wallis test was used to compare individual species' abundances between bladder cancer and normal samples. A total of 35 species were found to be differentially abundant between these disease states ($p < 0.05$) (Figure 3A). Most notably, *Caldanaerobacter subterraneus* was significantly enriched in the urine samples of patients with bladder cancer. Among others, the abundance of *Burkholderia ambifaria*, *Staphylococcus xylosus*, and *Klebsiella pneumoniae* was significantly lesser in these samples. The significance (Figure 3B) and fold-change (Figure 3C) distributions of species were plotted. A phylogenic tree was created to visualize the distribution of differentially abundant species by class or phylum (Figure 3D). A majority of the differentially abundant species were of the classes Betaproteobacteria and Gammaproteobacteria.

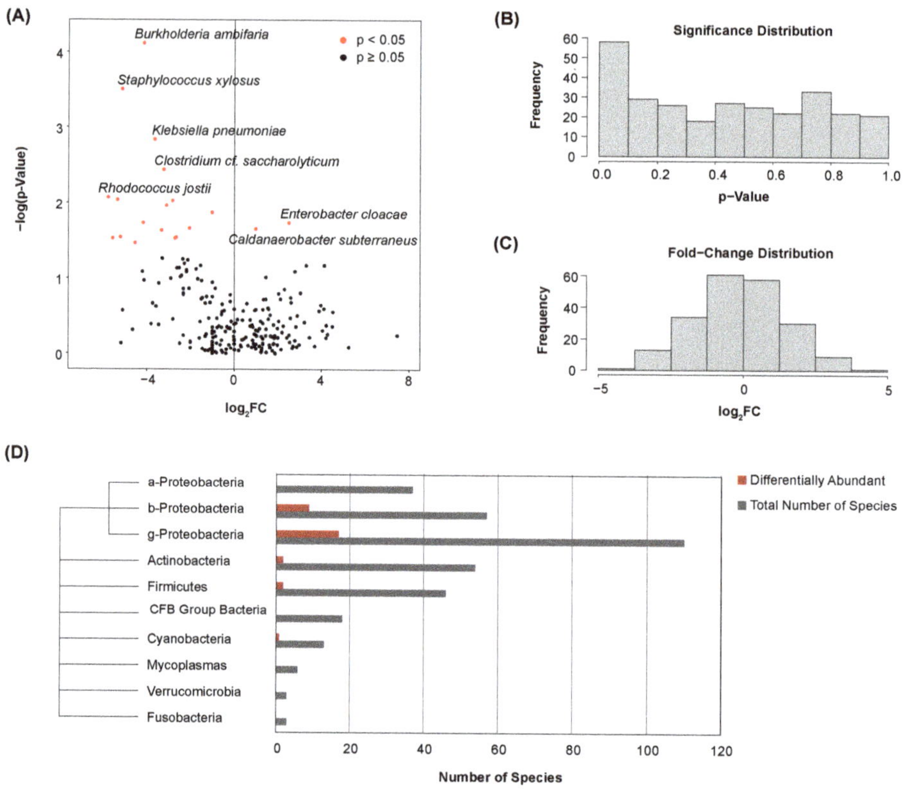

Figure 3. Differential abundance. (**A**) Volcano plot showing differential abundance of species between bladder cancer and normal samples. Points represent microbes. Thirty-five species were determined to be differentially abundant. (**B**) Histogram showing the significance distribution of species. (**C**) Histogram showing the fold-change distribution of species. (**D**) Phylogenic tree and bar chart of differentially abundant species by class or phylum.

3.4. Microbe-Associated Immune Dysregulation

Gene set enrichment analysis was conducted to determine whether select immune-associated pathways were enriched with respect to individual species' abundances. Twenty-two KEGG immune pathways were assessed for enrichment with each of the 35 differentially abundant species above (see Section 2). Nominal enrichment scores (NESs) and test statistics were calculated for each species–pathway combination. Several immune pathways show significant enrichment with respect to one or more of these species (Figure 4A), including antigen processing and presentation, cytosolic DNA sensing, and leukocyte transendothelial migration. Notably, samples with greater abundances of *Pseudomonas fluorescens* and *Pseudomonas putida* corresponded to the positive enrichment of these pathways. These species were less abundant in bladder cancer samples, with lesser abundance correlating to the downregulation of these pathways.

Spearman's correlations were further computed to assess these differentially abundant species for their implications in cytokine dysregulation. Correlation coefficients and test statistics were calculated of each species–cytokine combination. *Pseudomonas fluorescens* and *Pseudomonas aeruginosa* were significantly positively correlated to these cytokines' expressions, particularly for CCL3L1, IL1A, and IL4R (Figure 4B). Among others, numerous significant correlations were also observed of the species *Cutibacterium acnes*, *Cupriavidus metallidurans*, and *Stenotrophomonas maltophilia* to the expression of CCL3L1, IL1A, IL1B, IL1RAP, and IL4R.

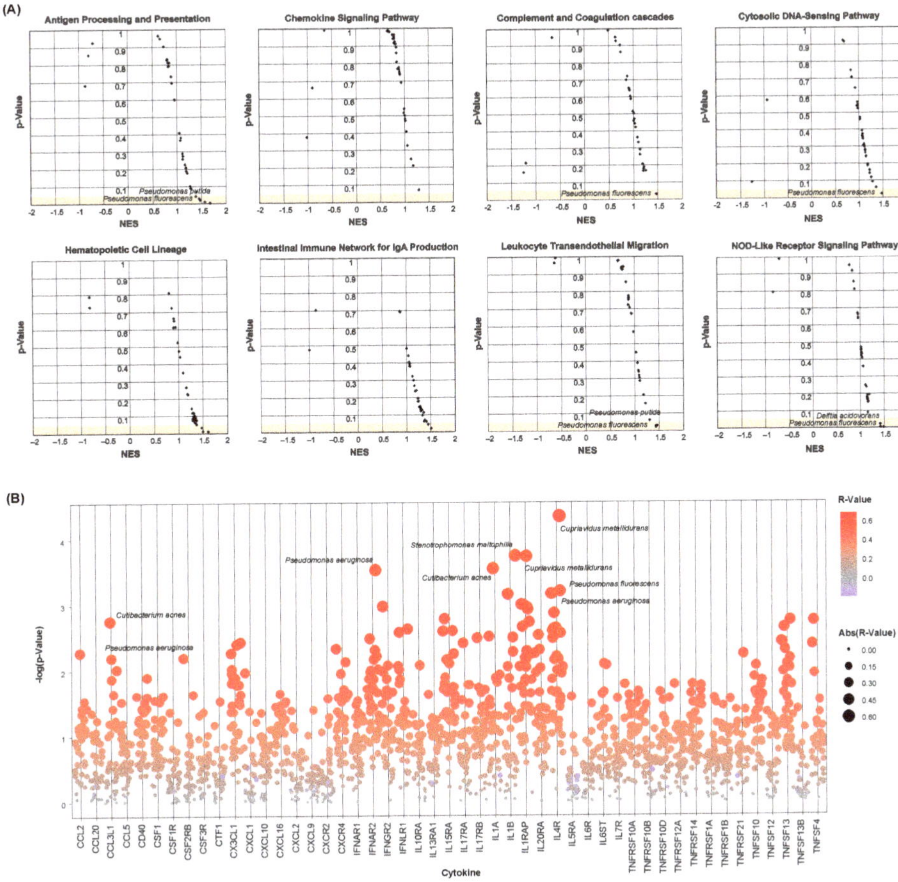

Figure 4. Microbial-associated immune dysregulation. (**A**) Scatter plots showing microbial-associated enrichment of select immune pathways. Nominal enrichment scores (NESs) and *p*-values are plotted. Each point represents a microbe–pathway combination. Only differentially abundant microbes were chosen for analysis. (**B**) Strip chart of microbe–cytokine correlations. *p*-values are plotted. Each point represents a microbe–cytokine combination, with sizes and colors indicating their correlation coefficients (R-value). Only differentially abundant microbes were chosen for analysis. Cytokines show positive correlation to a vast majority of the differentially abundant species.

3.5. Microbe-Associated Adherens Junction and WNT Signaling Enrichment

Due to their implications in the transition from non-muscle-invasive to muscle-invasive bladder cancer, EMT and the WNT signaling pathway were assessed for enrichment with respect to each of the 35 differentially abundant species above. The adherens junction KEGG pathway is composed of genes involved in intercellular adhesion interactions. It is closely associated with the genes involved in EMT, and thus was chosen to model this pathway [45]. Enrichment plots were created to visualize the running enrichment score of the 10 differentially abundant species of the greatest significance (Figure 5A). These pathways show positive enrichment with respect to a majority of these species, including *Pseudomonas fluorescens* and *Pseudomonas putida*. These species were less abundant in bladder cancer samples, with lesser abundance correlating to the downregulation of these pathways. Spearman's correlations were computed to further assess differentially abundant species for correlation to the expression of each of the genes in these pathways. Correlation coefficients and test statistics were calculated for each species–gene combination. Numerous species were of significant correlation to these genes' expression, with a vast majority of these correlations being positive (Figure 5B). The greater abundance of the species *Cupriavidus metallidurans* correlated to the increased expression of many of these genes, including ACTN1, CSNK2A1, NECTIN1, PTPRF, and RAC3 of the adherens junction pathway and CCND2, C2NKA1, FZD5, LRP6, RAC2, and RAC3 of the WNT signaling pathway.

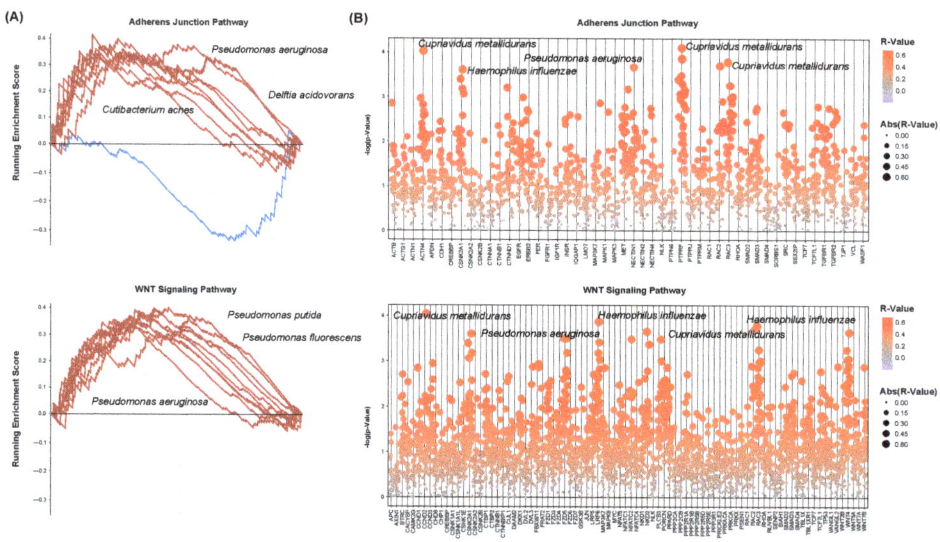

Figure 5. Microbial-associated adherens junction and signaling pathway dysregulation. (**A**) Enrichment plots showing the running enrichment score of select microbes to the adherens junction (top) and WNT signaling (bottom) pathways. Lines represent microbes. Only the ten microbes of the greatest significance in differential abundance are shown. Both pathways are positively enriched with respect to a majority of the microbes analyzed. (**B**) Strip charts of microbe–gene set correlations. Genes of the adherens junction (top) and WNT signaling (bottom) pathways are shown. *p*-values are plotted. Each point represents a microbe–gene combination, with sizes and colors indicating their correlation coefficients (R-value). Only differentially abundant microbes were chosen for analysis. Gene sets show positive correlation to a vast majority of the differentially abundant species.

3.6. Validation of Differential Abundance

We further attempted to validate whether the differentially abundant species identified above were of similar significance in a fourth dataset. After performing contamination correction (see Section 2), the Kruskal–Wallis test was again used to identify species that were of significantly altered abundance between the bladder cancer and normal urine samples. In total, 12 species were differentially abundant between these disease states ($p < 0.05$) (Figure 6A). Hypergeometric testing was used to quantify the extent of overlap between these 12 species and the 35 identified in the original datasets. At the genus-level, seven of these features were common to both datasets (Figure 6B). This yielded a test statistic of 7.86×10^{-7}, indicating a significant amount of overlap between the datasets. We present the following common genera for their potential as microbial urinary biomarkers of bladder cancer: *Escherichia*, *Acinetobacter*, and *Enterobacter*. Species of the genera *Escherichia* and *Acinetobacter* were consistently of lesser abundance in bladder cancer samples, and species of the genus *Enterobacter* were of greater abundance in bladder cancer samples.

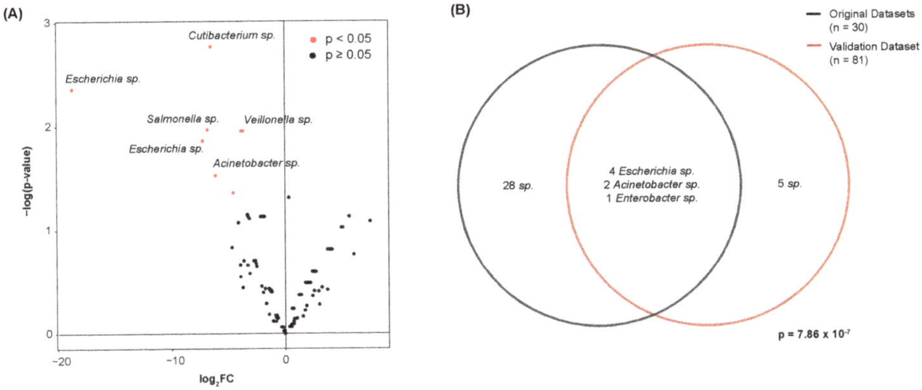

Figure 6. Validation of differentially abundant species by genus. (**A**) Volcano plot showing differential abundance of species between bladder cancer and normal samples. Points represent microbes. Twelve species were determined to be differentially abundant. (**B**) Venn diagram showing the number of differentially abundant species common to both the original datasets and the validation dataset. Species of the genera *Escherichia*, *Acinetobacter*, and *Enterobacter* were commonly differentially abundant. Hypergeometric testing revealed a significant amount of overlap between these datasets, with 35 species identified in the original datasets, 12 species identified in the validation dataset, and 602 noncontaminant species present in both datasets collectively.

4. Discussion

At a global level, bacterial abundance was found to vary significantly between bladder cancer and normal urine samples. Absolute and relative diversity values were generally lesser in the urine samples of patients with bladder cancer. A similar decrease in microbial diversity with bladder cancer has been reported previously, though studies lack consistency [46–48]. Through PCoA, we observed a global variation in microbiome composition between the urine samples of patients with bladder cancer and those of healthy individuals. Dysbiosis of the gut microbiome is known to be implicated in numerous human diseases [27,28], largely through differential immune modulation and metabolic interactions [29,30]. However, the extent to which this is true of the urinary microbiome is unclear. Regardless of the causal or resultant nature of this dysbiosis, the observed variations in the urinary microbiome may be highly useful in the diagnosis of bladder cancer. The detection of a urinary microbial profile distinct for patients with bladder cancer may provide an accurate, non-invasive means of diagnosis.

At a species level, we observed the differential abundance of specific taxa in bladder cancer urine samples. In total, 35 species were found to be differentially abundant between the samples' urinary microbiomes. A majority of these species were of the phyla Proteobacteria, Actinobacteria, Firmicutes, and Cyanobacteria. The differential abundance of these phyla has been identified by other studies of the urinary microbiome in bladder cancer [46–48]. At a genera level, we observed several consistencies in differential abundance, as well. Numerous species of the genus *Escherichia* were of lesser abundance in the bladder cancer samples. We also discovered a consistency in the enrichment of *Cupriavidus* in bladder cancer samples [47], and a decreased abundance of the genus *Acinetobacter*. After validation, we ultimately discovered that species of the following genera were consistently differentially abundant between bladder cancer and normal samples: *Escherichia*, *Acinetobacter*, and *Enterobacter*. Through further investigation, we may determine whether these genera and others are clinically relevant. We suspect that these genera may prove highly useful as biomarkers for this disease. Additional research on a greater number of patients is needed to confirm the implications of these genera and to determine their potential for use in a noninvasive diagnostic approach.

Alternatively, these findings might suggest the utility of microbial-based cancer therapies. The gut microbiome has been shown to influence the efficacy of many cancer therapies, including immunotherapy, chemotherapy, radiation therapy, and even surgery [49]. Studies have demonstrated the ability of fecal transplants and dietary interventions to increase a patient's likelihood of responding to anti-cancer treatments [50]. These interventions are designed to modulate the gut microbiome, and less is known regarding how they might affect the urinary microbiome. Nonetheless, these approaches prove highly promising. Given the relevance of the urinary microbiome as demonstrated above, additional research into microbial-based cancer therapies may similarly be of use for bladder cancers.

We further discovered the enrichment of specific immune pathways with respect to the differentially abundant species identified. Among others, *Pseudomonas fluorescens* and *Pseudomonas putida* consistently correlated to the enrichment of antigen processing and presentation pathways. These species were of decreased abundance in bladder cancer samples, corresponding to decreased antigen processing and presentation. Cancer cells are known to exhibit this trait as means of immune evasion, by which a reduction in antigen presentation prevents the activation of a host's immune response [51,52]. In this way, the reduced abundance of these species may contribute to a cancer's evasion of immune recognition. Similarly, cytosolic DNA sensing pathways were enriched with these species. A reduction in their abundance values in bladder cancer samples corresponded to a reduction in DNA sensing. The suppression of this pathway is also a known mechanism of immune evasion exhibited by cancer cells [53,54]. The lesser abundance of *Pseudomonas fluorescens* and *Pseudomonas putida*, as observed in bladder cancer samples, may provide cancer cells a greater means of evading immune recognition, ultimately promoting tumorigenesis. The microbial-associated enrichment of these pathways may act as a mechanistic link between the human microbiome and the pathogenesis of bladder cancer. Further investigation of these taxa and their specific metabolic interactions may prove useful toward understanding their implications in this disease.

As expected, these species were also found to correlate to differential cytokine expression. Among others, numerous significant correlations were observed between the species *Cutibacterium acnes*, *Cupriavidus metallidurans*, and *Stenotrophomonas maltophilia* and the cytokines CCL3L1, IL1A, IL1B, IL1RAP, and IL4R. Cytokine dysregulation is known to alter a local immune landscape through the differential recruitment of immune cells and the promotion of an inflammatory response [55]. The dysregulation of cytokine activity is heavily implicated in oncogenesis [55] and may mediate the effect of the urinary microbiome on bladder cancer development or progression. Through the immune modulatory relations demonstrated, the urinary microbiome may be implicated in the pathology of bladder cancers, with dysbiosis ultimately promoting a bladder cancer's development and progression.

EMT has been shown to be characteristic of the transition from non-muscle-invasive to muscle-invasive bladder cancer [17–19]. The genes involved in EMT are heavily associated with a decrease in cell adhesion, with many of them also being integral to the adherens junction pathway [20]. The destabilization of the adherens junction pathway is associated with increased cellular motility and metastasis resultant of decreased intercellular adhesion [56,57]. We observed the enrichment of the EMT pathway with respect to several microbial species. The decreased abundance of *Pseudomonas fluorescens* and *Pseudomonas putida* corresponded to decreased pathway activity, and thus decreased intercellular adhesion in bladder cancer samples. The observed decrease in these species' abundances may suggest their relation to EMT and to the pathology of bladder cancer as a whole. The adherens junction pathway has been previously implicated in many other cancer types, including colorectal cancer, breast cancer, and lung cancer [58–62]. Moreover, dysbiosis of the gut microbiome has also been shown to contribute to epithelial dysregulation [63]. We propose that the urinary microbiome may play a similar role in this pathway's regulation within the bladder. Functional metabolic analyses may further elucidate the urinary microbiome's implications in the adherens junction pathway and EMT.

The WNT pathway, too, has been shown to play an oncogenic role in bladder cancers [21,22]. It is thought to be involved in the transition from non-muscle-invasive to muscle-invasive bladder cancer and has been used as an important diagnostic and prognostic biomarker [21,22]. This pathway plays a central role in regulating cell differentiation, providing a suitable explanation as to its implications in cancer growth and metastasis [64]. We also observed the consistent upregulation of the WNT pathway with respect to several species' abundances. *Pseudomonas fluorescens* and *Pseudomonas putida* were of decreased abundance in bladder cancer samples, corresponding to the decreased activity of this pathway. These species may contribute to this pathway's dysregulation, ultimately yielding the decreased regulation of cell differentiation in bladder cancer samples. Various species have been implicated in the molecular alteration of the WNT glycoproteins, ultimately destabilizing its components [65]. Bacterial virulence factors, too, have been shown to modulate this pathway through an array of mechanisms, including the repression of WNT inhibitors, the blocking of WNT–Fzd ligands, and the dysregulation of WNT ligands' expressions [65]. We propose that the urinary microbiomes may dysregulate this pathway through similar means, consequently promoting cancer development and progression. Further metabolic analyses may confirm these hypotheses.

Moreover, the microbial-associated dysregulation of the adherens junction and WNT signaling pathways may mutually influence one another. Many genes are common between these pathways, perhaps explaining the observed similarities in their dysregulation. Genes of the WNT signaling pathway are known to interact with the β-catenin protein of the adherens junction cascades, resulting in the detachment of E-cadherin from a cell's cytoskeleton [66]. In this way, the microbial-associated dysregulation of these pathways may cyclically influence one another, driving a cancer toward the muscle-invasive subtype.

5. Conclusions

Ultimately, we have observed significant dysbiosis in the urinary microbiome of patients with bladder cancer. We discovered microbial-associated enrichment of immune pathways and cytokine activity, suggesting the potential immune modulatory relation of these species. The dysregulation of EMT and WNT/β-catenin signaling was also observed with these species, suggesting that the observed decreases in their abundances in bladder cancer samples may reflect the transition from the non-muscle-invasive to the muscle-invasive subtype. With these considerations, we may better understand the urinary microbiome for its implications in bladder cancer and for its implications in the acquisition of the muscle-invasive subtype. By further exploring the species that relate to this acquisition, we may be more equipped to develop urinary biomarker tests that are more capable of detecting less-advanced bladder cancers. Ultimately, the creation of a panel of urinary biomarker species may prove highly useful toward the non-invasive diagnosis of bladder cancer, ideally providing precision regardless of a cancer's stage or subtype.

In summary, our results suggest that the urinary microbiome may provide a non-invasive diagnostic tool of significant sensitivity and specificity, allowing for the earlier diagnosis of bladder cancer. Our results are limited due to the correlational nature of this study. We are unable to claim a causal relationship between dysbiosis of the urinary microbiome with bladder cancer pathogenesis. Due to the limited number of samples investigated, these results are further limited. Additional samples are necessary to confirm whether the differentially abundant species identified are clinically relevant, as is a greater variation in the disease progression of patients. Moreover, we acknowledge that potentially confounding variables might be present among these samples, including differences in the patients' types of bladder cancer, the patients' subtypes, the patients' genders, and the urine collection methods used [67]. This information was not available for each of the chosen datasets, preventing us from further stratifying our results. The sample collection and sequencing procedures used by these studies also inherently differed. We attempted to mitigate these differences through the above normalization procedures, though the potentially confounding effects should be noted. Lastly, species-level profiling performed with the use of a reference sequence database will only capture culturable species and may omit species otherwise present. This is common in most microbiome studies that employ direct sequence alignment.

Author Contributions: Conceptualization, W.T.L. and W.M.O.; formal analysis, M.U.; funding acquisition, W.M.O. and M.R.; investigation, M.U., T.C., R.X., D.J., W.T.L. and W.M.O.; methodology, M.U.; project administration, W.M.O. and M.R.; resources, W.M.O.; software, M.U.; supervision, W.M.O. and M.R.; visualization, M.U.; writing—original draft, M.U., T.C. and R.X.; writing—review and editing, M.U., T.C., R.X., D.J., W.T.L., W.M.O. and M.R. All authors have read and agreed to the published version of the manuscript.

Funding: This work was supported by the UC San Diego Academic Senate Grant RG096651 to W.M.O. and a VA Merit Award (1 I01 CX002401-01A2) to M.R.

Institutional Review Board Statement: Not applicable.

Informed Consent Statement: Not applicable.

Data Availability Statement: The data can be accessed through the NCBI BioProject Database under the accessions PRJNA657414, PRJNA872870, and PRJNA723026, and the Genome Sequencing Archive under the accession PRJCA003781.

Conflicts of Interest: The authors declare no conflicts of interest.

References

1. National Cancer Institute. *Cancer Stat Facts: Bladder Cancer*; National Cancer Institute: Bethesda, MD, USA, 2022.
2. Mossanen, M.; Kibel, A.S.; Goldman, R.H. Exploring exposure to Agent Orange and increased mortality due to bladder cancer. *Urol. Oncol.* **2017**, *35*, 627–632. [CrossRef] [PubMed]
3. Williams, S.B.; Janes, J.L.; Howard, L.E.; Yang, R.; De Hoedt, A.M.; Baillargeon, J.G.; Kuo, Y.F.; Tyler, D.S.; Terris, M.K.; Freedland, S.J. Exposure to Agent Orange and Risk of Bladder Cancer Among US Veterans. *JAMA Netw. Open* **2023**, *6*, e2320593. [CrossRef] [PubMed]
4. Odani, S.; Agaku, I.T.; Graffunder, C.M.; Tynan, M.A.; Armour, B.S. Tobacco product Use among military veterans—United States Military service members and Veterans. *Morb. Mortal. Wkly. Rep.* **2018**, *67*, 7–12. [CrossRef] [PubMed]
5. Freedman, N.D.; Silverman, D.T.; Hollenbeck, A.R.; Schatzkin, A.; Abnet, C.C. Association between smoking and risk of bladder cancer among men and women. *JAMA* **2011**, *306*, 737–745. [CrossRef]
6. Chang, S.S.; Boorjian, S.A.; Chou, R.; Clark, P.E.; Daneshmand, S.; Konety, B.R.; Pruthi, R.; Quale, D.Z.; Ritch, C.R.; Seigne, J.D.; et al. Diagnosis and Treatment of Non-Muscle Invasive Bladder Cancer: AUA/SUO Guideline. *J. Urol.* **2016**, *196*, 1021–1029. [CrossRef]
7. Sanli, O.; Dobruch, J.; Knowles, M.A.; Burger, M.; Alemozaffar, M.; Nielsen, M.E.; Lotan, Y. Bladder cancer. *Nat. Rev. Dis. Primers* **2017**, *3*, 17022. [CrossRef]
8. Fahmy, N.M.; Mahmud, S.; Aprikian, A.G. Delay in the surgical treatment of bladder cancer and survival: Systematic review of the literature. *Eur. Urol.* **2006**, *50*, 1176–1182. [CrossRef]
9. Davis, R.; Jones, J.S.; Barocas, D.A.; Castle, E.P.; Lang, E.K.; Leveillee, R.J.; Messing, E.M.; Miller, S.D.; Peterson, A.C.; Turk, T.M.; et al. Diagnosis, evaluation and follow-up of asymptomatic microhematuria (AMH) in adults: AUA guideline. *J. Urol.* **2012**, *188* (Suppl. 6), 2473–2481. [CrossRef]
10. Woldu, S.L.; Bagrodia, A.; Lotan, Y. Guideline of guidelines: Non-muscle-invasive bladder cancer. *BJU Int.* **2017**, *119*, 371–380. [CrossRef]
11. Raitanen, M.P.; Leppilahti, M.; Tuhkanen, K.; Forssel, T.; Nylund, P.; Tammela, T. Routine follow-up cystoscopy in detection of recurrence in patients being monitored for bladder cancer. *Ann. Chir. Gynaecol.* **2001**, *90*, 261–265.
12. Mowatt, G.; N'Dow, J.; Vale, L.; Nabi, G.; Boachie, C.; Cook, J.A.; Fraser, C.; Griffiths, T.R. Photodynamic diagnosis of bladder cancer compared with white light cystoscopy: Systematic review and meta-analysis. *Int. J. Technol. Assess. Health Care* **2011**, *27*, 3–10. [CrossRef]
13. Ramakumar, S.; Bhuiyan, J.; Besse, J.A.; Roberts, S.G.; Wollan, P.C.; Blute, M.L.; O'Kane, D.J. Comparison of screening methods in the detection of bladder cancer. *J. Urol.* **1999**, *161*, 388–394. [CrossRef] [PubMed]
14. Karakiewicz, P.I.; Benayoun, S.; Zippe, C.; Lüdecke, G.; Boman, H.; Sanchez-Carbayo, M.; Casella, R.; Mian, C.; Friedrich, M.G.; Eissa, S.; et al. Institutional variability in the accuracy of urinary cytology for predicting recurrence of transitional cell carcinoma of the bladder. *BJU Int.* **2006**, *97*, 997–1001. [CrossRef] [PubMed]

15. Mowatt, G.; Zhu, S.; Kilonzo, M.; Boachie, C.; Fraser, C.; Griffiths, T.R.; N'Dow, J.; Nabi, G.; Cook, J.; Vale, L. Systematic review of the clinical effectiveness and cost-effectiveness of photodynamic diagnosis and urine biomarkers (FISH, ImmunoCyt, NMP22) and cytology for the detection and follow-up of bladder cancer. *Health Technol. Assess.* **2010**, *14*, 1–331, iii–iv. [CrossRef] [PubMed]
16. Têtu, B. Diagnosis of urothelial carcinoma from urine. *Mod. Pathol.* **2009**, *22* (Suppl. 2), S53–S59. [CrossRef] [PubMed]
17. Guo, C.C.; Majewski, T.; Zhang, L.; Yao, H.; Bondaruk, J.; Wang, Y.; Zhang, S.; Wang, Z.; Lee, J.G.; Lee, S.; et al. Dysregulation of EMT Drives the Progression to Clinically Aggressive Sarcomatoid Bladder Cancer. *Cell Rep.* **2019**, *27*, 1781–1793.e4. [CrossRef]
18. Cao, R.; Yuan, L.; Ma, B.; Wang, G.; Qiu, W.; Tian, Y. An EMT-related gene signature for the prognosis of human bladder cancer. *J. Cell. Mol. Med.* **2020**, *24*, 605–617. [CrossRef] [PubMed]
19. Erin, N.; Grahovac, J.; Brozovic, A.; Efferth, T. Tumor microenvironment and epithelial mesenchymal transition as targets to overcome tumor multidrug resistance. *Drug Resist. Updates* **2020**, *53*, 100715. [CrossRef]
20. Kalluri, R.; Weinberg, R.A. The basics of epithelial-mesenchymal transition. *J. Clin. Investig.* **2009**, *119*, 1420–1428. [CrossRef]
21. Garg, M.; Maurya, N. WNT/β-catenin signaling in urothelial carcinoma of bladder. *World J. Nephrol.* **2019**, *8*, 83–94. [CrossRef]
22. Liu, J.; Xiao, Q.; Xiao, J.; Niu, C.; Li, Y.; Zhang, X.; Zhou, Z.; Shu, G.; Yin, G. Wnt/β-catenin signalling: Function, biological mechanisms, and therapeutic opportunities. *Signal Transduct. Target. Ther.* **2022**, *7*, 3. [CrossRef] [PubMed]
23. Debnath, P.; Huirem, R.S.; Dutta, P.; Palchaudhuri, S. Epithelial-mesenchymal transition and its transcription factors. *Biosci. Rep.* **2022**, *42*, BSR20211754. [CrossRef] [PubMed]
24. Gupta, I.; Pedersen, S.; Vranic, S.; Al Moustafa, A.E. Implications of Gut Microbiota in Epithelial-Mesenchymal Transition and Cancer Progression: A Concise Review. *Cancers* **2022**, *14*, 2964. [CrossRef] [PubMed]
25. Rogan, M.R.; Patterson, L.L.; Wang, J.Y.; McBride, J.W. Bacterial Manipulation of Wnt Signaling: A Host-Pathogen Tug-of-Wnt. *Front. Immunol.* **2019**, *10*, 2390. [CrossRef] [PubMed]
26. Barko, P.C.; McMichael, M.A.; Swanson, K.S.; Williams, D.A. The Gastrointestinal Microbiome: A Review. *J. Vet. Intern. Med.* **2018**, *32*, 9–25. [CrossRef]
27. Lynch, S.V.; Pedersen, O. The Human Intestinal Microbiome in Health and Disease. *N. Engl. J. Med.* **2016**, *375*, 2369–2379. [CrossRef]
28. Manos, J. The human microbiome in disease and pathology. *Apmis* **2022**, *130*, 690–705. [CrossRef]
29. Rooks, M.G.; Garrett, W.S. Gut microbiota, metabolites and host immunity. *Nat. Rev. Immunol.* **2016**, *16*, 341–352. [CrossRef]
30. Kayama, H.; Okumura, R.; Takeda, K. Interaction Between the Microbiota, Epithelia, and Immune Cells in the Intestine. *Annu. Rev. Immunol.* **2020**, *38*, 23–48. [CrossRef]
31. Sepich-Poore, G.D.; Zitvogel, L.; Straussman, R.; Hasty, J.; Wargo, J.A.; Knight, R. The microbiome and human cancer. *Science* **2021**, *371*, eabc4552. [CrossRef]
32. Cullin, N.; Azevedo Antunes, C.; Straussman, R.; Stein-Thoeringer, C.K.; Elinav, E. Microbiome and cancer. *Cancer Cell* **2021**, *39*, 1317–1341. [CrossRef] [PubMed]
33. Song, M.; Chan, A.T.; Sun, J. Influence of the Gut Microbiome, Diet, and Environment on Risk of Colorectal Cancer. *Gastroenterology* **2020**, *158*, 322–340. [CrossRef] [PubMed]
34. Rebersek, M. Gut microbiome and its role in colorectal cancer. *BMC Cancer* **2021**, *21*, 1325. [CrossRef]
35. Hilt, E.E.; McKinley, K.; Pearce, M.M.; Rosenfeld, A.B.; Zilliox, M.J.; Mueller, E.R.; Brubaker, L.; Gai, X.; Wolfe, A.J.; Schreckenberger, P.C. Urine is not sterile: Use of enhanced urine culture techniques to detect resident bacterial flora in the adult female bladder. *J. Clin. Microbiol.* **2014**, *52*, 871–876. [CrossRef] [PubMed]
36. Chipollini, J.; Wright, J.R.; Nwanosike, H.; Kepler, C.Y.; Batai, K.; Lee, B.R.; Spiess, P.E.; Stewart, D.B.; Lamendella, R. Characterization of urinary microbiome in patients with bladder cancer: Results from a single-institution, feasibility study. *Urol. Oncol.* **2020**, *38*, 615–621. [CrossRef]
37. Hourigan, S.K.; Zhu, W.; Wong, W.S.W.; Clemency, N.C.; Provenzano, M.; Vilboux, T.; Niederhuber, J.E.; Deeken, J.; Chung, S.; McDaniel-Wiley, K.; et al. Studying the urine microbiome in superficial bladder cancer: Samples obtained by midstream voiding versus cystoscopy. *BMC Urol.* **2020**, *20*, 5. [CrossRef]
38. Richards, K.A.; Ham, S.; Cohn, J.A.; Steinberg, G.D. Urinary tract infection-like symptom is associated with worse bladder cancer outcomes in the Medicare population: Implications for sex disparities. *Int. J. Urol.* **2016**, *23*, 42–47. [CrossRef]
39. Li, W.T.; Iyangar, A.S.; Reddy, R.; Chakladar, J.; Bhargava, V.; Sakamoto, K.; Ongkeko, W.M.; Rajasekaran, M. The Bladder Microbiome Is Associated with Epithelial-Mesenchymal Transition in Muscle Invasive Urothelial Bladder Carcinoma. *Cancers* **2021**, *13*, 3649. [CrossRef]
40. Hong, C.; Manimaran, S.; Shen, Y.; Perez-Rogers, J.F.; Byrd, A.L.; Castro-Nallar, E.; Crandall, K.A.; Johnson, W.E. PathoScope 2.0: A complete computational framework for strain identification in environmental or clinical sequencing samples. *Microbiome* **2014**, *2*, 33. [CrossRef]
41. Dobin, A.; Davis, C.A.; Schlesinger, F.; Drenkow, J.; Zaleski, C.; Jha, S.; Batut, P.; Chaisson, M.; Gingeras, T.R. STAR: Ultrafast universal RNA-seq aligner. *Bioinformatics* **2013**, *29*, 15–21. [CrossRef]
42. Fundel, K.; Haag, J.; Gebhard, P.M.; Zimmer, R.; Aigner, T. Normalization strategies for mRNA expression data in cartilage research. *Osteoarthr. Cartil.* **2008**, *16*, 947–955. [CrossRef] [PubMed]
43. Salter, S.J.; Cox, M.J.; Turek, E.M.; Calus, S.T.; Cookson, W.O.; Moffatt, M.F.; Turner, P.; Parkhill, J.; Loman, N.J.; Walker, A.W. Reagent and laboratory contamination can critically impact sequence-based microbiome analyses. *BMC Biol.* **2014**, *12*, 87. [CrossRef]

44. Yu, G.; Wang, L.G.; Han, Y.; He, Q.Y. clusterProfiler: An R package for comparing biological themes among gene clusters. *Omics* **2012**, *16*, 284–287. [CrossRef] [PubMed]
45. Peinado, H.; Quintanilla, M.; Cano, A. Transforming growth factor beta-1 induces snail transcription factor in epithelial cell lines: Mechanisms for epithelial mesenchymal transitions. *J. Biol. Chem.* **2003**, *278*, 21113–21123. [CrossRef] [PubMed]
46. Hrbáček, J.; Tláskal, V.; Čermák, P.; Hanáček, V.; Zachoval, R. Bladder cancer is associated with decreased urinary microbiota diversity and alterations in microbial community composition. *Urol. Oncol.* **2023**, *41*, 107.e15–107.e22. [CrossRef]
47. Liu, F.; Liu, A.; Lu, X.; Zhang, Z.; Xue, Y.; Xu, J.; Zeng, S.; Xiong, Q.; Tan, H.; He, X.; et al. Dysbiosis signatures of the microbial profile in tissue from bladder cancer. *Cancer Med.* **2019**, *8*, 6904–6914. [CrossRef]
48. Mansour, B.; Monyók, Á.; Makra, N.; Gajdács, M.; Vadnay, I.; Ligeti, B.; Juhász, J.; Szabó, D.; Ostorházi, E. Bladder cancer-related microbiota: Examining differences in urine and tissue samples. *Sci. Rep.* **2020**, *10*, 11042. [CrossRef]
49. Zhao, L.Y.; Mei, J.X.; Yu, G.; Lei, L.; Zhang, W.H.; Liu, K.; Chen, X.L.; Kołat, D.; Yang, K.; Hu, J.K. Role of the gut microbiota in anticancer therapy: From molecular mechanisms to clinical applications. *Signal Transduct. Target. Ther.* **2023**, *8*, 201. [CrossRef]
50. Fernandes, M.R.; Aggarwal, P.; Costa, R.G.F.; Cole, A.M.; Trinchieri, G. Targeting the gut microbiota for cancer therapy. *Nat. Rev. Cancer* **2022**, *22*, 703–722. [CrossRef]
51. Dhatchinamoorthy, K.; Colbert, J.D.; Rock, K.L. Cancer Immune Evasion through Loss of MHC Class I Antigen Presentation. *Front. Immunol.* **2021**, *12*, 636568. [CrossRef]
52. Kim, S.K.; Cho, S.W. The Evasion Mechanisms of Cancer Immunity and Drug Intervention in the Tumor Microenvironment. *Front. Pharmacol.* **2022**, *13*, 868695. [CrossRef]
53. Chen, Q.; Sun, L.; Chen, Z.J. Regulation and function of the cGAS-STING pathway of cytosolic DNA sensing. *Nat. Immunol.* **2016**, *17*, 1142–1149. [CrossRef]
54. Kwon, J.; Bakhoum, S.F. The Cytosolic DNA-Sensing cGAS-STING Pathway in Cancer. *Cancer Discov.* **2020**, *10*, 26–39. [CrossRef] [PubMed]
55. Lan, T.; Chen, L.; Wei, X. Inflammatory Cytokines in Cancer: Comprehensive Understanding and Clinical Progress in Gene Therapy. *Cells* **2021**, *10*, 100. [CrossRef] [PubMed]
56. Knights, A.J.; Funnell, A.P.; Crossley, M.; Pearson, R.C. Holding Tight: Cell Junctions and Cancer Spread. *Trends Cancer Res.* **2012**, *8*, 61–69. [PubMed]
57. Le Bras, G.F.; Taubenslag, K.J.; Andl, C.D. The regulation of cell-cell adhesion during epithelial-mesenchymal transition, motility and tumor progression. *Cell Adh. Migr.* **2012**, *6*, 365–373. [CrossRef]
58. Kinugasa, T.; Akagi, Y.; Ochi, T.; Tanaka, N.; Kawahara, A.; Ishibashi, Y.; Gotanda, Y.; Yamaguchi, K.; Shiratuchi, I.; Oka, Y.; et al. Increased claudin-1 protein expression in hepatic metastatic lesions of colorectal cancer. *Anticancer Res.* **2012**, *32*, 2309–2314.
59. Martin, T.A.; Mansel, R.E.; Jiang, W.G. Loss of occludin leads to the progression of human breast cancer. *Int. J. Mol. Med.* **2010**, *26*, 723–734. [CrossRef]
60. Elloul, S.; Bukholt Elstrand, M.; Nesland, J.M.; Tropé, C.G.; Kvalheim, G.; Goldberg, I.; Reich, R.; Davidson, B. Snail, Slug, and Smad-interacting protein 1 as novel parameters of disease aggressiveness in metastatic ovarian and breast carcinoma. *Cancer* **2005**, *103*, 1631–1643. [CrossRef]
61. Soini, Y. Tight junctions in lung cancer and lung metastasis: A review. *Int. J. Clin. Exp. Pathol.* **2012**, *5*, 126–136.
62. Kundu, S.T.; Gosavi, P.; Khapare, N.; Patel, R.; Hosing, A.S.; Maru, G.B.; Ingle, A.; Decaprio, J.A.; Dalal, S.N. Plakophilin3 downregulation leads to a decrease in cell adhesion and promotes metastasis. *Int. J. Cancer* **2008**, *123*, 2303–2314. [CrossRef]
63. Allam-Ndoul, B.; Castonguay-Paradis, S.; Veilleux, A. Gut Microbiota and Intestinal Trans-Epithelial Permeability. *Int. J. Mol. Sci.* **2020**, *21*, 6402. [CrossRef] [PubMed]
64. Sato, N.; Meijer, L.; Skaltsounis, L.; Greengard, P.; Brivanlou, A.H. Maintenance of pluripotency in human and mouse embryonic stem cells through activation of Wnt signaling by a pharmacological GSK-3-specific inhibitor. *Nat. Med.* **2004**, *10*, 55–63. [CrossRef] [PubMed]
65. Silva-García, O.; Valdez-Alarcón, J.J.; Baizabal-Aguirre, V.M. Wnt/β-Catenin Signaling as a Molecular Target by Pathogenic Bacteria. *Front. Immunol.* **2019**, *10*, 2135. [CrossRef] [PubMed]
66. Basu, S.; Cheriyamundath, S.; Ben-Ze'ev, A. Cell-cell adhesion: Linking Wnt/β-catenin signaling with partial EMT and stemness traits in tumorigenesis. *F1000Research* **2018**, *7*, 1488. [CrossRef]
67. Pohl, H.G.; Groah, S.L.; Pérez-Losada, M.; Ljungberg, I.; Sprague, B.M.; Chandal, N.; Caldovic, L.; Hsieh, M. The Urine Microbiome of Healthy Men and Women Differs by Urine Collection Method. *Int. Neurourol. J.* **2020**, *24*, 41–51. [CrossRef]

cancers

Review

Evolving Treatment Landscape of Frontline Therapy for Metastatic Urothelial Carcinoma: Current Insights and Future Perspectives

Whi-An Kwon [1,*] and Min-Kyung Lee [2,*]

1 Department of Urology, Myongji Hospital, Hanyang University College of Medicine, Goyang-si 10475, Republic of Korea
2 Department of Internal Medicine, Myongji Hospital, Hanyang University College of Medicine, Goyang-si 10475, Republic of Korea
* Correspondence: kein917@hanyang.ac.kr (W.-A.K.); min7949@naver.com (M.-K.L.)

Simple Summary: Metastatic urothelial carcinoma (mUC) has traditionally been treated with cisplatin-based chemotherapy, but nearly half of these patients cannot receive cisplatin owing to comorbidities. Although immune checkpoint inhibitors have become crucial alternatives, optimizing first-line therapies for mUC remains challenging. Recently, the combination of enfortumab vedotin and pembrolizumab has shown significantly improved survival and response rates in cisplatin-ineligible patients, marking a substantial shift in frontline treatment. This review evaluates the evolving landscape of mUC therapies, focusing on the clinical outcomes of innovative combination regimens.

Abstract: Cisplatin-based chemotherapy has long been the standard first-line (1L) treatment for metastatic urothelial carcinoma (mUC). However, up to 50% of patients with mUC may be ineligible for cisplatin owing to comorbidities, necessitating alternative primary treatment options. Immune checkpoint inhibitors (ICIs) have emerged as a vital alternative for those unable to receive cisplatin. Nevertheless, the prognosis of advanced UC remains dire and challenges persist in optimizing 1L therapy. Recent medical advancements have redirected attention towards innovative drug combinations for the primary treatment of mUC. The combination of enfortumab vedotin (EV) and pembrolizumab has shown significantly improved overall and progression-free survival rates compared to those with chemotherapy alone. This combination can be used as a 1L treatment for patients with mUC who are cisplatin-ineligible or require alternatives to standard chemotherapy. While platinum-based chemotherapy continues to be essential for many patients, the approval of EV and pembrolizumab as 1L treatments for cisplatin-ineligible patients signifies a major breakthrough in primary cancer care. These therapies offer enhanced outcomes in terms of survival and response rates and highlight the increasing relevance of ICI-containing regimens in frontline cancer care. This review provides an exhaustive overview of the current frontline treatment landscape of mUC and explores new therapeutic strategies, with the aim of facilitating clinical decision-making and guiding therapeutic strategies in patients with mUC.

Keywords: antibody-drug conjugates; cisplatin-based chemotherapy; enfortumab vedotin; frontline therapy; immune checkpoint inhibitors; metastatic urothelial carcinoma; platinum-based chemotherapy

1. Introduction

Significant advances have recently been made in the therapeutic landscape of metastatic urothelial carcinoma (mUC) (Figure 1) [1]. Bladder cancer (BC), the tenth most common malignancy worldwide, accounted for approximately 573,000 new cases and 213,000 deaths in 2020. Urothelial carcinoma (UC), the most prevalent histological subtype, particularly in the United States and Europe, presents as metastatic cancer in 5–10% of patients at diagnosis [2]. While approximately 75% of newly diagnosed cases are categorized as non-muscle-invasive BC, the remaining 25% are identified as muscle-invasive BC or metastatic disease. The prognosis of mUC is particularly dire, with >90% of those with metastatic disease succumbing to the illness within 5 years [3].

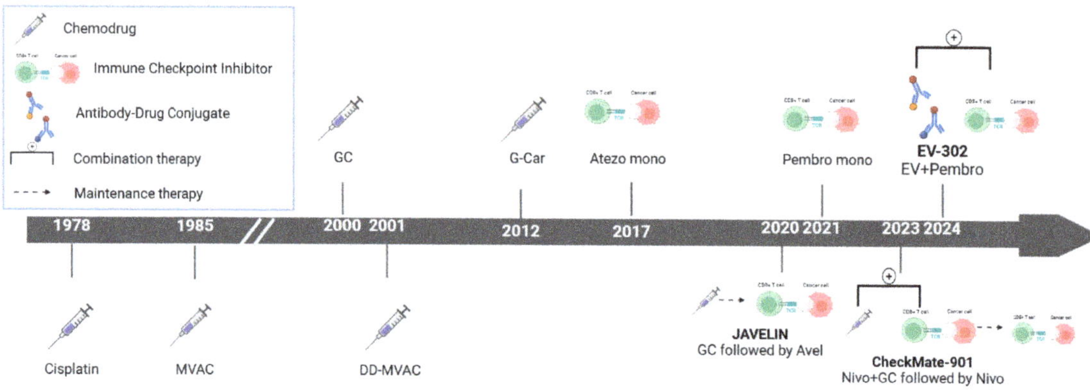

Figure 1. Evolution of frontline treatments for metastatic urothelial carcinoma. Since the approval of cisplatin in 1978, treatment options for urothelial cancer remained fairly static. While there were some modifications in chemotherapeutic regimens, such as dose-dense methotrexate, vinblastine, doxorubicin, and cisplatin (dd-MVAC), no fundamentally new treatment types emerged for decades. This situation changed in 2017 with the introduction of immune checkpoint inhibitors (ICIs), which marked a turning point in the management of metastatic urothelial carcinoma. Following the approval of the first ICIs, several new agents became available, including additional ICIs and antibody-drug conjugates. These developments were driven by pivotal phase III trials (JAVELIN, CheckMate-901, EV-302) that evaluated novel chemotherapies and other treatments. Atezo, atezolizumab; avel, avelumab; dd-MVAC, dose-dense methotrexate, vinblastine, doxorubicin and cisplatin; EV, enfortumab vedotin; GC, gemcitabine, cisplatin; G-Car, gemcitabine, carboplatin; nivo, nivolumab; pembro, pembrolizumab; mono, monotherapy.

Historically, the treatment of mUC has relied heavily on cisplatin-based chemotherapy regimens such as gemcitabine–cisplatin (GC) and methotrexate, vinblastine, doxorubicin, and cisplatin (MVAC), often supplemented with granulocyte colony-stimulating factor (G-CSF) for primary prophylaxis. These regimens yield a median (m) overall survival (OS) of approximately 14 months; however, up to 50% of patients are ineligible for cisplatin owing to comorbidities, poor performance status, or renal impairment. For these patients, alternatives include carboplatin and gemcitabine, as well as immune checkpoint inhibitors (ICIs) [4].

There has been a transformative shift in the treatment of mUC with the introduction of ICIs, antibody–drug conjugates (ADCs), and targeted therapies [5]. ICIs, such as pembrolizumab and atezolizumab, have gained regulatory approval for use in patients ineligible for cisplatin-based therapy, especially those with tumors expressing programmed death-ligand 1 (PD-L1), or those unsuitable for any form of platinum-based chemotherapy (PBC). Notably, pembrolizumab has demonstrated a significant survival benefit compared with second-line chemotherapy in patients who progress after PBC [6].

A significant advancement has been the molecular characterization of mUC, leading to the approval of targeted therapies, such as erdafitinib (fibroblast growth factor receptor (FGFR) inhibitor), for patients with FGFR-altered tumors [7]. These developments have broadened therapeutic options, particularly for patients who have progressed after or are ineligible for traditional chemotherapy.

Another notable milestone is the approval of avelumab as a switch maintenance therapy following first-line (1L) chemotherapy. This strategy may extend OS in patients responsive to initial treatment [8]. Recently, the results of the phase III EV-302 trial, which investigated the combination of enfortumab vedotin (EV) and pembrolizumab as the initial treatment, have challenged the established platinum-based treatment paradigm in mUC. The efficacy of this combination was further validated when the EV-302 trial successfully met its co-primary endpoints of OS and progression-free survival (PFS), marking a pivotal shift in the standard treatment of mUC [9].

Nevertheless, mUC management remains complex and challenging. Determining the optimal therapy for each patient, identifying appropriate treatment sequences, and exploring potential synergies among therapeutic agents are critical areas of ongoing research [10]. Real-world data suggest that only 30–40% of patients receiving primary therapy for mUC proceed to second-line treatment, underscoring the need for effective 1L treatments and improved strategies for subsequent lines of therapy [11].

In this review, we have explored the current therapeutic landscape of mUC, along with the challenges associated with optimizing treatment strategies and establishing effective treatment sequences, and the importance of personalized approaches in improving the survival outcome.

2. Types and Mechanisms of Drug Classes Used in the Frontline Treatment of mUC

2.1. Platinum-Based Chemotherapy

Platinum-based chemotherapy, such as cisplatin, primarily exerts its anticancer effects by forming DNA cross-links that disrupt the DNA double helix, thereby inhibiting critical processes such as DNA replication and transcription. This damage activates cellular stress responses, including DNA damage response pathways, leading to cell cycle arrest, and ultimately, apoptosis. Apoptosis is further enhanced by the activation of the intrinsic mitochondrial pathway and the tumor suppressor protein p53. Additionally, platinum compounds induce the production of reactive oxygen species, which further damage cellular components and amplify apoptosis. Although highly effective, platinum compounds also affect normal cells, leading to nephrotoxicity and neurotoxicity [12–14]. The multifaceted action of platinum-based drugs underscores their effectiveness in cancer treatment, particularly in BC; however, their efficacy needs to be balanced with adverse events (AEs).

2.2. ICIs

ICIs enhance the immune system's ability to recognize and eliminate tumor cells [15] by blocking specific immune checkpoint pathways that normally maintain self-tolerance and modulate immune responses [16]. Under physiological conditions, immune checkpoints are crucial for preventing autoimmunity and limiting immune responses to avoid excessive tissue damage. However, tumors often exploit these pathways to evade immune surveillance [17].

Two of the most well-studied immune checkpoints targeted by ICIs are cytotoxic T lymphocyte-associated protein 4 (CTLA-4) and programmed cell death protein 1 (PD-1), along with its ligand, PD-L1. CTLA-4 is expressed on activated T cells and functions as an inhibitory receptor by competing with the co-stimulatory receptor CD28 for binding to B7 molecules (B7-1/CD80 and B7-2/CD86) on antigen-presenting cells. The binding of CTLA-4 to B7 molecules transmits an inhibitory signal that reduces T cell activation and proliferation. By blocking the interaction between CTLA-4 and B7, CTLA-4 inhibitors, such as ipilimumab, enhance T cell activation, thereby promoting a robust immune response against cancer cells [18–20].

The PD-1/PD-L1 pathway plays a similar role in regulating immune responses. PD-1 is expressed on T, B, and natural killer cells. When PD-1 binds to its ligands PD-L1 or PD-L2, it delivers an inhibitory signal that dampens T cell activity, proliferation, and cytokine production. Tumor cells often upregulate PD-L1 to suppress T cell-mediated immune responses, effectively protecting themselves from immune attack. ICIs targeting this pathway, such as PD-1 inhibitors (nivolumab, pembrolizumab, etc.) or PD-L1 inhibitors (atezolizumab, durvalumab, etc.), block the interaction between PD-1 and its ligands, thereby maintaining T cell activity.

The therapeutic efficacy of ICIs is a consequence of their ability to "release the brakes" on the immune system, allowing for enhanced T cell activation and sustained anti-tumor responses. This mechanism is effective across various malignancies, including melanoma, non-small cell lung cancer, renal cell carcinoma, and UC [21–23].

2.3. ADCs

ADCs are a class of targeted cancer therapies that combine the specificity of monoclonal antibodies with the potent cytotoxic effects of chemotherapeutic agents [24]. They are able to selectively target and kill cancer cells while minimizing damage to normal tissues [24,25]. The monoclonal antibody component of the ADC recognizes and binds to a specific antigen overexpressed on the cancer cell-surface, ensuring that the ADC preferentially targets tumor cells while sparing most normal cells, which typically show low or no expression of the antigen. Once an ADC binds to the target antigen on the cancer cell surface, the entire complex is internalized through receptor-mediated endocytosis. After internalization, the ADC is trafficked to the lysosome, where the antibody-linked cytotoxic drug is released through various mechanisms, depending on the type of linker used in the ADC design. Linkers may be cleavable, breaking down owing to the acidic environment of the lysosome or through enzymatic action, or non-cleavable, where the drug is released only after the entire ADC is degraded. Once the cytotoxic drug is released inside the cancer cell, it interferes with critical cellular processes. Common payloads used in ADCs include highly potent chemotherapeutic agents, such as microtubule inhibitors (auristatins, maytansinoids, etc.) or DNA-damaging agents (e.g., calicheamicin). Microtubule inhibitors disrupt the microtubule network within the cell, preventing cell division and leading to apoptosis. DNA-damaging agents induce breaks in the DNA strand, leading to cell death through apoptosis or mitotic catastrophe.

The high potential systemic toxicity of these drugs is mitigated by the selective delivery mechanism of the ADC, concentrating the drug's effects within the tumor cells, thereby enhancing the treatment's therapeutic index [26,27]. This targeted approach enables ADCs to deliver highly potent drugs directly to cancer cells, improving treatment efficacy while limiting off-target effects [28].

Figure 2 illustrates the mechanisms of action of the major drug classes used in the frontline treatment of mUC, including PBC, ICIs, and ADCs.

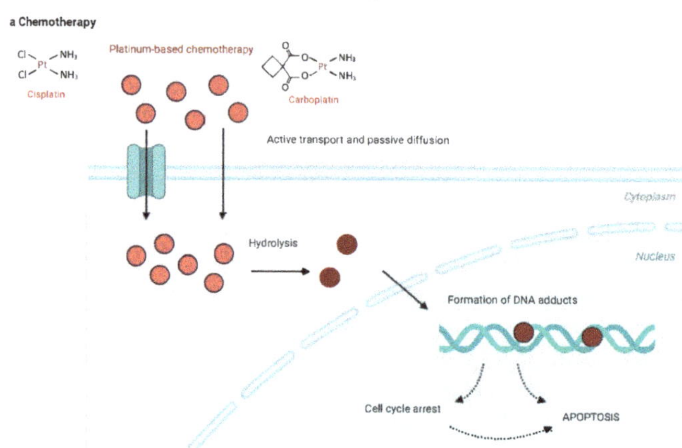

Figure 2. *Cont.*

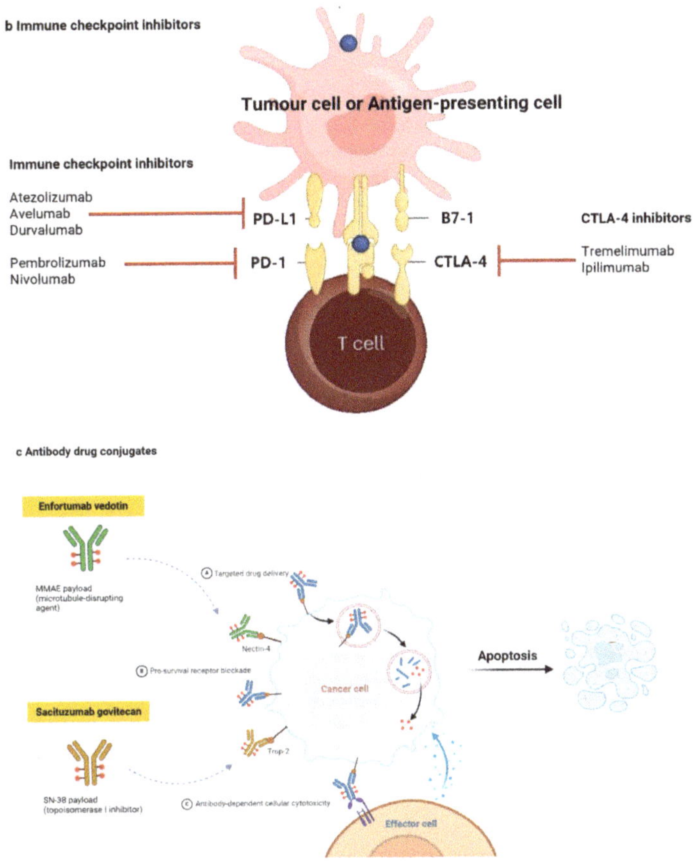

Figure 2. Drug classes and their mechanisms in the frontline treatment of metastatic urothelial carcinoma. (**a**) Platinum-based chemotherapy works by disrupting cell division. Platinum compounds bind to the DNA of cancer cells, creating cross-links that impede normal DNA replication and cell division. This DNA damage hampers the cancer cells' growth and spread. (**b**) Immuno-therapy boosts the patient's immune system to fight against cancer cells. It works by blocking immune checkpoint pathways, such as PD-1, PD-L1, and CTLA-4, which tumor cells use to evade immune detection. By inhibiting these pathways, immunotherapy enables the immune system to attack and eliminate cancer cells. (**c**) Antibody–drug conjugates (ADCs) consist of a cancer-specific antibody linked to a cytotoxic agent. Once the ADC attaches to the cancer cells, it is absorbed, and the toxic drug is released inside the cell, leading to cancer cell death. Enfortumab vedotin targets nectin-4, which is commonly overexpressed in urothelial cancer cells, while sacituzumab govitecan targets tumor cells through the anti-Trop-2 antibody. APC, antigen-presenting cell; CTLA-4, cytotoxic T-lymphocyte associated protein 4; MMAE, monomethyl auristatin; PD-1, programmed cell death protein 1; PD-L1, programmed death-ligand 1; PD-L2, programmed death-ligand 2; SN-38, 7-ethyl-10-hydroxycamptothecin.

3. Patient Selection

Selecting the appropriate frontline therapy for patients with mUC is crucial for optimizing treatment outcomes. This process involves a comprehensive assessment of clinical, molecular, and patient-specific factors. Most patients with mUC are older, with the majority aged >65 years and approximately half aged >70 years [29]. This population often presents with comorbidities that complicate the use of standard cisplatin-based chemotherapy [30].

Consequently, many such patients are ineligible for cisplatin-based therapy, traditionally defined by factors such as an Eastern Cooperative Oncology Group Performance Status (ECOG PS) of ≥2 [31]. Given the nephrotoxic nature of cisplatin, renal function assessment is essential, with a creatinine clearance (CrCl) ≥ 60 mL/min typically serving as the threshold for cisplatin eligibility [32]. Patients with renal impairment, indicated by a CrCl < 60 mL/min, are often considered unsuitable for cisplatin and receive alternative treatments, such as carboplatin-based regimens or ICIs [33].

While the cisplatin ineligibility criteria are relatively well-defined, the ineligibility criteria for carboplatin-based chemotherapy remain unclear, leading to variability in clinical practice [34]. The approval of ICIs for 1L treatment of platinum-ineligible patients underscores the need for a consistent definition of platinum ineligibility [4]. Consensus definitions suggest that patients with an ECOG PS ≥ 3, CrCl < 30 mL/min, peripheral neuropathy grade > 3, or New York Heart Association heart failure class > 3 should be considered ineligible for PBC [35]. Additionally, patients with an ECOG PS of 2 and CrCl < 30 mL/min may also be ineligible for PBC. However, these criteria may not capture all relevant factors, such as advanced age, poorly controlled diabetes, or inadequate bone marrow reserve, which could further contraindicate PBC [4].

The first formal attempts to define cisplatin eligibility in mUC were made in the 1990s. A survey by the European Organization for Research and Treatment of Cancer identified a CrCl ≥ 60 mL/min and World Health Organization performance status of 0 or 1 as key requirements for cisplatin use [36]. These criteria were refined in 2011 by Galsky et al., whose guidelines for cisplatin ineligibility are widely used in clinical practice [37]. However, the exact renal function thresholds for cisplatin eligibility remain unclear, with CrCl cutoffs ranging from <45 mL/min to <60 mL/min, depending on the context [38].

Furthermore, molecular biomarkers have gained importance in guiding frontline therapy decisions, particularly regarding immunotherapy [39]. Patients with high PD-L1 expression, especially those ineligible for cisplatin, are more likely to benefit from ICIs, such as pembrolizumab or atezolizumab. However, PD-L1 expression should not be the sole factor guiding treatment decisions but rather part of a broader clinical assessment [40]. The histological subtype of UC also influences treatment decisions. Variants such as micropapillary, sarcomatoid, or neuroendocrine differentiation may respond differently to standard therapies, requiring a more personalized approach. In such cases, strategies such as neoadjuvant chemotherapy or enrollment in clinical trials may offer better outcomes [41]. Data on ICIs and new therapies for micropapillary, sarcomatoid, and neuroendocrine UC are limited. ICIs showed a 28% overall response rate (ORR) in 25 patients, and EV achieved a 35% ORR in 41 patients with micropapillary components [42,43]. Advanced sarcomatoid UC exhibits higher PD-L1 expression with 35–40% response rates to ICIs [42]; however, low nectin-4 expression may limit EV and pembrolizumab efficacy [44]. For neuroendocrine UC, single-agent anti-PD-1/PD-L1 inhibitors, as well as lurbinectedin and sacituzumab govitecan have demonstrated some efficacy in small studies [45–48], but the effectiveness of dual checkpoint blockade is uncertain [49,50], and low nectin-4 expression may limit EV's benefits [43,44].

Patient preferences and quality of life are also critical in selecting frontline therapy. Having a thorough discussion with patients regarding the potential benefits and risks of each treatment option, specifically the impact on daily life and long-term prognosis, is essential [29]. This ensures that the chosen treatment aligns with the patient's values and goals. Moreover, eligibility for clinical trials can provide access to novel therapies that may not be widely available [51].

Finally, the presence of specific genomic alterations, such as FGFR3 mutations, can guide the selection of targeted therapies, although these are currently used only in the second-line setting. Ongoing research may expand their use in frontline therapy, further personalizing the treatment approach for mUC [52].

Selecting frontline therapy for mUC requires a multifaceted evaluation, including performance status, renal function, comorbidities, molecular biomarkers, histological subtype, and patient preferences. A personalized approach is essential to optimize treatment outcomes of patients with mUC.

Table 1 provides an overview of the key factors involved in selecting the appropriate frontline therapy for patients with mUC.

Table 1. Key factors involved in selecting the appropriate frontline therapy for patients with mUC.

Criteria	Category	Frontline Therapy Options
Cisplatin Eligibility [4,31,34]	Cisplatin-Eligible (eGFR $\geq$ 60 mL/min/1.73 m^2)	- Gemcitabine + Cisplatin (standard of care) - Dose-dense MVAC (Methotrexate, Vinblastine, Doxorubicin, and Cisplatin) - Avelumab maintenance therapy after a response or stable disease following 4–6 cycles of chemotherapy.
	Cisplatin-Ineligible (eGFR < 60 mL/min/1.73 m^2)	- Gemcitabine + Carboplatin (standard alternative) - Atezolizumab or Pembrolizumab (in patients with high PD-L1 expression or those who are not candidates for any platinum therapy) - Avelumab maintenance therapy following stable disease or response to chemotherapy.
PD-L1 Expression	High or intermediate (if platinum-Ineligible, Atezolizumab: SP142 assay, PD-L1–stained tumor-infiltrating immune cells covering $\geq$5% of the tumor area, Pembrolizumab: TPS $\geq$ 1%) [53,54]	- Atezolizumab or Pembrolizumab.
	Low or negative PD-L1 (Cisplatin-Ineligible)	- Gemcitabine + Carboplatin.
Performance Status (ECOG)	ECOG 0-1	- These patients typically tolerate platinum-based chemotherapy well, and cisplatin-based regimens are the standard. If cisplatin-ineligible, carboplatin-based regimens or PD-L1-targeted immunotherapy can be considered, especially in PD-L1 positive patients.
	ECOG 2	- For patients with moderate performance status (ECOG 2), carboplatin-based chemotherapy is preferred, as cisplatin may be too toxic. Immunotherapy is another option, especially in patients with high PD-L1 expression.
	ECOG $\geq$ 3	- Patients with poor performance status are generally not good candidates for chemotherapy. Atezolizumab or pembrolizumab monotherapy may be considered, especially in those with high PD-L1 expression. Supportive care or clinical trials are also options.
Other Factors	Comorbidities (e.g., cardiovascular disease)	- Patients with significant comorbidities that make cisplatin too toxic are typically treated with carboplatin-based chemotherapy or immunotherapy. Atezolizumab or pembrolizumab may be used for those who are cisplatin-ineligible and PD-L1 positive.
Molecular Profiling	FGFR2/3 alterations (approved criteria: Four-point mutations: R248C, S249C, G370C, Y373C, and Five fusions: FGFR2-BICC1, FGFR2-CASP7, FGFR3-TACC3 (variants V1 and V3), FGFR3-BAIAP2L1) [7,55]	- Patients with FGFR mutations who have progressed on platinum-based chemotherapy may be eligible for erdafitinib, an FGFR inhibitor, but this is not used in frontline therapy. However, molecular profiling can inform future treatment lines.

Abbreviation: TPS, tumor proportion score.

4. Clinical Development

4.1. Chemotherapy

Cisplatin-based chemotherapy has long been the cornerstone of managing mUC, with an ORR of approximately 50%, PFS of up to 7 months, and mOS of 13–15 months [56,57]. Historically, the MVAC regimen was favored due to its superior OS compared to cisplatin monotherapy and other combinations like cisplatin, cyclophosphamide, and doxorubicin. However, application of MVAC has been limited by severe toxicities, including grade $\geq$ 3 leukopenia, neutropenic fever, mucositis, and gastrointestinal AEs, with a drug-associated mortality rate of 3–4% [57,58].

In a crucial phase III trial, the GC regimen showed long-term OS and PFS outcomes similar to those of MVAC but better tolerability regarding AEs and quality of life, leading many oncologists to prefer GC over MVAC [58]. Subsequently, high-dose-intensity chemotherapy with dose-dense (dd) MVAC plus G-CSF every 2 weeks demonstrated reduced toxicity and improved response rates compared to the conventional 4-week MVAC schedule [59,60]. Another phase III study reported similar outcomes between ddGC and ddMVAC, further supporting the use of either regimen based on patient tolerance [61].

For cisplatin-ineligible patients, carboplatin-based regimens have been employed. However, outcomes with carboplatin-based combinations are generally inferior to those with cisplatin-based regimens, although evidence is based on underpowered trials [62]. Recently, the DANUBE, IMvigor130, and JAVELIN-100 trials confirmed the superiority of cisplatin over carboplatin in platinum-eligible patients [63–65]. Split-dose administration of cisplatin has been considered for patients with borderline renal function, offering a potentially less nephrotoxic alternative while maintaining efficacy [66]. However, the VEFORA GETUG-AFU V06 study, comparing split-dose cisplatin with standard-dose carboplatin, was halted owing to excessive toxicities in the cisplatin arm [67].

Regarding chemotherapy cycles, consensus guidelines recommend 2–6 cycles of PBC [53]. Post hoc analysis from the JAVELIN Bladder 100 trial suggested that survival benefits from maintenance avelumab are consistent regardless of whether patients received 4, 5, or 6 cycles of chemotherapy [68]. Advances in treatment have diminished the role of second- and later-line chemotherapy regimens, which previously offered limited benefits over best supportive care (BSC) [69].

4.2. Immunotherapy

4.2.1. 1L Monotherapy for Platinum-Ineligible Patients

ICIs such as atezolizumab and pembrolizumab have been extensively evaluated as monotherapy for cisplatin-ineligible patients with mUC 4. The phase II IMvigor210 trial evaluated atezolizumab as a 1L therapy in 119 patients with locally advanced or metastatic (la/m) UC who were ineligible for cisplatin-based chemotherapy [70]. The trial reported an ORR of 23%, with 9% patients achieving a complete response (CR) (mOS, 15.9 months). The revised ORRs by PD-L1 subgroup were 28% (95% confidence interval [CI]: 14–47) in IC2/3, 24% (95% CI: 15–35) in IC1/2/3, 21% (95% CI: 10–35) in IC1, and 21% (95% CI: 9–36) in IC0. Atezolizumab demonstrated a manageable safety profile, with grade 3 or 4 treatment-related AEs occurring in 16% patients. However, in May 2018, the Food and Drug Administration (FDA) issued a safety alert after early data from the IMvigor130 trial, and another study, suggested decreased survival of patients receiving atezolizumab as 1L monotherapy compared to those receiving PBC [71]. Consequently, the FDA restricted the use of atezolizumab as a 1L treatment to patients who were either ineligible for cisplatin-based chemotherapy with high PD-L1 expression ($\geq$5% of immune cells) or those ineligible for any PBC, regardless of PD-L1 status [71]. The IMvigor130 trial, a multicenter phase III study [64], did not find a significant OS advantage for atezolizumab monotherapy over chemotherapy alone. Consequently, the manufacturer voluntarily withdrew the 1L indication for atezolizumab in mUC in November 2022 [11]. Nevertheless, the National Comprehensive Cancer Network (NCCN) Panel continues to recommend atezolizumab as a 1L option for patients ineligible for cisplatin-containing chemotherapy with tumors expressing PD-L1 or those ineligible for any PBC regardless of the PD-L1 status (category 2B recommendation) [53].

Subsequently, pembrolizumab was evaluated as 1L monotherapy for cisplatin-ineligible patients in the phase II KEYNOTE-052 trial [72], where it demonstrated an ORR of 24%, with 5% patients achieving a CR. Long-term outcomes remained consistent, with an ORR of 28.6% and mOS of 11.3 months. In patients with a PD-L1 combined positive score (CPS) $\geq$ 10, the ORR was 47.3%, with 20.0% patients achieving CR; for those with a PD-L1 CPS < 10, the ORR was 20.3%. The mOS was 18.5 months (95% CI, 12.2–28.5 months) in the CPS $\geq$ 10 group and 9.7 months (95% CI, 7.6–11.5 months) in the CPS < 10 group. However, similar to atezolizumab, the FDA issued a safety alert for pembrolizumab in May 2018 based on early findings from the KEYNOTE-361 trial that suggested decreased survival of patients receiving pembrolizumab monotherapy compared to those receiving PBC [73]. Therefore, the FDA restricted the use of pembrolizumab as a 1L treatment to patients who were ineligible for cisplatin-containing chemotherapy and had high PD-L1 expression (CPS $\geq$ 10) or those ineligible for any PBC regardless of the PD-L1 status [6]. The indication was further limited to patients ineligible for any PBC, with the NCCN Panel continuing to recommend pembrolizumab as a 1L treatment for cisplatin-ineligible patients regardless of the PD-L1 status, and specifically endorsing its use for those ineligible for any PBC [53].

Overall, while both atezolizumab and pembrolizumab provide new therapeutic options for cisplatin-ineligible patients with mUC, their use as 1L monotherapies has been restricted owing to concerns over OS, particularly in patients with low PD-L1 expression. The NCCN's continued endorsement of these therapies, albeit with specific limitations, underscores the importance of careful patient selection in the management of mUC.

4.2.2. 1L Combination Therapy

Combinations of ICIs and chemotherapy have generally yielded less favorable outcomes than anticipated [74]. For instance, the phase III trials IMvigor130 and KEYNOTE-361 evaluated the efficacy of atezolizumab and pembrolizumab, respectively, either as monotherapies or in combination with PBC, compared to chemotherapy alone [64,75]. The KEYNOTE-361 trial showed negligible improvements in PFS or OS when pembrolizumab was combined with PBC compared to chemotherapy alone in patients with mUC. Similarly, the final survival analysis from the IMvigor130 study did not demonstrate a significant OS advantage for the combination of atezolizumab with platinum and gemcitabine over chemotherapy alone in patients with mUC [76]. Nevertheless, exploratory data suggest a potential benefit of atezolizumab monotherapy in 1L cisplatin-ineligible patients with high PD-L1 expression, although the results were not statistically significant. Interestingly, a potentially greater benefit was observed when atezolizumab was combined with cisplatin instead of carboplatin, suggesting the need to determine the optimal chemotherapy regimen.

The phase III DANUBE trial further explored ICI combinations by evaluating durvalumab, an anti-PD-L1 agent, either as a monotherapy or in combination with tremelimumab, an anti-CTLA-4 agent, against standard chemotherapy in patients with mUC [63]. Unfortunately, the trial failed to meet its co-primary endpoints, which included OS comparisons between durvalumab monotherapy and chemotherapy in patients with high PD-L1 expression, as well as that between the durvalumab–tremelimumab combination and chemotherapy in the overall population. However, the promising activity observed in the PD-L1-high population led to the revision of the NILE protocol, which now focuses on untreated patients with mUC and high PD-L1 expression. The results of this global phase III trial are highly anticipated and may redefine treatment approaches for this subset of patients [77].

Contrastingly, the multinational phase III CheckMate 901 study demonstrated the efficacy of adding nivolumab to GC chemotherapy in 608 patients with previously untreated or unresectable mUC [78]. In this study, 251 patients who received the nivolumab combination continued with maintenance nivolumab for up to 2 years. After a median follow-up of 33.6 months, the results showed that the nivolumab plus GC combination significantly improved mOS compared to GC alone (21.7 vs. 18.9 months; hazard ratio [HR], 0.78; 95% CI, 0.63–0.96; $p = 0.02$). Although the median PFS (mPFS) was similar between the two groups (7.9 vs. 7.6 months; $p = 0.001$), the PFS curves began to diverge over time, with a higher percentage of patients remaining progression-free at 12 months in the nivolumab combination group (34.2% vs. 21.8%). Furthermore, the ORR was notably higher in the nivolumab combination group (57.6% vs. 43.1%), with a CR rate of 21.7% compared to 11.8% in the chemotherapy-alone group. Among patients with tumor PD-L1 expression $\geq$1%, the nivolumab combination demonstrated a better HR compared to gemcitabine–cisplatin alone. The HR for OS and PFS as assessed by a central review were 0.75 (95% CI, 0.53–1.06) and 0.60 (95% CI, 0.41–0.81), respectively. However, the combination therapy was associated with a higher incidence of grade $\geq$ 3 treatment-related AEs (TRAEs), occurring in 61.8% of patients compared to 51.7% in the chemotherapy-alone group. These findings led to the regimen being designated as a category 1 recommendation by the NCCN Panel [53]. The results of the CheckMate-901 trial stand in contrast to those of earlier phase III trials, such as the KEYNOTE-361 and IMvigor130, which did not show significant improvements in either OS or PFS when ICIs such as pembrolizumab or atezolizumab were added to PBC for 1L treatment of mUC. Differences in the immunomodulatory effects of cisplatin and carboplatin may partially explain the discrepancies between these trials [78]. Exploratory analyses of both KEYNOTE-361 and IMvigor130 suggested that combining ICIs with cisplatin-based therapy, but not carboplatin-based therapy, resulted in better outcomes. Specifically, the outcomes were better when patients with pretreated tumors with higher PD-L1 expression were treated with GC than with gemcitabine–carboplatin [79]. Furthermore, single-cell RNA sequencing of circulating immune cells in the IMvigor130 trial revealed that GC, but not gemcitabine–carboplatin, upregulated immune-related transcriptional programs, including those involved in antigen presentation [80]. Therefore, cisplatin-based chemotherapy may have particularly favorable immunogenic effects when combined with ICIs in mUC treatment, as observed in the CheckMate-901 trial, highlighting the importance of chemotherapy selection for optimizing the efficacy of combination therapies in mUC.

4.2.3. Maintenance Therapy

Avelumab as maintenance therapy following 1L PBC is considered a significant advancement in mUC treatment [81]. This regimen is based on findings from the phase III JAVELIN Bladder 100 trial 62, which demonstrated that avelumab significantly prolongs OS compared to BSC alone in patients who achieved either a response or stable disease after 1L chemotherapy. Specifically, the trial showed an mOS of 21.4 months for patients treated with avelumab, compared to 14.3 months for those who received BSC alone, corresponding to an HR of 0.69 (95% CI, 0.56–0.86; $p = 0.001$). This OS benefit was consistent across all prespecified subgroups, including patients with PD-L1-positive tumors.

In the PD-L1-positive population, the avelumab group had significantly longer OS compared to the control group, with a 1-year survival rate of 79.1% (95% CI, 72.1–84.5) versus 60.4% (95% CI, 52.0–67.7) in the control group (stratified HR, 0.56; 95% CI, 0.40–0.79; $p < 0.001$). Among patients with PD-L1-negative tumors, the mOS was 18.8 months (95% CI, 13.3–22.5) in the avelumab group compared to 13.7 months (95% CI, 10.8–17.8) in the control group (stratified HR, 0.85; 95% CI, 0.62–1.18). Additionally, avelumab was also associated with a longer PFS compared to BSC alone. Importantly, preplanned subgroup analyses demonstrated that the OS benefit of avelumab was significant regardless of previous treatment with cisplatin or carboplatin or the response to chemotherapy. Despite a higher incidence of subsequent treatments in the control group, including with ICIs, the 12-month OS was substantially higher in the avelumab arm (71%) compared to that in the BSC arm (58%). The incidence of grade $\geq$ 3 AEs was higher in the avelumab group (47.4%) compared to that in the BSC group (25.2%). Yet, the long-term safety profile of avelumab remained manageable, with the most common TRAEs being pruritus, hypothyroidism, fatigue, diarrhea, and asthenia. Based on the findings of the JAVELIN Bladder 100 trial, the NCCN assigned a category 1 recommendation to avelumab maintenance therapy for patients with mUC who do not experience disease progression after 1L PBC 65. Subsequent extended follow-up data, with a median duration of 38 months, confirmed the durability of the OS and PFS benefits of avelumab, with an OS of 23.8 months versus 15.0 months (HR 0.76; 95% CI, 0.631–0.915; $p = 0.0036$) and PFS of 5.5 months versus 2.1 months (HR 0.54; 95% CI, 0.457–0.645; $p < 0.0001$) [82].

Real-world studies conducted in Italy (READY study) and France (AVENANCE study) have further validated the clinical benefits and manageable safety profile of avelumab as a 1L maintenance therapy for patients with mUC [83,84]. These studies reported 12-month OS rates of 65.4–69.2% and mPFS of 5.7–8.1 months, consistent with the findings of the JAVELIN Bladder 100 trial.

Following the results of the CheckMate-901 trial, nivolumab has also emerged as a viable maintenance therapy option for patients with mUC who respond to nivolumab plus 1L cisplatin-based chemotherapy. The trial demonstrated that nivolumab plus GC significantly improved outcomes in these patients, leading the NCCN to recommend nivolumab as an alternative maintenance therapy alongside avelumab [53]. This expanded recommendation gives clinicians more flexibility when selecting an appropriate maintenance therapy based on patient-specific factors.

While both avelumab and nivolumab maintenance therapies have significantly improved the outcomes of patients with mUC, ongoing phase II and phase III trials are exploring combinations of these agents with other therapies as 1L maintenance treatments. The optimal second-line therapy for patients with disease progression during or after maintenance therapy with either avelumab or nivolumab is still under investigation, and enrollment in clinical trials is strongly recommended [85].

4.3. EV Combination Therapy

The combination of the ICI pembrolizumab with the ADC EV has been explored extensively for mUC treatment 10. Initial studies were conducted within certain phase Ib/II EV-103 cohorts, mainly focusing on cisplatin-ineligible patients with previously untreated la/mUC [86]. In cohort A, 45 patients received the combination therapy, resulting in an ORR of 73.3% and CR of 15.6%. However, the treatment was associated with significant AEs, including peripheral sensory neuropathy (55.6%), fatigue (51.1%), and alopecia (48.9%), with 64.4% of patients experiencing grade $\geq$ 3 AEs, and one treatment-related death. Cohort K of the EV-103 trial randomized cisplatin-ineligible patients to receive either EV alone or in combination with pembrolizumab. The combination therapy achieved a confirmed ORR of 64.5% (95% CI, 52.7–75.1%) compared to 45.2% (95% CI, 33.5–57.3%) for EV monotherapy. The median duration of response was not reached for the combination, whereas it was 13.2 months for the monotherapy.

The combination was further evaluated in the phase III EV-302 trial in 886 patients with previously untreated la/mUC [9]. Patients were randomized to receive either EV plus pembrolizumab or standard chemotherapy with gemcitabine in combination with either cisplatin or carboplatin. After a median follow-up of 17.2 months, the combination therapy significantly improved PFS and OS. Specifically, the mPFS was 12.5 months with the combination versus 6.3 months with chemotherapy (HR, 0.45; 95% CI, 0.38–0.54; $p < 0.001$), and the mOS was 31.5 months versus 16.1 months (HR, 0.47; 95% CI, 0.38–0.58; $p < 0.001$). Additionally, the confirmed ORR was 67.7% for the combination compared to 44.4% for chemotherapy, with CR in 29.1% of patients in the combination group versus 12.5% in the chemotherapy group. Notably, grade $\geq$ 3 TRAEs occurred in 55.9% of patients receiving the combination therapy, compared to 69.5% of those receiving chemotherapy.

The impressive outcomes from the EV-302 trial led to the combination of EV and pembrolizumab being recognized as the preferred 1L systemic therapy for patients with advanced UC or mUC, regardless of cisplatin eligibility. This regimen has received a category 1 designation from the NCCN panel, solidifying its status as a new standard of care in this setting [53].

EV-302 and JAVELIN Paradigm Versus CheckMate-901

The role of GC/nivo (gemcitabine/cisplatin with nivolumab) and the JAVELIN paradigm in the management of mUC is being reevaluated in light of the impressive results of EV/pembro (enfortumab vedotin with pembrolizumab) [9]. The usefulness of GC/nivo in cisplatin-eligible patients is because of several factors. Firstly, cisplatin-based combination therapies have historically cured 5–15% of patients [58,60]. The long-term CR observed in approximately 22% of patients receiving GC/nivo supports the possibility of achieving a cure in a subset of patients [78]. While EV/pembro may also lead to cure, long-term follow-up is required to confirm this potential. Secondly, compared to EV/pembro, GC/nivo offers a finite duration of chemotherapy, providing advantages of reduced toxicity and improved quality of life during treatment [9,78]. Additionally, GC/nivo is more cost-effective compared to EV/pembro, making it a financially viable option for many healthcare systems and patients [87,88]. Moreover, GC/nivo may be considered for patients with uncontrolled diabetes mellitus or liver dysfunction owing to the specific safety and tolerability considerations associated with EV [78,89,90].

The identification of predictive biomarkers for CR is crucial for implementing precision medicine in mUC. Disease confined to lymph nodes is a favorable prognostic factor for both cisplatin-based chemotherapy and PD-1 inhibition, suggesting the aggressive use of GC/nivo in this patient group [91,92]. Additionally, ERCC2 mutations, previously validated for predicting pathological CR with neoadjuvant cisplatin-based chemotherapy, may serve as biomarkers for predicting CR with cisplatin-based therapy [93].

Given that aggressive multi-agent combination therapies are feasible only in selected patients in real-world settings, all 1L regimens, including EV/pembro, GC/nivo, and the JAVELIN paradigm, have legitimate roles in clinical practice [53].

Despite the availability of maintenance immunotherapy, its implementation in real-world practice is limited. In the EV-302 study, only 32.2% patients received a PD-1/L1 inhibitor as maintenance therapy after PBC, and only 20% patients in the GC arm of the CheckMate-901 study received a PD-1/L1 inhibitor before progression. The suboptimal application of the JAVELIN paradigm may be attributed to attrition from disease progression, persistent toxicities, poor ECOG performance status (PS), frailty, comorbidities, and patient decisions [85]. Therefore, potent 1L regimens that provide early and durable benefits, such as EV/pembro and GC/nivo, both of which induce rapid responses within 2–3 months, are expected to replace the JAVELIN paradigm for most patients. Nonetheless, in frail or vulnerable cisplatin-ineligible patients (including potentially some with ECOG PS 2), employing the JAVELIN paradigm of carboplatin/gemcitabine followed by maintenance avelumab may be a safer option.

Table 2 summarizes the key clinical trials on frontline therapy for mUC, highlighting the interventions, outcomes, and AEs associated with each treatment strategy.

Table 2. Key clinical trials in frontline therapy for mUC.

Trial	Intervention Arm	Control Arm	Median PFS in the Intervention Arm (Months)	Median PFS in the Control Arm (Months)	Hazard Ratio (HR) (95% CI)	p-Value	Median OS in the Intervention Arm (Months)	Median OS in the Control Arm (Months)	Hazard Ratio (HR) (95% CI)	p-Value	Adverse Events
De Santis et al. 2009 [62]	Gemcitabine/ Carboplatin	Methotrexate/ Carboplatin/ Vinblastine	Not available	Not available			9.3	8.1			
Sternberg et al. 2006 [60]	High-dose intensity M-VAC + G-CSF	Classic M-VAC	Not available	Not available			15.9	14.2		0.075	Reduced toxicity with dose-dense M-VAC
GC vs. MVAC [57]	Gemcitabine + Cisplatin	MVAC	7.0	7.5	Similar HR	0.8	14.0	15.2	Similar HR	0.6	GC better tolerability, lower toxicity (Grade 3+ AE)
KEYNOTE-901 [78]	Nivolumab + GC	Gemcitabine-cisplatin	7.9	7.6	0.78 (0.63–0.96)	0.02	21.7	18.9	0.78 (0.63–0.96)	0.02	Grade 3+ TRAEs 61.8% vs. 51.7%
JAVELIN-100 [82]	Avelumab (maintenance)	Best Supportive Care	5.5	2.1	0.69 (0.56–0.86)	0.001	21.4	14.3	0.69 (0.56–0.86)	0.001	Grade 3+ TRAEs 47% vs. 25%
DANUBE [63]	Durvalumab + tremelimumab	Chemotherapy	6.7	6.9	0.85 (0.71–1.02)	0.075	15.1	12.1	0.85 (0.72–1.02)	0.054	Grade 3+ TRAEs 61% vs. 50%
IMvigor130 [64]	Atezolizumab + chemo	Chemotherapy alone	8.2	6.3	0.82 (0.70–0.96)	0.007	16.0	13.4	0.83 (0.69–1.00)	0.027	Grade 3+ TRAEs 81% vs. 76%
IMvigor210 [70]	Atezolizumab (monotherapy)	No control (single-arm)	2.7	N/A	N/A	N/A	7.9	N/A	N/A	N/A	Grade 3–4 TRAEs 16%
EV-103 [94]	EV + Pembrolizumab	No control (single-arm)	12.3	N/A	N/A	N/A	26.1	N/A	N/A	N/A	Grade 3–4 TRAEs 54%
EV-302 [9]	EV + Pembrolizumab	Standard chemotherapy	12.5	6.3	0.45 (0.38–0.54)	<0.001	31.5	16.1	0.47 (0.38–0.58)	<0.001	Grade 3+ TRAEs 55.9% vs. 69.5%
KEYNOTE-052 [72]	Pembrolizumab (monotherapy)	No control (single-arm)	2.1	N/A	N/A	N/A	11.3	N/A	N/A	N/A	Grade 3–4 TRAEs 16%
KEYNOTE-361 [75]	Pembrolizumab + chemo	Chemotherapy alone	8.3	7.1	0.78 (0.65–0.93)	0.003	17.0	14.3	0.86 (0.72–1.02)	0.04	Grade 3–4 TRAEs 67% vs. 63%

Abbreviations: CI, Confidence Interval; GC, Gemcitabine+Cisplatin; Ev, Enfortumab Vedotin; G-CSF: Granulocyte-Colony Stimulating Factor; HR: Hazard Ratio; M-VAC: Methotrexate, Vinblastine, Doxorubicin, and Cisplatin; N/A: Not Available; OS: Overall Survival; PFS: Progression-Free Survival; TRAE: Treatment-Related Adverse Events.

4.4. Real-World 1L Treatment Patterns and Survival Rates for la/mUC

Several retrospective studies have analyzed real-world 1L treatment patterns and OS in patients with la/mUC in the United States and Germany [95–97]. These regions were chosen owing to their high incidence of UC and availability of comprehensive healthcare data that support real-world analysis.

A large-scale analysis of Medicare fee-for-service claims from 2015 to 2022 involving 13,104 U.S. patients with UC revealed that PBC remains the most commonly administered 1L treatment. Specifically, 19.7% patients received cisplatin and 28.4% received carboplatin. ICI monotherapy was also prevalent, being administered to 34.8% of patients, particularly those with comorbidities such as renal disease (39.9%), chronic obstructive pulmonary disease (36.1%), and diabetes (32.2%). Despite cisplatin-treated patients showing the longest median OS at 17.0 months, overall outcomes were generally poor across all treatment groups, largely due to disease progression, limited efficacy of available treatments, and patient comorbidities that impacted tolerability and response [97].

Following the FDA approval of avelumab maintenance therapy in June 2020, a study utilized the U.S. Oncology Network electronic health records from December 2019 to September 2022 and assessed 1072 patients with la/mUC (median age: 73 years, 74.9% male). The 1L treatments included ICI monotherapy (43.8%), PBC alone (37.3%), and PBC followed by avelumab maintenance (10.4%). Notably, ICI monotherapy was frequently used even in patients eligible for PBC. Patients receiving PBC with subsequent avelumab maintenance exhibited the longest median OS (20 months for cisplatin plus avelumab and 18.4 months for carboplatin plus avelumab), supporting avelumab maintenance as a standard option for those without disease progression on PBC. Thus, incorporating maintenance therapy into clinical practice may potentially extend patient survival, especially in those responding well to initial PBC [96].

In Germany, the CONVINCE retrospective multicenter study evaluated 188 patients treated between 2019 and 2021 (median age: 70 years, 72.3% male). The majority (76.1%) received PBC, predominantly combined with gemcitabine, while 19.1% received ICI monotherapy, mainly atezolizumab or pembrolizumab. A small group received other non-PBC treatments. The study found high adherence to treatment guidelines recommending PBC as the 1L therapy. The emerging use of ICI therapies, including avelumab maintenance, indicates potential for improved patient outcomes and necessity for further real-world research to assess their integration into clinical practice [95].

Collectively, these studies demonstrate that while PBC remains the standard 1L treatment associated with longer OS in patients with la/mUC, the OS rates are suboptimal, primarily due to disease biology, treatment tolerability, and patient-specific factors such as comorbidities. The increasing adoption of ICI therapies and maintenance treatments such as avelumab may enhance outcomes. However, the substantial use of ICI monotherapy, even among patients who could tolerate PBC, suggests opportunities to optimize treatment strategies. These findings underscore an unmet need for more effective 1L therapies to improve survival of patients with la/mUC.

4.5. Survival Benefits of the Different Therapeutic Protocols

Among cisplatin-eligible patients, gemcitabine plus cisplatin, the historical standard, achieved a mOS of 13.8 months [57]. The addition of nivolumab (CheckMate 901) improved the OS to 21.7 months [78]. EV plus pembrolizumab (EV-302) reported the longest OS at 31.5 months [9].

For cisplatin-ineligible patients, gemcitabine plus carboplatin resulted in a median OS of 9.3 months [98], highlighting the limitations of carboplatin-based chemotherapy, which is generally less effective owing to its lower potency and reduced ability to form DNA cross-links compared to cisplatin. Pembrolizumab monotherapy (KEYNOTE-052), approved for platinum-ineligible patients, demonstrated an OS of 11.3 months but remains less effective than combination therapies [72].

Avelumab maintenance therapy (JAVELIN 100), following disease control with PBC, significantly prolonged survival [65]. The median OS was 25.8 months for patients receiving carboplatin during induction and 31.5 months for those receiving cisplatin. This highlights the specific role of avelumab in maintaining disease control and extending OS, particularly in patients who initially respond to platinum-based induction therapy.

However, outcomes for cisplatin-ineligible patients remain suboptimal, as reflected by the poorer OS with carboplatin-based or immunotherapy monotherapies, emphasizing the need for further research, including the development of novel targeted therapies and improved ADCs, and exploring combination regimens with better response rates.

5. Future Perspectives and Discussion

The evolving landscape of frontline therapy for mUC presents significant advancements, with many ongoing Phase III and II clinical trials actively contributing to the refinement of future treatment paradigms (Table 3). Recent developments have introduced promising therapeutic agents and combination therapies for mUC, such as EV with pembrolizumab, which may potentially enhance patient outcomes. However, challenges persist in determining the optimal sequencing, duration, and combination of these therapies, as well as in identifying predictive biomarkers to guide clinical decision-making.

Table 3. Recent ongoing first-line phase III/II clinical trials in patients with advanced UC.

Study	Cisplatin-Eligibility	Experimental Arm	Status	Phase	Enrolment (n)	Patients	Primary End Point
NCT03682068 (NILE)	cisplatin-eligible	Durvalumab + SoC (CT) or durvalumab + tremelimumab + SoC vs. SoC	Active, not recruiting	III	1292	La/mUC	OS
NCT03036098	cisplatin-eligible	Nivolumab + ipilimumab or + SoC CT vs. SoC	Active, not recruiting	III	1307	La/mUC	OS, PFS
NCT05302284	cisplatin-eligible	RC48-ADC + toripalimab vs. CT alone	Recruiting	III	452	La/mUC with HER2 expressing	OS, PFS
NCT03967977	cisplatin-eligible	Cis/Car + G + tislelizumab vs. Cis/Car + G + placebo	Recruiting	III	420	La/mUC	OS
NCT02567409	cisplatin-eligible	Cis + G ± M6620	Active, not recruiting	II	91 actuals	mUC	PFS
NCT04486781	cisplatin/platinum-ineligible	Pembrolizumab + sEphB4-HSA	Recruiting	II	38	mUC patients CT ineligible or refused	ORR
NCT03237780	cisplatin/platinum-ineligible	Eribulin mesylate + atezolizumab vs. atezolizumab alone	Active, not recruiting	II	72	La/mUC	AEs. ORR
NCT04601857	cisplatin/platinum-ineligible	Futibatinib + pembrolizumab	Active, not recruiting	II	46	La/mUC	ORR
NCT05645692	cisplatin/platinum-ineligible	RO7247669 ± tiragolumab vs. atezolizumab	Active, not recruiting	II	240	La/mUC	ORR

5.1. Challenges in Optimizing EV Plus Pembrolizumab for Frontline mUC Treatment

The combination of EV with pembrolizumab in the frontline setting has shown promise as a potential standard of care for all patients, regardless of their eligibility for PBC. This raises the possibility of reserving chemotherapy and targeted agents for later lines of treatment, adding complexity to treatment decisions [85]. However, several questions remain, such as the optimal duration of therapy, sequencing of treatments, and potential for EV rechallenge after discontinuation owing to toxicity. Additionally, the role of EV plus pembrolizumab versus EV alone in patients who have previously received adjuvant immunotherapy is worth investigating [99,100]. Clinical trials are exploring these questions, including alternative dosing schedules and maintenance strategies, such as reducing the dosing frequency of EV or implementing maintenance pembrolizumab after an initial course of EV plus pembrolizumab [101].

As the mUC treatment landscape continues to evolve, the sequencing of therapies is becoming increasingly complex. The potential widespread adoption of EV plus pembrolizumab as frontline therapy may shift the use of chemotherapy and other targeted agents to subsequent lines, necessitating a re-evaluation of the current treatment paradigms, particularly for patients who experience disease progression after 1L therapy [9,102]. However, questions remain regarding the role of chemotherapy after progression on EV plus pembrolizumab. Ongoing trials are examining the efficacy of various sequences, such as gemcitabine–carboplatin following EV plus pembrolizumab, and combinations of newer agents such as sacituzumab govitecan with pembrolizumab [103,104].

5.2. Biomarkers of Response

Identifying predictive biomarkers is crucial for frontline mUC treatment to guide therapeutic decisions. Predicting which patients will benefit most from specific regimens, such as EV plus pembrolizumab, GC with nivolumab followed by maintenance, or other chemo-immunotherapy combinations, is essential for optimizing outcomes [105]. Considerable progress has been made in this area, particularly with biomarkers related to immunotherapy, such as PD-L1 expression, microsatellite instability, defective mismatch repair phenotype, and tumor mutational burden [106]. A recent meta-analysis of 14 studies showed that PD-L1-positive UC is associated with higher response rates and improved survival outcomes in patients treated with ICIs. Although PD-L1 positivity suggests a better prognosis, it is not a reliable predictive biomarker for ICI response [40].

Emerging biomarkers, including circulating tumor DNA (ctDNA) and gut microbiota, have shown promise but require further validation [107]. The STING trial underscored the feasibility and reliability of plasma ctDNA in identifying actionable targets and selecting genotype-specific therapies in mUC [108].

5.3. Managing Toxicities in Frontline Therapy

The emergence of EV plus pembrolizumab as a frontline treatment is associated with challenges in managing the associated toxicities. Peripheral neuropathy and skin reactions are among the most-reported AEs of EV, requiring careful management, especially in patients with comorbidities such as diabetes. Additionally, a recently reported case of lung toxicity emphasizes the need for close pulmonary monitoring during EV treatment [109]. While these toxicities are generally manageable, they can lead to treatment interruptions or discontinuation [9,110]. Given the increasing use of EV plus pembrolizumab, there is a growing focus on optimizing dosing schedules to minimize toxicity while maintaining efficacy. Ongoing clinical trials are exploring fixed-duration EV therapy followed by pembrolizumab maintenance as a potential approach to improve the quality of life of patients [111].

5.4. Combining Low-Risk Dietary and Metabolic Therapies with Standard Cancer Treatments to Enhance Efficacy and Mitigate Toxicity

The therapeutic effectiveness of standard cancer therapies, such as ICIs and ADCs, is limited by severe AEs. Therefore, there is a need for low risk combined therapies that enhance the immune system. Plant-based dietary nutrients, such as ginger derivatives, show anti-tumor effects and can mitigate ICI-related AEs [112]. High-dose ascorbic acid has significant potential but is underutilized [113–115]. Metabolic interventions such as fasting, avoiding sugar to starve tumor cells, and increasing tumor pH to inhibit growth have been considered [116]. Combining these measures with standard treatments has the potential to improve efficacy and reduce toxicity.

5.5. *Clinical Significance of Newer Treatments Other than EV-302*

The currently recommended treatment algorithm (Figure 3) for mUC outlines strategies based on cisplatin eligibility and patient-specific factors and incorporates recent evidence to guide therapeutic decisions. For patients with visceral and/or bone metastasis, upper tract UC, high-risk cardiac disease, or good performance status, regardless of cisplatin eligibility, EV/pembro is recommended because of improved survival outcomes. In cisplatin-eligible patients with comorbidities such as poorly controlled diabetes or retinal/corneal abnormalities, GC/nivo followed by maintenance nivolumab or GC followed by maintenance avelumab is advised, enabling a tailored approach based on disease response and tolerability. For cisplatin-ineligible patients with peripheral neuropathy (Grade $\geq$ 2) or other vulnerabilities, gemcitabine–carboplatin followed by maintenance avelumab remains the standard of care. Finally, for patients who are platinum-ineligible, pembrolizumab monotherapy is the primary option, particularly for those who cannot tolerate platinum-based regimens. This algorithm reflects a personalized approach, optimizing the use of combination therapies such as EV/pembro and maintenance strategies with avelumab or nivolumab, while addressing the unmet needs of patients with significant comorbidities or platinum ineligibility.

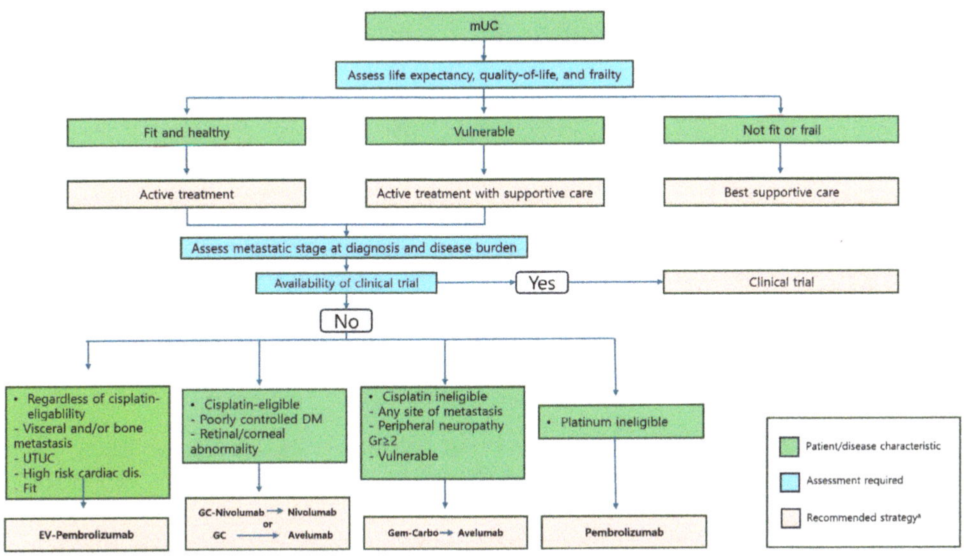

Figure 3. Recommended treatment approaches for frontline patients with mUC. All treatment decisions should be made only after thoroughly discussing the benefits and risks with the patient and/or their caregiver. Abbreviations: DM, diabetes mellitus; EV, enfortumab vedotin; GC, gemcitabine–cisplatin; gem–carbo, gemcitabine–carboplatin.

6. Conclusions

The evolving landscape of frontline mUC treatment is marked by a shift from traditional PBC to more innovative and targeted therapies, such as EV plus pembrolizumab and GC plus nivolumab followed by nivolumab maintenance. These regimens have significantly improved survival outcomes, offering effective 1L options for a broader range of patients, including those previously ineligible for cisplatin-based treatments. As EV plus pembrolizumab becomes increasingly favored owing to its substantial impact on PFS and OS, managing its associated toxicities, such as neuropathy and other AEs, remains a critical challenge. Similarly, the GC plus nivolumab combination, with its potential for durable responses, particularly in node-only disease, offers new hope for curative outcomes.

Future efforts should focus on optimizing treatment strategies, identifying biomarkers, and further understanding the drug resistance mechanisms. As new frontline therapies are integrated into clinical practice, their long-term impact on outcomes and quality of life of patients will continue to shape the future of mUC treatment.

Author Contributions: Conceptualization, W.-A.K. and M.-K.L.; writing—original draft preparation, W.-A.K.; writing—review and editing, W.-A.K. and M.-K.L. supervision, W.-A.K. All authors have read and agreed to the published version of the manuscript.

Funding: This work was supported by the National Research Foundation of Korea (NRF) grant funded by the Korean government (MSIT) (2022R1F1A061069), and the Technology Innovation Program (20008924), funded by the Ministry of Trade, Industry and Energy (MOTIE, Korea).

Institutional Review Board Statement: Not applicable.

Informed Consent Statement: Not applicable.

Data Availability Statement: No new data were created.

Conflicts of Interest: The authors declare no conflicts of interest.

References

1. Nadal, R.; Valderrama, B.P.; Bellmunt, J. Progress in systemic therapy for advanced-stage urothelial carcinoma. *Nat. Rev. Clin. Oncol.* **2023**, *21*, 8–27. [CrossRef] [PubMed]
2. Sung, H.; Ferlay, J.; Siegel, R.L.; Laversanne, M.; Soerjomataram, I.; Jemal, A.; Bray, F. Global Cancer Statistics 2020: GLOBOCAN Estimates of Incidence and Mortality Worldwide for 36 Cancers in 185 Countries. *CA Cancer J. Clin.* **2021**, *71*, 209–249. [CrossRef] [PubMed]
3. Witjes, J.A.; Bruins, H.M.; Cathomas, R.; Compérat, E.M.; Cowan, N.C.; Gakis, G.; Hernández, V.; Espinós, E.L.; Lorch, A.; Neuzillet, Y.; et al. European Association of Urology Guidelines on Muscle-invasive and Metastatic Bladder Cancer: Summary of the 2020 Guidelines. *Eur. Urol.* **2020**, *79*, 82–104. [CrossRef] [PubMed]
4. Moussa, M.J.; Campbell, M.T.; Alhalabi, O. Revisiting Treatment of Metastatic Urothelial Cancer: Where Do Cisplatin and Plat-inum Ineligibility Criteria Stand? *Biomedicines* **2024**, *12*, 519. [CrossRef] [PubMed]
5. Kwon, W.-A.; Lee, S.-Y.; Jeong, T.Y.; Kim, H.H.; Lee, M.-K. Antibody-Drug Conjugates in Urothelial Cancer: From Scientific Rationale to Clinical Development. *Cancers* **2024**, *16*, 2420. [CrossRef]
6. Suzman, D.L.; Agrawal, S.; Ning, Y.-M.; Maher, V.E.; Fernandes, L.L.; Karuri, S.; Tang, S.; Sridhara, R.; Schroeder, J.; Goldberg, K.B.; et al. FDA Approval Summary: Atezolizumab or Pembrolizumab for the Treatment of Patients with Advanced Urothelial Carcinoma Ineligible for Cisplatin-Containing Chemotherapy. *Oncologist* **2018**, *24*, 563–569. [CrossRef]
7. Benjamin, D.J.; Hsu, R. Treatment approaches for FGFR-altered urothelial carcinoma: Targeted therapies and immunotherapy. *Front. Immunol.* **2023**, *14*, 1258388. [CrossRef]
8. Miyake, M.; Shimizu, T.; Oda, Y.; Tachibana, A.; Ohmori, C.; Itami, Y.; Kiba, K.; Tomioka, A.; Yamamoto, H.; Ohnishi, K.; et al. Switch-maintenance avelumab immunotherapy following first-line chemotherapy for patients with advanced, unresectable or metastatic urothelial carcinoma: The first Japanese real-world evidence from a multicenter study. *Jpn. J. Clin. Oncol.* **2022**, *53*, 253–262. [CrossRef]
9. Powles, T.; Valderrama, B.P.; Gupta, S.; Bedke, J.; Kikuchi, E.; Hoffman-Censits, J.; Iyer, G.; Vulsteke, C.; Park, S.H.; Shin, S.J.; et al. Enfortumab Vedotin and Pembrolizumab in Untreated Advanced Urothelial Cancer. *N. Engl. J. Med.* **2024**, *390*, 875–888. [CrossRef]
10. Yu, P.; Zhu, C.; You, X.; Gu, W.; Wang, X.; Wang, Y.; Bu, R.; Wang, K. The combination of immune checkpoint inhibitors and antibody-drug conjugates in the treatment of urogenital tumors: A review insights from phase 2 and 3 studies. *Cell Death Dis.* **2024**, *15*, 433. [CrossRef]
11. Thomas, V.M.; Jo, Y.; Tripathi, N.; Roy, S.; Chigarira, B.; Narang, A.; Gebrael, G.; Chehade, C.H.; Sayegh, N.; Fortuna, G.G.; et al. Treatment Patterns and Attrition with Lines of Therapy for Advanced Urothelial Carcinoma in the US. *JAMA Netw. Open* **2024**, *7*, e249417. [CrossRef] [PubMed]
12. Dasari, S.; Tchounwou, P.B. Cisplatin in cancer therapy: Molecular mechanisms of action. *Eur. J. Pharmacol.* **2014**, *740*, 364–378. [CrossRef] [PubMed]
13. Forgie, B.N.; Prakash, R.; Telleria, C.M. Revisiting the Anti-Cancer Toxicity of Clinically Approved Platinating Derivatives. *Int. J. Mol. Sci.* **2022**, *23*, 15410. [CrossRef]
14. Sazonova, E.V.; Kopeina, G.S.; Imyanitov, E.N.; Zhivotovsky, B. Platinum drugs and taxanes: Can we overcome resistance? *Cell Death Discov.* **2021**, *7*, 155. [CrossRef]
15. Shiravand, Y.; Khodadadi, F.; Kashani, S.M.A.; Hosseini-Fard, S.R.; Hosseini, S.; Sadeghirad, H.; Ladwa, R.; O'byrne, K.; Kulasinghe, A. Immune Checkpoint Inhibitors in Cancer Therapy. *Curr. Oncol.* **2022**, *29*, 3044–3060. [CrossRef] [PubMed]

16. Meng, L.; Wu, H.; Wu, J.; Ding, P.; He, J.; Sang, M.; Liu, L. Mechanisms of immune checkpoint inhibitors: Insights into the regulation of circular RNAS involved in cancer hallmarks. *Cell Death Dis.* **2024**, *15*, 3. [CrossRef]
17. Cai, X.; Zhan, H.; Ye, Y.; Yang, J.; Zhang, M.; Li, J.; Zhuang, Y. Current Progress and Future Perspectives of Immune Checkpoint in Cancer and Infectious Diseases. *Front. Genet.* **2021**, *12*, 785153. [CrossRef]
18. Qin, S.; Xu, L.; Yi, M.; Yu, S.; Wu, K.; Luo, S. Novel immune checkpoint targets: Moving beyond PD-1 and CTLA-4. *Mol. Cancer* **2019**, *18*, 155. [CrossRef]
19. Wojtukiewicz, M.Z.; Rek, M.M.; Karpowicz, K.; Górska, M.; Polityńska, B.; Wojtukiewicz, A.M.; Moniuszko, M.; Radziwon, P.; Tucker, S.C.; Honn, K.V. Inhibitors of immune checkpoints—PD-1, PD-L1, CTLA-4—New opportunities for cancer patients and a new challenge for internists and general practitioners. *Cancer Metastasis Rev.* **2021**, *40*, 949–982. [CrossRef]
20. Martins, F.; Sofiya, L.; Sykiotis, G.P.; Lamine, F.; Maillard, M.; Fraga, M.; Shabafrouz, K.; Ribi, C.; Cairoli, A.; Guex-Crosier, Y.; et al. Adverse effects of immune-checkpoint inhibitors: Epidemiology, management and surveillance. *Nat. Rev. Clin. Oncol.* **2019**, *16*, 563–580. [CrossRef]
21. Han, Y.; Liu, D.; Li, L. PD-1/PD-L1 pathway: Current researches in cancer. *Am. J. Cancer Res.* **2020**, *10*, 727–742. [PubMed]
22. Gao, M.; Shi, J.; Xiao, X.; Yao, Y.; Chen, X.; Wang, B.; Zhang, J. PD-1 regulation in immune homeostasis and immunotherapy. *Cancer Lett.* **2024**, *588*, 216726. [CrossRef] [PubMed]
23. Ghosh, C.; Luong, G.; Sun, Y. A snapshot of the PD-1/PD-L1 pathway. *J. Cancer* **2021**, *12*, 2735–2746. [CrossRef] [PubMed]
24. Fu, Z.; Li, S.; Han, S.; Shi, C.; Zhang, Y. Antibody drug conjugate: The "biological missile" for targeted cancer therapy. *Signal Transduct. Target. Ther.* **2022**, *7*, 93. [CrossRef]
25. Parit, S.; Manchare, A.; Gholap, A.D.; Mundhe, P.; Hatvate, N.; Rojekar, S.; Patravale, V. Antibody-Drug Conjugates: A promising breakthrough in cancer therapy. *Int. J. Pharm.* **2024**, *659*, 124211. [CrossRef]
26. Nguyen, T.D.; Bordeau, B.M.; Balthasar, J.P. Mechanisms of ADC Toxicity and Strategies to Increase ADC Tolerability. *Cancers* **2023**, *15*, 713. [CrossRef]
27. Marei, H.E.; Cenciarelli, C.; Hasan, A. Potential of antibody–drug conjugates (ADCs) for cancer therapy. *Cancer Cell Int.* **2022**, *22*, 255. [CrossRef]
28. Aggarwal, D.; Yang, J.; Salam, A.; Sengupta, S.; Al-Amin, Y.; Mustafa, S.; Khan, M.A.; Huang, X.; Pawar, J.S. Antibody-drug conjugates: The paradigm shifts in the targeted cancer therapy. *Front. Immunol.* **2023**, *14*, 1203073. [CrossRef]
29. Hemenway, G.; Anker, J.F.; Riviere, P.; Rose, B.S.; Galsky, M.D.; Ghatalia, P. Advancements in Urothelial Cancer Care: Optimizing Treatment for Your Patient. *Am. Soc. Clin. Oncol. Educ. Book* **2024**, *44*, e432054. [CrossRef]
30. Bellmunt, J.; Mottet, N.; De Santis, M. Urothelial carcinoma management in elderly or unfit patients. *Eur. J. Cancer Suppl.* **2016**, *14*, 1–20. [CrossRef]
31. Galsky, M.D.; Ma, E.; Shah-Manek, B.; Mills, R.; Ha, L.; Krebsbach, C.; Blouin, E.; Tayama, D.; Ogale, S. Cisplatin Ineligibility for Patients with Metastatic Urothelial Carcinoma: A Survey of Clinical Practice Perspectives Among US Oncologists. *Bladder Cancer* **2019**, *5*, 281–288. [CrossRef]
32. Motwani, S.S.; Sandhu, S.K.; Kitchlu, A. Cisplatin Nephrotoxicity: Novel Insights into Mechanisms and Preventative Strategies. *Semin. Nephrol.* **2023**, *42*, 151341. [CrossRef] [PubMed]
33. Powles, T.; Bellmunt, J.; Comperat, E.; De Santis, M.; Huddart, R.; Loriot, Y.; Necchi, A.; Valderrama, B.; Ravaud, A.; Shariat, S.; et al. ESMO Clinical Practice Guideline interim update on first-line therapy in advanced urothelial carcinoma. *Ann. Oncol.* **2024**, *35*, 485–490. [CrossRef] [PubMed]
34. Gupta, S.; Andreev-Drakhlin, A.; Fajardo, O.; Fassò, M.; Garcia, J.A.; Wee, C.; Schröder, C. Platinum ineligibility and survival outcomes in patients with advanced urothelial carcinoma receiving first-line treatment. *JNCI J. Natl. Cancer Inst.* **2023**, *116*, 547–554. [CrossRef] [PubMed]
35. Gupta, S.; Bellmunt, J.; Plimack, E.R.; Sonpavde, G.P.; Grivas, P.; Apolo, A.B.; Pal, S.K.; Siefker-Radtke, A.O.; Flaig, T.W.; Galsky, M.D.; et al. Defining "platinum-ineligible" patients with metastatic urothelial cancer (mUC). *J. Clin. Oncol.* **2022**, *40*, 4577. [CrossRef]
36. de Wit, R. Overview of bladder cancer trials in the European Organization for Research and Treatment. *Cancer* **2003**, *97*, 2120–2126. [CrossRef]
37. Galsky, M.D.; Hahn, N.M.; Rosenberg, J.; Sonpavde, G.; Hutson, T.; Oh, W.K.; Dreicer, R.; Vogelzang, N.; Sternberg, C.; Bajorin, D.F.; et al. A consensus definition of patients with metastatic urothelial carcinoma who are unfit for cisplatin-based chemotherapy. *Lancet Oncol.* **2011**, *12*, 211–214. [CrossRef]
38. Côté, G.; Alqaisi, H.; Chan, C.T.; Jiang, D.M.; Kandel, C.; Pelletier, K.; Wald, R.; Sridhar, S.S.; Kitchlu, A. Kidney and Cancer Outcomes with Standard Versus Alternative Chemotherapy Regimens for First-Line Treatment of Metastatic Urothelial Carcinoma. *Kidney360* **2023**, *4*, e1203–e1211. [CrossRef]
39. Yang, F.; Wang, J.F.; Wang, Y.; Liu, B.; Molina, J.R. Comparative Analysis of Predictive Biomarkers for PD-1/PD-L1 Inhibitors in Cancers: Developments and Challenges. *Cancers* **2021**, *14*, 109. [CrossRef]
40. Maiorano, B.A.; Di Maio, M.; Cerbone, L.; Maiello, E.; Procopio, G.; Roviello, G.; MeetURO Group; Accettura, C.; Aieta, M.; Alberti, M.; et al. Significance of PD-L1 in Metastatic Urothelial Carcinoma Treated with Immune Checkpoint Inhibitors. *JAMA Netw. Open* **2024**, *7*, e241215. [CrossRef]

41. Claps, F.; Biasatti, A.; Di Gianfrancesco, L.; Ongaro, L.; Giannarini, G.; Pavan, N.; Amodeo, A.; Simonato, A.; Crestani, A.; Cimadamore, A.; et al. The Prognostic Significance of Histological Subtypes in Patients with Mus-cle-Invasive Bladder Cancer: An Overview of the Current Literature. *J. Clin. Med.* **2024**, *13*, 4349. [CrossRef] [PubMed]
42. Miller, N.J.; Khaki, A.R.; Diamantopoulos, L.N.; Bilen, M.A.; Santos, V.; Agarwal, N.; Morales-Barrera, R.; Devitt, M.; Nelson, A.; Hoimes, C.J.; et al. Histological Subtypes and Response to PD-1/PD-L1 Blockade in Advanced Urothelial Cancer: A Retrospective Study. *J. Urol.* **2020**, *204*, 63–70. [CrossRef]
43. Jindal, T.; Jiang, C.Y.; Alhalabi, O.; Nguyen, C.B.; Nizam, A.; Basu, A.; Bilen, M.A.; Zakharia, Y.; Milowsky, M.I.; Brown, J.R.; et al. Outcomes with enfortumab vedotin in patients with advanced urothelial carcinoma and histology variants: Analysis of the UNITE study. *J. Clin. Oncol.* **2024**, *42*, 652. [CrossRef]
44. Hoffman-Censits, J.H.; Lombardo, K.A.B.; Parimi, V.; Kamanda, S.; Choi, W.; Hahn, N.M.; McConkey, D.J.; McGuire, B.M.B.; Bivalacqua, T.J.; Kates, M.; et al. Expression of Nectin-4 in Bladder Urothelial Carcinoma, in Morphologic Variants, and Nonurothelial Histotypes. *Appl. Immunohistochem. Mol. Morphol.* **2021**, *29*, 619–625. [CrossRef] [PubMed]
45. Nizam, A.; Jindal, T.; Jiang, C.Y.; Alhalabi, O.; Davidsohn, M.P.; Bakaloudi, D.R.; Talukder, R.; Nguyen, C.B.; Oh, E.; Taylor, A.K.; et al. Outcomes with sacituzumab govitecan (SG) in patients (pts) with advanced urothelial carcinoma (aUC) and variant histologies (VH): Analysis of the UNITE study. *J. Clin. Oncol.* **2024**, *42*, 667. [CrossRef]
46. Moussa, M.J.; Naqvi, S.A.A.; Khandelwal, J.; Campbell, M.T.; Aparicio, A.; Siddiqui, B.A.; Bryce, A.H.; Singh, P.; Alhalabi, O. Clinical efficacy of lurbinectedin in metastatic neuroendocrine carcinomas of the genitourinary tract: Multi-institutional real-world experience. *J. Clin. Oncol.* **2024**, *42*, 601. [CrossRef]
47. Guo, C.C.; Lee, S.; Lee, J.G.; Chen, H.; Zaleski, M.; Choi, W.; McConkey, D.J.; Wei, P.; Czerniak, B. Molecular profile of bladder cancer progression to clinically aggressive subtypes. *Nat. Rev. Urol.* **2024**, *21*, 391–405. [CrossRef]
48. Hoffman-Censits, J.; Choi, W.; Bivalacqua, T.J.; Pierorazio, P.; Kates, M.; Lombardo, K.; Parini, V.; McConkey, D.; Trabulsi, E.J.; Hahn, N.; et al. Small Cell Bladder Cancer Response to Second-line and Beyond Checkpoint Inhibitor Therapy: Retrospective Experience. *Clin. Genitourin. Cancer* **2020**, *19*, 176–181. [CrossRef]
49. McGregor, B.A.; Campbell, M.T.; Xie, W.; Farah, S.; Bilen, M.A.; Schmidt, A.L.; Sonpavde, G.P.; Kilbridge, K.L.; Choudhury, A.D.; Mortazavi, A.; et al. Results of a multicenter, phase 2 study of nivolumab and ipilimumab for patients with advanced rare genitourinary malignancies. *Cancer* **2020**, *127*, 840–849. [CrossRef]
50. Sarfaty, M.; Whiting, K.; Teo, M.Y.; Lee, C.; Peters, V.; Durocher, J.; Regazzi, A.M.; McCoy, A.S.; Hettich, G.; Jungbluth, A.A.; et al. A phase II trial of durvalumab and tremelimumab in metastatic, non-urothelial carcinoma of the urinary tract. *Cancer Med.* **2020**, *10*, 1074–1083. [CrossRef]
51. Kamat, A.M.; Apolo, A.B.; Babjuk, M.; Bivalacqua, T.J.; Black, P.C.; Buckley, R.; Campbell, M.T.; Compérat, E.; Efstathiou, J.A.; Grivas, P.; et al. Definitions, End Points, and Clinical Trial Designs for Bladder Cancer: Recommendations from the Society for Immunotherapy of Cancer and the International Bladder Cancer Group. *J. Clin. Oncol.* **2023**, *41*, 5437–5447. [CrossRef]
52. Ascione, C.M.; Napolitano, F.; Esposito, D.; Servetto, A.; Belli, S.; Santaniello, A.; Scagliarini, S.; Crocetto, F.; Bianco, R.; Formisano, L. Role of FGFR3 in bladder cancer: Treatment landscape and future challenges. *Cancer Treat. Rev.* **2023**, *115*, 102530. [CrossRef] [PubMed]
53. National Comprehensive Cancer Network (NCCN) Guidelines Version 4.2024 "Bladder Cancer". Available online: https://www.nccn.org/guidelines/guidelines-detail?category=1&id=1417 (accessed on 13 September 2024).
54. Reck, M.; Rodríguez-Abreu, D.; Robinson, A.G.; Hui, R.; Csőszi, T.; Fülöp, A.; Gottfried, M.; Peled, N.; Tafreshi, A.; Cuffe, S.; et al. Pembrolizumab versus Chemotherapy for PD-L1–Positive Non–Small-Cell Lung Cancer. *N. Engl. J. Med.* **2016**, *375*, 1823–1833. [CrossRef] [PubMed]
55. Wang, S.; Burgess, M.; Major, C.; English, A.; Sweeney, M.; Hartmann, A. Identifying fibroblast growth factor receptor genetic alterations using RNA-based assays in patients with metastatic or locally advanced, surgically unresectable, urothelial carcinoma who may benefit from erdafitinib treatment. *J. Pathol. Clin. Res.* **2020**, *6*, 207–214. [CrossRef] [PubMed]
56. Lenis, A.T.; Lec, P.M.; Chamie, K. Bladder cancer: A review. *JAMA* **2020**, *324*, 1980–1991. [CrossRef]
57. Von Der Maase, H.; Hansen, S.W.; Roberts, J.T.; Dogliotti, L.; Oliver, T.; Moore, M.J.; Bodrogi, I.; Albers, P.; Knuth, A.; Lippert, C.M.; et al. Gemcitabine and Cisplatin Versus Methotrexate, Vinblastine, Doxorubicin, and Cisplatin in Advanced or Metastatic Bladder Cancer: Results of a Large, Randomized, Multinational, Multicenter, Phase III Study. *J. Clin. Oncol.* **2000**, *18*, 3068–3077. [CrossRef]
58. von der Maase, H.; Sengelov, L.; Roberts, J.T.; Ricci, S.; Dogliotti, L.; Oliver, T.; Moore, M.J.; Zimmermann, A.; Arning, M. Long-Term Survival Results of a Randomized Trial Comparing Gemcitabine Plus Cisplatin, With Methotrexate, Vinblastine, Doxorubicin, Plus Cisplatin in Patients with Bladder Cancer. *J. Clin. Oncol.* **2005**, *23*, 4602–4608. [CrossRef]
59. Sternberg, C.N.; de Mulder, P.H.; Schornagel, J.H.; Théodore, C.; Fossa, S.D.; van Oosterom, A.T.; Witjes, F.; Spina, M.; van Groeningen, C.J.; de Balincourt, C.; et al. Randomized Phase III Trial of High–Dose-Intensity Methotrexate, Vinblastine, Doxorubicin, and Cisplatin (MVAC) Chemotherapy and Recombinant Human Granulocyte Colony-Stimulating Factor Versus Classic MVAC in Advanced Urothelial Tract Tumors: European Organization for Research and Treatment of Cancer Protocol No. 30924. *J. Clin. Oncol.* **2001**, *19*, 2638–2646. [CrossRef]
60. Sternberg, C.; de Mulder, P.; Schornagel, J.; Theodore, C.; Fossa, S.; van Oosterom, A.; Witjes, J.; Spina, M.; van Groeningen, C.; Duclos, B.; et al. Seven year update of an EORTC phase III trial of high-dose intensity M-VAC chemotherapy and G-CSF versus classic M-VAC in advanced urothelial tract tumours. *Eur. J. Cancer* **2006**, *42*, 50–54. [CrossRef]

61. Bamias, A.; Dafni, U.; Karadimou, A.; Timotheadou, E.; Aravantinos, G.; Psyrri, A.; Xanthakis, I.; Tsiatas, M.; Koutoulidis, V.; Constantinidis, C.; et al. Prospective, open-label, randomized, phase III study of two dose-dense regimens MVAC versus gemcitabine/cisplatin in patients with inoperable, metastatic or relapsed urothelial cancer: A Hellenic Cooperative Oncology Group study (HE 16/03). *Ann. Oncol.* **2012**, *24*, 1011–1017. [CrossRef]
62. De Santis, M.; Bellmunt, J.; Mead, G.; Kerst, J.M.; Leahy, M.; Maroto, P.; Skoneczna, I.; Marreaud, S.; de Wit, R.; Sylvester, R. Randomized Phase II/III Trial Assessing Gemcitabine/Carboplatin and Methotrexate/Carboplatin/Vinblastine in Patients with Advanced Urothelial Cancer "Unfit" for Cisplatin-Based Chemotherapy: Phase II—Results of EORTC Study 30986. *J. Clin. Oncol.* **2009**, *27*, 5634–5639. [CrossRef]
63. Powles, T.; Castellano, D.; Loriot, Y.; Ogawa, O.; Park, S.H.; De Giorgi, U.; Bögemann, M.; Bamias, A.; Gurney, H.; Fradet, Y.; et al. Durvalumab alone and durvalumab plus tremelimumab versus chemotherapy in previously untreated patients with unresectable, locally advanced or metastatic urothelial carcinoma (DANUBE): A randomised, open-label, multicentre, phase 3 trial. *Lancet Oncol.* **2020**, *21*, 1574–1588. [CrossRef] [PubMed]
64. Galsky, M.D.; Arija, J.Á.A.; Bamias, A.; Davis, I.D.; De Santis, M.; Kikuchi, E.; Garcia-Del-Muro, X.; De Giorgi, U.; Mencinger, M.; Izumi, K.; et al. Atezolizumab with or without chemotherapy in metastatic urothelial cancer (IMvigor130): A multicentre, randomised, placebo-controlled phase 3 trial. *Lancet* **2020**, *395*, 1547–1557. [CrossRef] [PubMed]
65. Powles, T.; Park, S.H.; Voog, E.; Caserta, C.; Valderrama, B.P.; Gurney, H.; Kalofonos, H.; Radulović, S.; Demey, W.; Ullén, A.; et al. Avelumab Maintenance Therapy for Advanced or Metastatic Urothelial Carcinoma. *N. Engl. J. Med.* **2020**, *383*, 1218–1230. [CrossRef] [PubMed]
66. Osterman, C.K.; Babu, D.S.; Geynisman, D.M.; Lewis, B.; Somer, R.A.; Balar, A.V.; Zibelman, M.R.; Guancial, E.A.; Antinori, G.; Yu, S.; et al. Efficacy of Split Schedule Versus Conventional Schedule Neoadjuvant Cisplatin-Based Chemotherapy for Muscle-Invasive Bladder Cancer. *Oncologist* **2019**, *24*, 688–690. [CrossRef]
67. Mourey, L.; Flechon, A.; Tosi, D.; Lacourtoisie, S.A.; Joly, F.; Guillot, A.; Loriot, Y.; Dauba, J.; Roubaud, G.; Rolland, F.; et al. Vefora, GETUG-AFU V06 study: Randomized multicenter phase II/III trial of fractionated cisplatin (CI)/gemcitabine (G) or carboplatin (CA)/g in patients (pts) with advanced urothelial cancer (UC) with impaired renal function (IRF)—Results of a planned interim analysis. *J. Clin. Oncol.* **2020**, *38*, 461. [CrossRef]
68. Grivas, P.; Grande, E.; Davis, I.; Moon, H.; Grimm, M.-O.; Gupta, S.; Barthélémy, P.; Thibault, C.; Guenther, S.; Hanson, S.; et al. Avelumab first-line maintenance treatment for advanced urothelial carcinoma: Review of evidence to guide clinical practice. *ESMO Open* **2023**, *8*, 102050. [CrossRef]
69. Zhang, T.; Tan, A.; Shah, A.Y.; Iyer, G.; Morris, V.; Michaud, S.; Sridhar, S.S. Reevaluating the role of platinum-based chemotherapy in the evolving treatment landscape for patients with advanced urothelial carcinoma. *Oncologist* **2024**, oyae215. [CrossRef]
70. Balar, A.V.; Galsky, M.D.; Rosenberg, J.E.; Powles, T.; Petrylak, D.P.; Bellmunt, J.; Loriot, Y.; Necchi, A.; Hoffman-Censits, J.; Perez-Gracia, J.L.; et al. Atezolizumab as first-line treatment in cisplatin-ineligible patients with locally advanced and metastatic urothelial carcinoma: A single-arm, multicentre, phase 2 trial. *Lancet* **2017**, *389*, 67–76, Erratum in *Lancet* **2017**, *390*, 848. [CrossRef]
71. Powles, T.; Walker, J.; Williams, J.A.; Bellmunt, J. The evolving role of PD-L1 testing in patients with metastatic urothelial carcinoma. *Cancer Treat. Rev.* **2019**, *82*, 101925. [CrossRef]
72. Vuky, J.; Balar, A.V.; Castellano, D.; O'donnell, P.H.; Grivas, P.; Bellmunt, J.; Powles, T.; Bajorin, D.; Hahn, N.M.; Savage, M.J.; et al. Long-Term Outcomes in KEYNOTE-052: Phase II Study Investigating First-Line Pembrolizumab in Cisplatin-Ineligible Patients with Locally Advanced or Metastatic Urothelial Cancer. *J. Clin. Oncol.* **2020**, *38*, 2658–2666. [CrossRef] [PubMed]
73. Ghatalia, P.; Zibelman, M.; Geynisman, D.M.; Plimack, E.R. First-line Immunotherapy in Metastatic Urothelial Carcinoma. *Eur. Urol. Focus* **2019**, *6*, 45–47. [CrossRef] [PubMed]
74. Rhea, L.P.; Aragon-Ching, J.B. Advances and Controversies with Checkpoint Inhibitors in Bladder Cancer. *Clin. Med. Insights Oncol.* **2021**, *15*, 11795549211044963. [CrossRef] [PubMed]
75. Powles, T.; Matsubara, N.; Cheng, S.Y.-S.; Fradet, Y.; Oudard, S.; Vulsteke, C.; Barrera, R.M.; Gunduz, S.; Loriot, Y.; Rodriguez-Vida, A.; et al. Pembrolizumab alone or combined with chemotherapy versus chemotherapy as first-line therapy for advanced urothelial carcinoma (KEYNOTE-361): A randomised, open-label, phase 3 trial. *Lancet Oncol.* **2021**, *22*, 931–945. [CrossRef]
76. Grande, E.; Bamias, A.; Galsky, M.D.; Kikuchi, E.; Davis, I.D.; Arranz, J.A.; Rezazadeh, A.; Garcia del Muro, X.; Park, S.H.; De Giorgi, U.; et al. *Overall Survival (OS) by Response to First-Line (1L) Induction Treatment with Atezoli-Zumab (Atezo)+ Platinum/Gemcitabine (plt/gem) vs Placebo+ plt/gem in Patients (pts) with Metastatic Urothelial Carcinoma (mUC): Updated Data from the IMvigor130 OS Final Analysis*; American Society of Clinical Oncology: Orlando, FL, USA, 2023.
77. Galsky, M.D.; Necchi, A.; Sridhar, S.S.; Ogawa, O.; Angra, N.; Hois, S.; Xiao, F.; Goluboff, E.; Bellmunt, J. A phase III, randomized, open-label, multicenter, global study of first-line durvalumab plus standard of care (SoC) chemotherapy and durvalumab plus tremelimumab, and SoC chemotherapy versus SoC chemotherapy alone in unresectable locally advanced or metastatic urothelial cancer (NILE). *J. Clin. Oncol.* **2021**, *39*, TPS504. [CrossRef]
78. van der Heijden, M.S.; Sonpavde, G.; Powles, T.; Necchi, A.; Burotto, M.; Schenker, M.; Sade, J.P.; Bamias, A.; Beuzeboc, P.; Bedke, J.; et al. Nivolumab plus Gemcitabine–Cisplatin in Advanced Urothelial Carcinoma. *N. Engl. J. Med.* **2023**, *389*, 1778–1789. [CrossRef]
79. Houssiau, H.; Seront, E. Improving the role of immune checkpoint inhibitors in the management of advanced urothelial carcinoma, where do we stand? *Transl. Oncol.* **2022**, *19*, 101387. [CrossRef]

80. Galsky, M.D.; Guan, X.; Banchereau, R.; Wang, L.; Zhu, J.; Yu, H.; Rishipathak, D.; Hajaj, E.; Herbst, R.; Davis, I.; et al. 658MO Cisplatin (cis)-related immunomodulation and efficacy with atezolizumab (atezo) + cis- vs carboplatin (carbo)-based chemotherapy (chemo) in metastatic urothelial cancer (mUC). *Ann. Oncol.* **2021**, *32*, S682–S683. [CrossRef]
81. Kwon, W.-A.; Seo, H.K. Emerging agents for the treatment of metastatic urothelial cancer. *Investig. Clin. Urol.* **2021**, *62*, 243–255. [CrossRef]
82. Powles, T.; Park, S.H.; Caserta, C.; Valderrama, B.P.; Gurney, H.; Ullén, A.; Loriot, Y.; Sridhar, S.S.; Sternberg, C.N.; Bellmunt, J.; et al. Avelumab First-Line Maintenance for Advanced Urothelial Carcinoma: Results from the JAVELIN Bladder 100 Trial After ≥2 Years of Follow-Up. *J. Clin. Oncol.* **2023**, *41*, 3486–3492. [CrossRef]
83. Bracarda, S.; Antonuzzo, L.; Maruzzo, M.; Santini, D.; Tambaro, R.; Buti, S.; Carrozza, F.; Calabrò, F.; Di Lorenzo, G.; Fornarini, G.; et al. Subgroup analyses from READY: Real-world data from an Italian compassionate use program (CUP) of avelumab first-line maintenance (1LM) treatment for locally advanced or metastatic urothelial carcinoma (la/mUC). *J. Clin. Oncol.* **2024**, *42*, 558. [CrossRef]
84. Barthelemy, P.; Loriot, Y.; Voog, E.; Eymard, J.C.; Ravaud, A.; Flechon, A.; Jaillon, C.A.; Chasseray, M.; Lorgis, V.; Hilgers, W.; et al. Full analysis from AVENANCE: A real-world study of avelumab first-line (1L) maintenance treatment in patients (pts) with advanced urothelial carcinoma (aUC). *J. Clin. Oncol.* **2023**, *41*, 471. [CrossRef]
85. Srinivasalu, V.K.; Robbrecht, D. Advancements in First-Line Treatment of Metastatic Bladder Cancer: EV-302 and Checkmate-901 Insights and Future Directions. *Cancers* **2024**, *16*, 2398. [CrossRef] [PubMed]
86. O'Donnell, P.H.; Milowsky, M.I.; Petrylak, D.P.; Hoimes, C.J.; Flaig, T.W.; Mar, N.; Moon, H.H.; Friedlander, T.W.; McKay, R.R.; Bilen, M.A.; et al. Enfortumab Vedotin with or Without Pembrolizumab in Cisplatin-Ineligible Patients with Previously Untreated Locally Advanced or Metastatic Urothelial Cancer. *J. Clin. Oncol.* **2023**, *41*, 4107–4117. [CrossRef]
87. Lin, Y.-T.; Wang, C.; He, X.-Y.; Yao, Q.-M.; Chen, J. Comparative cost-effectiveness of first-line pembrolizumab plus chemotherapy vs. chemotherapy alone in persistent, recurrent, or metastatic cervical cancer. *Front. Immunol.* **2024**, *14*, 1345942. [CrossRef]
88. Li, A.; Wu, M.; Xie, O.; Xiang, H.; Meng, K.; Tan, C.; Wang, L.; Wan, X. Cost-effectiveness of First-Line Enfortumab Vedotin in Addition to Pembrolizumab for Metastatic Urothelial Carcinoma in the United States. *Front. Immunol.* **2024**, *15*, 1464092. [CrossRef]
89. Rosenberg, J.E.; O'Donnell, P.H.; Balar, A.V.; McGregor, B.A.; Heath, E.I.; Yu, E.Y.; Galsky, M.D.; Hahn, N.M.; Gartner, E.M.; Pinelli, J.M.; et al. Pivotal Trial of Enfortumab Vedotin in Urothelial Carcinoma After Platinum and Anti-Programmed Death 1/Programmed Death Ligand 1 Therapy. *J. Clin. Oncol.* **2019**, *37*, 2592–2600. [CrossRef]
90. Tang, M.; Garg, A.; Bonate, P.L.; Rosenberg, J.E.; Matsangou, M.; Kadokura, T.; Yamada, A.; Choules, M.; Pavese, J.; Nagata, M.; et al. Clinical Pharmacology of the Antibody–Drug Conjugate Enfortumab Vedotin in Advanced Urothelial Carcinoma and Other Malignant Solid Tumors. *Clin. Pharmacokinet.* **2024**, *63*, 423–438. [CrossRef]
91. Bajorin, D.F.; Dodd, P.M.; Mazumdar, M.; Fazzari, M.; McCaffrey, J.A.; Scher, H.I.; Herr, H.; Higgins, G.; Boyle, M.G. Long-Term Survival in Metastatic Transitional-Cell Carcinoma and Prognostic Factors Predicting Outcome of Therapy. *J. Clin. Oncol.* **1999**, *17*, 3173–3181. [CrossRef]
92. Sonpavde, G.; Manitz, J.; Gao, C.; Tayama, D.; Kaiser, C.; Hennessy, D.; Makari, D.; Gupta, A.; Abdullah, S.E.; Niegisch, G.; et al. Five-Factor Prognostic Model for Survival of Post-Platinum Patients with Metastatic Urothelial Carcinoma Receiving PD-L1 Inhibitors. *J. Urol.* **2020**, *204*, 1173–1179. [CrossRef]
93. Liu, D.; Plimack, E.R.; Hoffman-Censits, J.; Garraway, L.A.; Bellmunt, J.; Van Allen, E.; Rosenberg, J.E. Clinical Validation of Chemotherapy Response Biomarker *ERCC2* in Muscle-Invasive Urothelial Bladder Carcinoma. *JAMA Oncol.* **2016**, *2*, 1094–1096. [CrossRef] [PubMed]
94. Gupta, S.; Rosenberg, J.E.; McKay, R.R.; Flaig, T.W.; Petrylak, D.P.; Hoimes, C.J.; Friedlander, T.W.; Bilen, M.A.; Srinivas, S.; Burgess, E.F.; et al. Study EV-103 dose escalation/cohort A: Long-term outcome of enfortumab vedotin + pembrolizumab in first-line (1L) cisplatin-ineligible locally advanced or metastatic urothelial carcinoma (la/mUC) with nearly 4 years of follow-up. *J. Clin. Oncol.* **2023**, *41*, 4505. [CrossRef]
95. Machtens, S.; Schlack, K.; Kubin, T.; Ruhnke, M.; Schulte, C.; Eisen, A.; Osowski, U.; Guenther, S.; Kearney, M.; Lipp, R.; et al. Real-world treatment (tx) patterns and clinical outcomes in patients (pts) with locally advanced or metastatic urothelial carcinoma (la/mUC) in Germany: Results of a retrospective observational study (CONVINCE). *J. Clin. Oncol.* **2024**, *42*, 551. [CrossRef]
96. Bupathi, M.; Sura, S.; Ike, C.; Morris, V.A.; Conkling, P.R.; Todoroff, K.; Bhanegaonkar, A. Real-world (rw) treatment (tx) patterns and clinical outcomes in patients (pts) with locally advanced/metastatic urothelial carcinoma (la/mUC): Insights from The US Oncology Network electronic health record (EHR). *J. Clin. Oncol.* **2024**, *42*, e16551. [CrossRef]
97. Chen, R.C.; Mucha, L.; Nimke, D.; Young, C.; Yang, H.; Liu, Q.; Greatsinger, A.; Zhang, A.; Wright, P.; Quicquaro, C.M. Real-world first-line treatment patterns and outcomes in patients with locally advanced or metastatic urothelial carcinoma in the United States. *J. Clin. Oncol.* **2024**, *42*, e23287. [CrossRef]
98. De Santis, M.; Bellmunt, J.; Mead, G.; Kerst, J.M.; Leahy, M.; Maroto, P.; Gil, T.; Marreaud, S.; Daugaard, G.; Skoneczna, I.; et al. Randomized Phase II/III Trial Assessing Gemcitabine/Carboplatin and Methotrexate/Carboplatin/Vinblastine in Patients with Advanced Urothelial Cancer Who Are Unfit for Cisplatin-Based Chemotherapy: EORTC Study 30986. *J. Clin. Oncol.* **2012**, *30*, 191–199. [CrossRef] [PubMed]
99. Bellmunt, J.; Nadal, R. Enfortumab vedotin and pembrolizumab combination as a relevant game changer in urothelial carcinoma: What is left behind? *Med* **2024**, *5*, 490–492. [CrossRef] [PubMed]

100. Santoni, M.; Takeshita, H.; Massari, F.; Bamias, A.; Cerbone, L.; Fiala, O.; Mollica, V.; Buti, S.; Santoni, A.; Bellmunt, J. Pembrolizumab plus enfortumab vedotin in urothelial cancer. *Nat. Rev. Urol.* **2024**, *21*, 387–388. [CrossRef]
101. Patel, D.M.; Mateen, R.; Qaddour, N.; Carrillo, A.; Verschraegen, C.; Yang, Y.; Li, Z.; Sundi, D.; Mortazavi, A.; Collier, K.A. A Comprehensive Review of Immunotherapy Clinical Trials for Metastatic Urothelial Carcinoma: Immune Checkpoint Inhibitors Alone or in Combination, Novel Antibodies, Cellular Therapies, and Vaccines. *Cancers* **2024**, *16*, 335. [CrossRef]
102. Tan, W.S.; Tan, M.-Y.; Alhalabi, O.; Campbell, M.T.; Kamat, A.M.; Gao, J. Evolving systemic management of urothelial cancers. *Curr. Opin. Oncol.* **2023**, *35*, 186–199. [CrossRef]
103. Grivas, P.; Pouessel, D.; Park, C.H.; Barthelemy, P.; Bupathi, M.; Petrylak, D.P.; Agarwal, N.; Gupta, S.; Fléchon, A.; Ramamurthy, C.; et al. Sacituzumab Govitecan in Combination with Pembrolizumab for Patients with Metastatic Urothelial Cancer That Progressed After Platinum-Based Chemotherapy: TROPHY-U-01 Cohort 3. *J. Clin. Oncol.* **2024**, *42*, 1415–1425. [CrossRef] [PubMed]
104. Tonni, E.; Oltrecolli, M.; Pirola, M.; Tchawa, C.; Roccabruna, S.; D'Agostino, E.; Matranga, R.; Piombino, C.; Pipitone, S.; Baldessari, C.; et al. New Advances in Metastatic Urothelial Cancer: A Narrative Review on Recent Developments and Future Perspectives. *Int. J. Mol. Sci.* **2024**, *25*, 9696. [CrossRef] [PubMed]
105. Parent, P.; Marcq, G.; Adeleke, S.; Turpin, A.; Boussios, S.; Rassy, E.; Penel, N. Predictive biomarkers for immune checkpoint inhibitor response in urothelial cancer. *Ther. Adv. Med. Oncol.* **2023**, *15*, 17588359231192402. [CrossRef]
106. Queiroz, M.M.; de Souza, Z.S.; Gongora, A.B.L.; Barbosa, F.d.G.; Buchpiguel, C.A.; de Castro, M.G.; de Macedo, M.P.; Coelho, R.F.; Soko, E.S.; Camargo, A.A.; et al. Emerging biomarkers in metastatic urothelial carcinoma: Tumour mutational burden, PD-L1 expression and APOBEC polypeptide-like signature in a patient with complete response to anti-programmed cell death protein-1 inhibitor. *Ecancermedicalscience* **2021**, *15*, 1306. [CrossRef]
107. Zhou, Y.; Tao, L.; Qiu, J.; Xu, J.; Yang, X.; Zhang, Y.; Tian, X.; Guan, X.; Cen, X.; Zhao, Y. Tumor biomarkers for diagnosis, prognosis and targeted therapy. *Signal Transduct. Target. Ther.* **2024**, *9*, 132. [CrossRef]
108. Rodriguez, J.; Baldini, C.; Bayle, A.; Pages, A.; Danlos, F.X.; Vasseur, D.; Rouleau, E.; Lacroix, L.; de Castro, B.A.; Goldschmidt, V.; et al. Impact of Clonal Hematopoiesis–Associated Mutations in Phase I Patients Treated for Solid Tumors: An Analysis of the STING Trial. *JCO Precis. Oncol.* **2024**, *8*, e2300631. [CrossRef]
109. Desimpel, G.; Zammit, F.; Lejeune, S.; Grisay, G.; Seront, E. Lung Toxicity Occurring During Enfortumab Vedotin Treatment: From a Priming Case Report to a Retrospective Analysis. *Pharmaceuticals* **2024**, *17*, 1547. [CrossRef] [PubMed]
110. Brower, B.; McCoy, A.; Ahmad, H.; Eitman, C.; Bowman, I.A.; Rembisz, J.; Milowsky, M.I. Managing potential adverse events during treatment with enfortumab vedotin + pembrolizumab in patients with advanced urothelial cancer. *Front. Oncol.* **2024**, *14*, 1326715. [CrossRef]
111. Pretelli, G.; Mati, K.; Motta, L.; Stathis, A. Antibody-drug conjugates combinations in cancer treatment. *Explor. Target. Anti-Tumor Ther.* **2024**, *5*, 714–741. [CrossRef]
112. Zadorozhna, M.; Mangieri, D. Mechanisms of Chemopreventive and Therapeutic Proprieties of Ginger Extracts in Cancer. *Int. J. Mol. Sci.* **2021**, *22*, 6599. [CrossRef]
113. Isola, S.; Gammeri, L.; Furci, F.; Gangemi, S.; Pioggia, G.; Allegra, A. Vitamin C Supplementation in the Treatment of Autoim-mune and Onco-Hematological Diseases: From Prophylaxis to Adjuvant Therapy. *Int. J. Mol. Sci.* **2024**, *25*, 7284. [CrossRef] [PubMed]
114. Klenner, F.R. Observations on the dose and administration of ascorbic acid when employed beyond the range of a vitamin in human pathology. *J. Appl. Nutr.* **1971**, *23*, 61–68.
115. Klenner, F.R. Significance of high daily intake of ascorbic acid in preventive medicine. In *A Physician's Handbook on Orthomolecular Medicine*; Elsevier: Amsterdam, The Netherlands, 1977; pp. 51–59.
116. Cunha, A.; Silva, P.M.A.; Sarmento, B.; Queirós, O. Targeting Glucose Metabolism in Cancer Cells as an Approach to Overcoming Drug Resistance. *Pharmaceutics* **2023**, *15*, 2610. [CrossRef] [PubMed]

cancers

MDPI

Article

Prognostic Significance of the Cribriform Pattern in Prostate Cancer: Clinical Outcomes and Genomic Alterations

Mutlay Sayan [1,*], Yetkin Tuac [2], Mahmut Akgul [3], Grace K. Pratt [1], Mary D. Rowan [1], Dilara Akbulut [4], Samet Kucukcolak [5], Elza Tjio [6], Shalini Moningi [1], Jonathan E. Leeman [1], Peter F. Orio [1], Paul L. Nguyen [1], Anthony V. D'Amico [1] and Cagdas Aktan [7]

1 Department of Radiation Oncology, Dana Farber Cancer Institute, Brigham and Women's Hospital, Harvard Medical School, Boston, MA 02215, USA
2 Department of Statistics, Ankara University, 06100 Ankara, Türkiye
3 Department of Pathology and Laboratory Medicine, Albany Medical Center, Albany, NY 12208, USA
4 Center for Cancer Research, Laboratory of Pathology, National Institutes of Health, Bethesda, MD 20892, USA
5 Department of Pathology and Laboratory Medicine, Rutgers University, New Brunswick, NJ 08901, USA
6 Histopathology Department, Harrogate District Hospital, Harrogate HG2 7SX, UK
7 Department of Medical Biology, Faculty of Medicine, Bandirma Onyedi Eylul University, 10250 Balikesir, Türkiye
* Correspondence: msayan@bwh.harvard.edu

Simple Summary: Prostate cancer is a condition with varying outcomes, and understanding its progression is vital for treatment. Our research focused on a specific pattern observed in tumor cells, known as cribriform pattern 4 (CP4), which can indicate how aggressive a cancer might be. By studying patients who had undergone surgery to remove the prostate gland, we found that those with CP4 tended to have a higher risk of cancer recurrence. Additionally, we discovered certain genes that behaved differently in patients with CP4, suggesting unique genetic changes associated with this pattern. Our findings suggest that patients with CP4 might need more intense treatment after surgery and could help doctors decide on the best course of action. Importantly, our research provides new insights that could lead to better management of prostate cancer, aiming to improve patient outcomes.

Abstract: Purpose: Given the diverse clinical progression of prostate cancer (PC) and the evolving significance of histopathological factors in its management, this study aimed to explore the impact of cribriform pattern 4 (CP4) on clinical outcomes in PC patients and examine its molecular characteristics. Methods: This retrospective study analyzed data from The Cancer Genome Atlas (TCGA) database and included PC patients who underwent radical prostatectomy (RP) and had pathology slides available for the assessment of CP4. A multivariable competing risk regression analysis was used to assess the association between CP4 and progression-free survival (PFS) while adjusting for established PC prognostic factors. The frequency of genomic alterations was compared between patients with and without CP4 using the Fisher's exact test. Results: Among the 394 patients analyzed, 129 (32.74%) had CP4. After a median follow-up of 40.50 months (IQR: 23.90, 65.60), the presence of CP4 was significantly associated with lower PFS (AHR, 1.84; 95% CI, 1.08 to 3.114; p = 0.023) after adjusting for covariates. Seven hub genes—KRT13, KRT5, KRT15, COL17A1, KRT14, KRT16, and TP63—had significantly lower mRNA expression levels in patients with CP4 compared to those without. Conclusions: PC patients with CP4 have distinct genomic alterations and are at a high risk of disease progression following RP. Therefore, these patients may benefit from additional post-RP treatments and should be the subject of a prospective randomized clinical trial.

Keywords: prostate cancer; cribriform pattern; genomic alterations; radical prostatectomy; progression-free survival

1. Introduction

Risk stratification plays a critical role in the management of prostate cancer (PC) as it directly impacts treatment strategies. A key element in this process is histopathology, which has seen significant evolution over the years. The Gleason score, first introduced in 1977, remains a cornerstone in this domain, though its definitions and criteria have been continuously refined [1]. The most recent update to the Gleason scoring system mandates that all cribriform glands be classified as Gleason pattern 4 [2]. Consequently, the clinical implications of cribriform pattern 4 (CP4) in PC have gained a growing interest in recent years, particularly due to its association with adverse clinical outcomes [3–10]. A comprehensive meta-analysis highlighted these concerns, revealing that the presence of CP4 is associated with increased risks for biochemical recurrence (hazard ratio [HR]: 2.14; $p < 0.01$) and cancer-specific mortality (HR: 3.30; $p < 0.01$), as well as increased likelihood of extra-prostatic extension (odds ratio [OR] 1.96; $p < 0.0001$), seminal vesicle invasion (OR: 2.89; $p < 0.01$), and positive surgical margins (OR: 1.88; $p < 0.0007$) [11]. These findings emphasize the critical role of CP4 in prognosticating the course of PC and highlight the need for continued research in this area.

The current standard of care for patients with PC following radical prostatectomy (RP) involves salvage radiation therapy (RT) when the prostate-specific antigen (PSA) level reaches 0.1 ng/mL. Identifying specific growth patterns such as CP4 is becoming increasingly crucial, as they hold potential to refine post-prostatectomy treatment strategies. While the clinical relevance of CP4 in PC is evolving, the understanding of its molecular characteristics remains limited. In this study, we analyze the impact of CP4 on progression-free survival (PFS), adjusting for recognized PC prognostic factors, and explore CP4 molecular characteristics. This research aims to identify patients who may benefit from adjuvant therapies, thereby guiding the development of future randomized clinical trials.

2. Materials and Methods

2.1. Patient Characteristics

This retrospective study involved an analysis of patient data from The Cancer Genome Atlas (TCGA) database. The selection criteria included patients diagnosed with PC, who had undergone RP and had digitized hematoxylin-and-eosin (HE)-stained slides with clearly identifiable tumor sections available for review. Demographic and clinical data, including age at diagnosis, pathologic tumor stage, margin status, Gleason score, and pre-RP PSA levels, were collected due to their established significance in predicting PC prognosis and treatment outcomes. The follow-up period was defined from the date of RP to the last available follow-up or death.

A pathological review of the RP specimens was undertaken by a team of three pathologists with experience in genitourinary pathology (MA, ET, SK). The primary objective was to identify cases with CP4. This entailed a thorough review of the pathology slides, with a special emphasis on identifying the presence and characteristics of cribriform architectural structures. Distinguishing between CP4 and intraductal carcinoma in our study was primarily based on the difference in their morphologic features, as described in previous literature [12,13].

2.2. Statistical Methods

2.2.1. Comparison of the Distribution of Clinical Factors Stratified by Cribriform Pattern 4

This study followed a prespecified statistical analysis plan. Descriptive statistics provided an overview of the clinical and treatment characteristics of 394 patients, categorized based on whether they exhibited CP4 or not. The comparison of these characteristics utilized the Pearson's chi-squared test for categorical variables and the Wilcoxon two-sample test for analyzing distribution differences in continuous variables, such as age and PSA levels [14]. Additionally, the distribution of the follow-up times was assessed using the reverse Kaplan–Meier method and evaluated for significance with a log-rank p-value [15].

2.2.2. Covariate-Adjusted Hazard Ratios and Estimates of Progression-Free Survival

The primary endpoint of this study was PFS, defined as the time from RP to the first evidence of disease progression or death from any cause [16–18]. Univariable and multivariable competing risk regression analysis using the Fine–Gray mode was applied to assess whether a significant association existed between the presence of CP4 and PFS [19]. The covariates included in the model were age at the time of diagnosis, pre-RP PSA, pathologic tumor stage, Gleason score, and margin status. Time 0 was the date of RP. For the purpose of illustration, covariate-adjusted estimates of PFS following RP, stratified by the presence or absence of CP4, were calculated using the Kaplan–Meier method [20]. The p-values for the adjusted Kaplan–Meier plots were calculated using the log-rank test. The threshold for statistical significance was established at $p < 0.05$. All statistical analyses were performed with R (version 4.2.3).

2.2.3. Molecular Characterization and Genomic Alterations Analysis

The expression levels of mRNAs from the TCGA dataset were examined, and genes meeting the criteria of an absolute log fold change ($|\text{logFC}|$) > 1 or <−1, along with a q-value < 0.05, were identified as differentially expressed genes (DEGs) in patients with and without CP4 [21].

Following the identification of DEGs, a protein–protein interaction (PPI) network was constructed using the STRING tool [22], and the results were visualized using Cytoscape software v310.1 [23]. A topological analysis was performed on each gene to identify hub genes, which are genes highly interconnected within the PPI network. Subsequently, Molecular Complex Detection (MCODE) plugin was applied to identify significant modules within the PPI network, using module detection criteria that included a node score cutoff of 0.2, a K-core value of 2, and a degree cutoff of 2 [24]. As a result, seven hub genes (KRT13, KRT5, KRT15, COL17A1, KRT14, KRT16, TP63) were identified. Subsequently, the frequency of genomic alterations was compared between patients with and without a CP4 using the Fisher's exact test.

3. Results

3.1. Comparison of the Distribution of Clinical Factors Stratified by Cribriform Pattern 4

Among the 394 patients analyzed, 129 (32.74%) had CP4. The characteristics of these patients, stratified by the presence of CP4, are presented in Table 1. Compared to those without CP4, the patients with CP4 had a longer median follow-up [46.37 months (IQR: 24.13, 76.97) versus 37.27 months (IQR: 22.87, 62.90), $p = 0.001$], a higher pre-RP PSA [8.10 ng/mL (IQR: 5.20, 14.40) versus 7.00 ng/mL (IQR: 5.00, 9.9), $p = 0.007$], and a higher Gleason score (52% versus 27%, $p = 0.001$) and were more likely to have T3a or higher stage PC (76% versus 53%, $p < 0.001$).

Table 1. Comparison of the distribution of clinical and treatment factors stratified by the presence of the cribriform pattern.

	CP4 (n = 129)	Non-CP4 (n = 265)	p
Age (years), median (IQR)	62 (57, 66)	61 (55, 66)	0.174
Pre-RP PSA, ng/mL, median (IQR)	8.10 (5.20, 14.40)	7.00 (5.00, 9.9)	0.007
Prostatectomy tumor stage, No. (%)			<0.001
T2	30 (24%)	124 (47%)	
T3a or higher	97 (76%)	138 (53%)	
Prostatectomy Gleason score, No. (%)			<0.001
7 or less	60 (48%)	188 (73%)	
8–10	66 (52%)	69 (27%)	

Table 1. *Cont.*

	CP4 (n = 129)	Non-CP4 (n = 265)	p
Prostatectomy margin status, No. (%)			0.200
Negative	92 (72%)	167 (66%)	
Positive	35 (28%)	87 (34%)	
Prostatectomy nodal status, No. (%)			0.300
Negative (N0)	99 (81%)	181 (86%)	
Positive (N1)	23 (19%)	30 (14%)	
* Follow-up (month), median (IQR)	46.37 (24.13, 76.97)	37.27 (22.87, 62.90)	0.001

Abbreviations: CP4, cribriform pattern 4; non-CP4, non-cribriform pattern 4; RP, radical prostatectomy; PSA, prostate-specific antigen; IQR, interquartile range.* reverse KM method is used to estimate time of median follow-up.

3.2. Covariate-Adjusted Hazard Ratios and Estimates of Progression-Free Survival

After a median follow-up of 40.50 months (IQR: 23.90, 65.60), the outcomes included biochemical recurrence in 79 men (20.05%), locoregional recurrence in 5 (1.26%), distant metastasis in 2 (0.50%), new primary tumors in 2 (0.50%), and 4 deaths (1.01%). As shown in Table 2, the presence of CP4 was associated with a significantly lower PFS (AHR, 1.84; 95% CI, 1.08 to 3.11; p = 0.023) after adjusting for known covariates. As illustrated in Figure 1, men with CP4 had significantly lower estimates of adjusted PFS compared to those without it ($p < 0.001$), with the adjusted 10-year PFS estimate being 85.72% (95% CI, 74.79% to 98.24%) for men with CP4 versus 93.01% (95% CI, 87.79% to 98.54%) for those without.

Table 2. Covariate-adjusted hazard ratios for progression-free survival.

Covariates	Univariable			Multivariable		
	HR	95% CI	p	AHR	95% CI	p
Age (years)	0.993	0.967–1.019	0.601	0.977	0.950–1.005	0.109
Baseline PSA, ng/mL						
<4	0.990	0.409–2.398	0.984	0.616	0.233–1.626	0.327
4–10	Reference	Reference		Reference	Reference	
>10	1.463	0.917–2.335	0.110	0.741	0.431–1.275	0.279
Prostatectomy tumor stage, No.						
T2	Reference	Reference		Reference	Reference	
T3a or higher	4.949	2.450–9.999	<0.001	3.903	1.693–8.995	0.001
Prostatectomy Gleason score						
7 or less	Reference	Reference		Reference	Reference	
8–10	3.461	2.198–5.472	<0.001	2.279	1.342–3.870	0.002
Prostatectomy margin status						
Negative	Reference	Reference		Reference	Reference	
Positive	1.604	1.017–2.530	0.042	1.117	0.642–1.945	0.693
Cribriform pattern 4						
Non-CP4	Reference	Reference		Reference	Reference	
CP4	2.210	1.429–3.417	<0.001	1.837	1.080–3.114	0.023

Abbreviations: HR, hazard ratio; CI, confidence interval; AHR, adjusted hazard ratio; CP4, cribriform pattern 4; non-CP4, non-cribriform pattern 4.

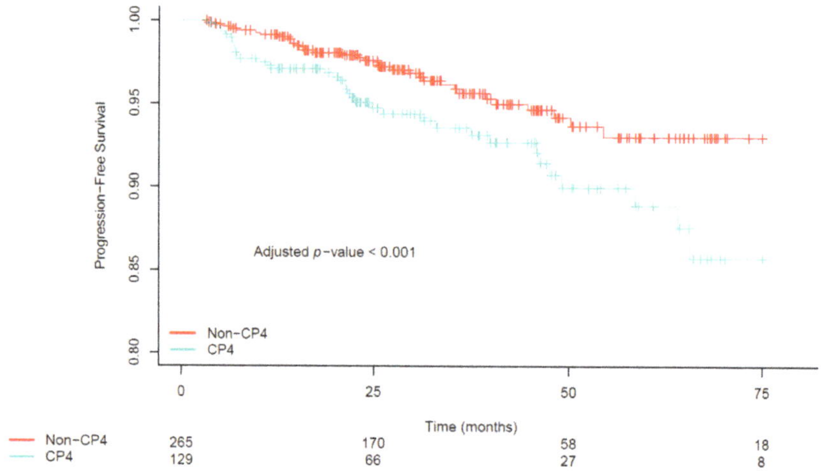

Figure 1. Covariate-adjusted estimates of progression-free survival stratified by the presence of cribriform pattern 4. Abbreviations: CP4, cribriform pattern 4; non-CP4, non-cribriform pattern 4.

3.3. Genetic and Molecular Profiles Stratified by the Cribriform Pattern

The expression levels of two specific mRNAs were significantly elevated in patients with CP4, while 90 other mRNAs exhibited significantly reduced expression levels in these patients compared to those without CP4 (Figure 2a). Furthermore, seven hub genes, namely, KRT13, KRT5, KRT15, COL17A1, KRT14, KRT16, and TP63, exhibited significantly lower mRNA expression levels in patients with CP4 compared to those without (Figure 2b–h).

The FRG1BP gene displayed the highest mutation frequency in both groups, with 50 mutations affecting 26.1% of the patients with CP4 and 69 mutations affecting 16.6% of the patients without CP4. Among the hub genes, only genomic alterations in COL17A1 significantly differed between patients with CP4 and those without (Figure 3).

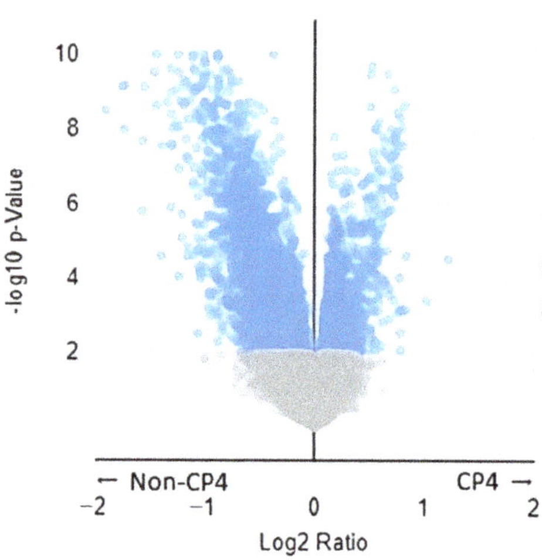

(a)

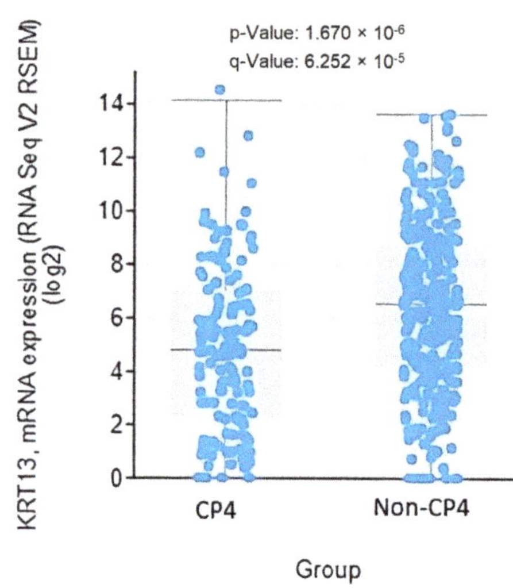

(b)

Figure 2. *Cont.*

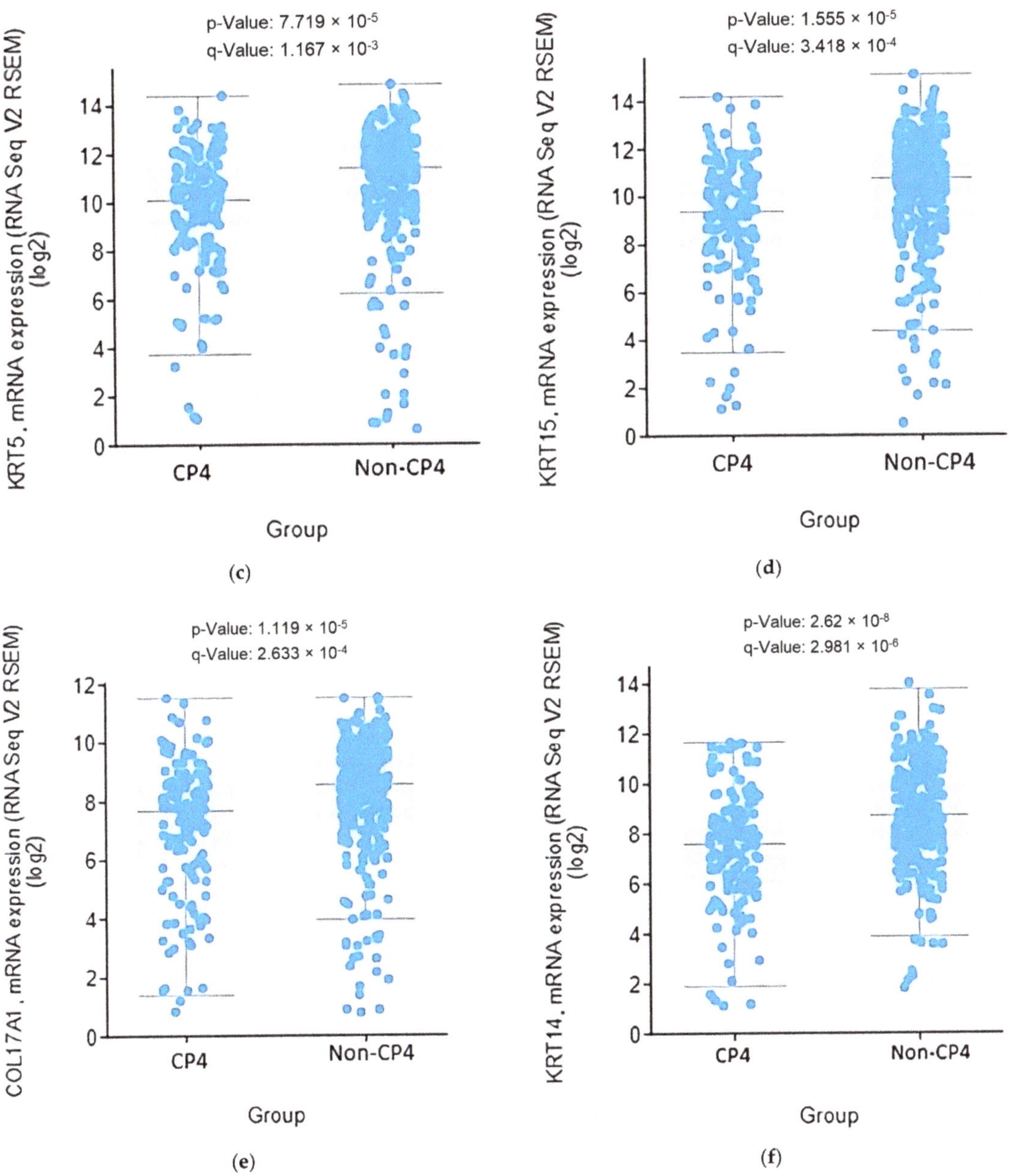

Figure 2. *Cont.*

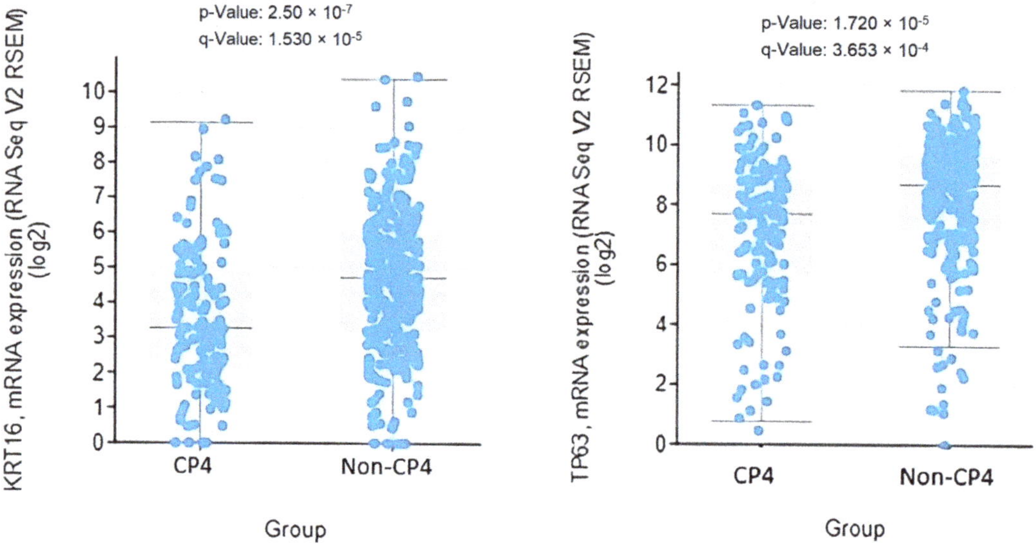

(g) (h)

Figure 2. The mRNA expression level of (**a**) the differentially expressed genes (DEGs) and (**b**–**h**) the seven hub genes stratified by the presence of cribriform pattern 4. Abbreviations: CP4, cribriform pattern 4; non-CP4, non-cribriform pattern 4.

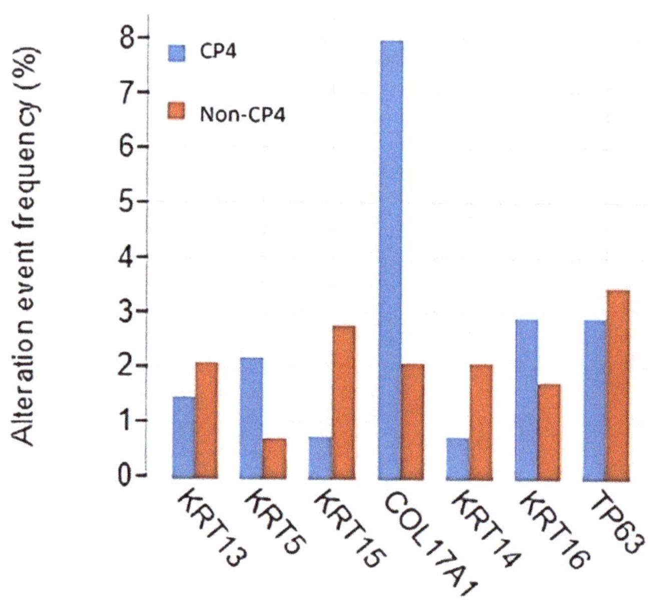

Figure 3. Genomic alterations in the seven hub genes stratified by the presence of cribriform pattern 4. Abbreviations: CP4, cribriform pattern 4; non-CP4, non-cribriform pattern 4.

4. Discussion

In this study, we found that the presence of CP4 in PC patients undergoing RP was associated with reduced PFS, even when accounting for known PC prognostic factors, and was also linked to distinct genomic alterations. The clinical significance of these findings is that they allow for identifying a subset of patients with adverse histopathological characteristics who are at a higher risk of reduced PFS and have unique genomic alterations. This information is valuable for the selection of candidates for future prospective randomized clinical trials designed to explore additional treatments following RP.

In recent years, specific morphologic features, such as CP4, have been increasingly recognized as significant predictors of prognosis in PC patients, highlighting their importance in the stratification of disease aggressiveness. Oufattole et al. highlighted that the presence of CP4 or comedo/solid components in Gleason score 9–10 PC is associated with higher rates of lymphovascular invasion and biochemical recurrence, suggesting that the CP4 morphology is an independent predictor of a higher risk of biochemical recurrence [25]. Similarly, Okubo et al. demonstrated that the presence of CP4 in prostate biopsy specimens is an independent risk factor for lymph node metastasis, showing the prognostic significance of this morphologic feature even when partially present [26]. Moreover, Shimodaira et al. revealed that in patients with Gleason score 8 PC, the area and percentage of CP4 are independent predictors of biochemical recurrence after robot-assisted radical prostatectomy [27]. These findings collectively demonstrate the prognostic significance of CP4 in prostate cancer, reinforcing its role in guiding post-surgical management and highlighting the need for a meticulous histopathological evaluation to identify CP4. Furthermore, the study by Di Mauro et al. showed the critical role of pre-operative assessments, revealing that the PIRADS scores at multiparametric MRI are significant predictors of CP4 in patients undergoing RP, thereby reinforcing the necessity of incorporating advanced imaging findings to enhance the prognostic accuracy for PC patients with CP4 [28]. Our analysis supports these conclusions, demonstrating the association of CP4 with reduced PFS, thereby emphasizing the value of including this morphologic feature in the prognostic assessment of PC patients.

The current standard of care for patients who have undergone RP involves initiating salvage RT once the PSA level reaches 0.1 ng/mL. This approach is supported by a meta-analysis of three prospective randomized controlled trials, focusing on PFS as the primary endpoint [29]. However, concerns have been raised regarding the potential impact of immortal time bias on the results of the meta-analysis, suggesting that a subgroup of high-risk patients might benefit from adjuvant RT [30]. Supporting this, evidence from a large multi-national and multi-institutional study indicated a significant reduction in all-cause mortality with the use of adjuvant RT over salvage RT, particularly in patients with a pathological Gleason score of 8–10 and stage-pT3 or -pT4 PC [31]. Furthermore, the ongoing NRG-GU008 randomized control trial is exploring treatment intensification with abiraterone and apalutamide following RP in patients with pathologically node-positive disease and detectable PSA [32]. Patients with CP4 post-RP may also benefit from adjuvant RT or treatment intensification, highlighting the need for their inclusion in future randomized trials.

Our findings contribute to the limited but growing body of literature on the molecular characteristics of PC with CP4. Notably, the distinct molecular features observed in our study, such as the differential expression and mutation frequency of genes like FRG1BP and alterations in COL17A1, align with and extend previous research by Elfandy et al., who reported unique genetic, transcriptional, and epigenetic features distinguishing CP4 from non-cribriform pattern 4 (non-CP4) tumors [33]. These features include increased somatic copy number variations, mutations in SPOP and ATM, and pathway enrichments, which collectively suggest a distinct molecular phenotype for CP4 PC that closely resembles that of metastatic PC and is associated with progression to lethal disease [33]. Similarly, our study echoes the findings of Böttcher et al., who reported that CP4 is linked to increased genomic instability, highlighting CP4 role as a pathological substrate for progressive molecular tumor derangement [34]. Together, these findings emphasize CP4 significance in the molecular landscape of PC, highlighting its potential as a marker of aggressive disease and a target for future therapeutic strategies.

Several points require further discussion. First, histologic interpretations in this study were based on one or two virtual slides. Considering the pathology review committee's limited access to the entire prostatectomy specimens, it is possible that patients classified as lacking evidence of cribriform pattern 4 could, in fact, present this pattern in unreviewed sections of the specimens. Despite this limitation, a significant association was observed between the presence of CP4 and reduced PFS. Second, it is important to emphasize that although men with CP4 are more likely to present with higher pre-RP PSA levels and Gleason scores and advanced-stage disease (T3a or higher), these variables were carefully considered and adjusted for in the multivariable model. Third, the TCGA database lacks detailed longitudinal PSA measurements and imaging results post-RP, necessitating our PFS assessment to be based solely on available dates of diagnosis, treatment, and significant clinical events. Fourth, the absence of data on adjuvant treatments in our dataset represents a limitation, potentially impacting the interpretation of the PFS outcomes. Finally, as this is a retrospective study, the results are hypothesis-generating and warrant further investigation in a prospective cohort study.

5. Conclusions

The association of CP4 with reduced PFS in PC patients undergoing RP highlights the importance of identifying patients at increased risk of disease progression. These findings advocate for the potential benefits of adjuvant treatment in this subgroup, emphasizing the need for further investigation through prospective randomized clinical trials. Moreover, the distinct genetic and molecular characteristics of CP4 further solidify its role as a critical marker of aggressive PC, reinforcing the importance of targeted treatment strategies and comprehensive molecular profiling in future clinical trials.

Author Contributions: Conceptualization, M.S., Y.T. and C.A.; methodology, M.S., Y.T., M.A., D.A., S.K., E.T., A.V.D. and C.A.; data curation, Y.T., G.K.P. and M.D.R.; writing—original draft preparation, M.S. and C.A.; writing—review and editing, M.S., Y.T., M.A., G.K.P., M.D.R., D.A., S.K., E.T., S.M., J.E.L., P.F.O., P.L.N., A.V.D. and C.A.; supervision, M.S. and C.A. All authors have read and agreed to the published version of the manuscript.

Funding: This research received no external funding.

Institutional Review Board Statement: The study was conducted according to the guidelines of the Declaration of Helsinki and met the exception criteria from review by the Institutional Review Board of the Dana-Farber Cancer Institute, exception number, 491519, exception date, 2 February 2024.

Informed Consent Statement: Since the data are anonymized, and patient privacy is fully safeguarded, the ethics committee exempted this retrospective study from the requirement of obtaining written informed consent from the patients.

Data Availability Statement: The original contributions presented in the study are included in the article. Further inquiries can be directed to the corresponding author.

Acknowledgments: We would like to acknowledge the patients and their families for participating in this research.

Conflicts of Interest: The authors declare that the research was conducted without any commercial or financial relationships that could be construed as potential conflicts of interest.

References

1. Bailar, J.C., 3rd; Mellinger, G.T.; Gleason, D.F. Survival rates of patients with prostatic cancer, tumor stage, and differentiation—Preliminary report. *Cancer Chemother. Rep.* **1966**, *50*, 129–136.
2. Epstein, J.I.; Amin, M.B.; Reuter, V.E.; Humphrey, P.A. Contemporary Gleason Grading of Prostatic Carcinoma: An Update with Discussion on Practical Issues to Implement the 2014 International Society of Urological Pathology (ISUP) Consensus Conference on Gleason Grading of Prostatic Carcinoma. *Am. J. Surg. Pathol.* **2017**, *41*, e1–e7. [CrossRef] [PubMed]

3. Iczkowski, K.A.; Torkko, K.C.; Kotnis, G.R.; Wilson, R.S.; Huang, W.; Wheeler, T.M.; Abeyta, A.M.; La Rosa, F.G.; Cook, S.; Werahera, P.N.; et al. Digital quantification of five high-grade prostate cancer patterns, including the cribriform pattern, and their association with adverse outcome. *Am. J. Clin. Pathol.* **2011**, *136*, 98–107. [CrossRef] [PubMed]
4. Kir, G.; Sarbay, B.C.; Gümüş, E.; Topal, C.S. The association of the cribriform pattern with outcome for prostatic adenocarcinomas. *Pathol.-Res. Pract.* **2014**, *210*, 640–644. [CrossRef] [PubMed]
5. Kweldam, C.F.; Wildhagen, M.F.; Steyerberg, E.W.; Bangma, C.H.; van der Kwast, T.H.; van Leenders, G.J. Cribriform growth is highly predictive for postoperative metastasis and disease-specific death in Gleason score 7 prostate cancer. *Mod. Pathol.* **2015**, *28*, 457–464. [CrossRef] [PubMed]
6. Trudel, D.; Downes, M.R.; Sykes, J.; Kron, K.J.; Trachtenberg, J.; van der Kwast, T.H. Prognostic impact of intraductal carcinoma and large cribriform carcinoma architecture after prostatectomy in a contemporary cohort. *Eur. J. Cancer* **2014**, *50*, 1610–1616. [CrossRef]
7. Hollemans, E.; Verhoef, E.I.; Bangma, C.H.; Rietbergen, J.; Helleman, J.; Roobol, M.J.; van Leenders, G. Large cribriform growth pattern identifies ISUP grade 2 prostate cancer at high risk for recurrence and metastasis. *Mod. Pathol.* **2019**, *32*, 139–146. [CrossRef] [PubMed]
8. Hollemans, E.; Verhoef, E.I.; Bangma, C.H.; Rietbergen, J.; Osanto, S.; Pelger, R.C.M.; van Wezel, T.; van der Poel, H.; Bekers, E.; Helleman, J.; et al. Cribriform architecture in radical prostatectomies predicts oncological outcome in Gleason score 8 prostate cancer patients. *Mod. Pathol.* **2021**, *34*, 184–193. [CrossRef]
9. Kweldam, C.F.; Kümmerlin, I.P.; Nieboer, D.; Verhoef, E.I.; Steyerberg, E.W.; van der Kwast, T.H.; Roobol, M.J.; van Leenders, G.J. Disease-specific survival of patients with invasive cribriform and intraductal prostate cancer at diagnostic biopsy. *Mod. Pathol.* **2016**, *29*, 630–636. [CrossRef]
10. Masoomian, M.; Downes, M.R.; Sweet, J.; Cheung, C.; Evans, A.J.; Fleshner, N.; Maganti, M.; van der Kwast, T. Concordance of biopsy and prostatectomy diagnosis of intraductal and cribriform carcinoma in a prospectively collected data set. *Histopathology* **2019**, *74*, 474–482. [CrossRef]
11. Russo, G.I.; Soeterik, T.; Puche-Sanz, I.; Broggi, G.; Lo Giudice, A.; De Nunzio, C.; Lombardo, R.; Marra, G.; Gandaglia, G. Oncological outcomes of cribriform histology pattern in prostate cancer patients: A systematic review and meta-analysis. *Prostate Cancer Prostatic Dis.* **2023**, *26*, 646–654. [CrossRef] [PubMed]
12. Guo, C.C.; Epstein, J.I. Intraductal carcinoma of the prostate on needle biopsy: Histologic features and clinical significance. *Mod. Pathol.* **2006**, *19*, 1528–1535. [CrossRef] [PubMed]
13. Zhou, M. High-grade prostatic intraepithelial neoplasia, PIN-like carcinoma, ductal carcinoma, and intraductal carcinoma of the prostate. *Mod. Pathol.* **2018**, *31*, S71–S79. [CrossRef] [PubMed]
14. Hollander, M.; Wolfe, D.A.; Chicken, E. *Nonparametric Statistical Methods*; John Wiley & Sons: Hoboken, NJ, USA, 2013.
15. Schemper, M.; Smith, T.L. A note on quantifying follow-up in studies of failure time. *Control. Clin. Trials* **1996**, *17*, 343–346. [CrossRef] [PubMed]
16. Fleming, T.R. Surrogate endpoints and FDA's accelerated approval process. *Health Aff.* **2005**, *24*, 67–78. [CrossRef] [PubMed]
17. Broglio, K.R.; Berry, D.A. Detecting an overall survival benefit that is derived from progression-free survival. *J. Natl. Cancer Inst.* **2009**, *101*, 1642–1649. [CrossRef] [PubMed]
18. Burzykowski, T.; Buyse, M.; Piccart-Gebhart, M.J.; Sledge, G.; Carmichael, J.; Lück, H.J.; Mackey, J.R.; Nabholtz, J.M.; Paridaens, R.; Biganzoli, L.; et al. Evaluation of tumor response, disease control, progression-free survival, and time to progression as potential surrogate end points in metastatic breast cancer. *J. Clin. Oncol.* **2008**, *26*, 1987–1992. [CrossRef]
19. Fine, J.P.; Gray, R.J. A proportional hazards model for the subdistribution of a competing risk. *J. Am. Stat. Assoc.* **1999**, *94*, 496–509. [CrossRef]
20. Kaplan, E.L.; Meier, P. Nonparametric estimation from incomplete observations. *J. Am. Stat. Assoc.* **1958**, *53*, 457–481. [CrossRef]
21. De Bruijn, I.; Kundra, R.; Mastrogiacomo, B.; Tran, T.N.; Sikina, L.; Mazor, T.; Li, X.; Ochoa, A.; Zhao, G.; Lai, B.; et al. Analysis and Visualization of Longitudinal Genomic and Clinical Data from the AACR Project GENIE Biopharma Collaborative in cBioPortal. *Cancer Res.* **2023**, *83*, 3861–3867. [CrossRef]
22. Szklarczyk, D.; Franceschini, A.; Wyder, S.; Forslund, K.; Heller, D.; Huerta-Cepas, J.; Simonovic, M.; Roth, A.; Santos, A.; Tsafou, K.P.; et al. STRING v10: Protein-protein interaction networks, integrated over the tree of life. *Nucleic Acids Res.* **2015**, *43*, D447–D452. [CrossRef]
23. Shannon, P.; Markiel, A.; Ozier, O.; Baliga, N.S.; Wang, J.T.; Ramage, D.; Amin, N.; Schwikowski, B.; Ideker, T. Cytoscape: A software environment for integrated models of biomolecular interaction networks. *Genome Res.* **2003**, *13*, 2498–2504. [CrossRef]
24. Bader, G.D.; Hogue, C.W. An automated method for finding molecular complexes in large protein interaction networks. *BMC Bioinform.* **2003**, *4*, 2. [CrossRef] [PubMed]
25. Oufattole, J.; Dey, T.; D'Amico, A.V.; van Leenders, G.; Acosta, A.M. Cribriform morphology is associated with higher risk of biochemical recurrence after radical prostatectomy in patients with Grade Group 5 prostate cancer. *Histopathology* **2023**, *82*, 1089–1097. [CrossRef] [PubMed]
26. Okubo, Y.; Sato, S.; Hasegawa, C.; Koizumi, M.; Suzuki, T.; Yamamoto, Y.; Yoshioka, E.; Ono, K.; Washimi, K.; Yokose, T.; et al. Cribriform pattern and intraductal carcinoma of the prostate can have a clinicopathological impact, regardless of their percentage and/or number of cores. *Hum. Pathol.* **2023**, *135*, 99–107. [CrossRef] [PubMed]

27. Shimodaira, K.; Inoue, R.; Hashimoto, T.; Satake, N.; Shishido, T.; Namiki, K.; Harada, K.; Nagao, T.; Ohno, Y. Significance of the cribriform morphology area ratio for biochemical recurrence in Gleason score 4 + 4 prostate cancer patients following robot-assisted radical prostatectomy. *Cancer Med.* **2024**, *13*, e7086. [CrossRef] [PubMed]
28. Di Mauro, E.; Di Bello, F.; Califano, G.; Morra, S.; Creta, M.; Celentano, G.; Abate, M.; Fraia, A.; Pezone, G.; Marino, C.; et al. Incidence and Predicting Factors of Histopathological Features at Robot-Assisted Radical Prostatectomy in the mpMRI Era: Results of a Single Tertiary Referral Center. *Medicina* **2023**, *59*, 625. [CrossRef] [PubMed]
29. Vale, C.L.; Fisher, D.; Kneebone, A.; Parker, C.; Pearse, M.; Richaud, P.; Sargos, P.; Sydes, M.R.; Brawley, C.; Brihoum, M.; et al. Adjuvant or early salvage radiotherapy for the treatment of localised and locally advanced prostate cancer: A prospectively planned systematic review and meta-analysis of aggregate data. *Lancet* **2020**, *396*, 1422–1431. [CrossRef] [PubMed]
30. MacDuffie, E.; D'Amico, A.V. Adjuvant vs Salvage Radiation Therapy for High-Risk Prostate Cancer Following Radical Prostatectomy. *JAMA Oncol.* **2020**, *6*, 1165–1166. [CrossRef] [PubMed]
31. Tilki, D.; Chen, M.H.; Wu, J.; Huland, H.; Graefen, M.; Wiegel, T.; Böhmer, D.; Mohamad, O.; Cowan, J.E.; Feng, F.Y.; et al. Adjuvant Versus Early Salvage Radiation Therapy for Men at High Risk for Recurrence Following Radical Prostatectomy for Prostate Cancer and the Risk of Death. *J. Clin. Oncol.* **2021**, *39*, 2284–2293. [CrossRef]
32. Chen, R.C.; Karrison, T.; Lawton, C.A.; Hall, W.A.; Borno, H.; Rosu, M.; Jani, A.B.; Schuster, D.M.; Seider, M.J.; Efstathiou, J.A.; et al. INNOVATE (NRG-GU008): A randomized phase III trial of salvage radiotherapy and androgen deprivation therapy (ADT) with/without abiraterone and apalutamide for patients with node-positive prostate cancer after radical prostatectomy. *J. Clin. Oncol.* **2021**, *39*, TPS179. [CrossRef]
33. Elfandy, H.; Armenia, J.; Pederzoli, F.; Pullman, E.; Pertega-Gomes, N.; Schultz, N.; Viswanathan, K.; Vosoughi, A.; Blattner, M.; Stopsack, K.H.; et al. Genetic and Epigenetic Determinants of Aggressiveness in Cribriform Carcinoma of the Prostate. *Mol. Cancer Res.* **2019**, *17*, 446–456. [CrossRef] [PubMed]
34. Böttcher, R.; Kweldam, C.F.; Livingstone, J.; Lalonde, E.; Yamaguchi, T.N.; Huang, V.; Yousif, F.; Fraser, M.; Bristow, R.G.; van der Kwast, T.; et al. Cribriform and intraductal prostate cancer are associated with increased genomic instability and distinct genomic alterations. *BMC Cancer* **2018**, *18*, 8. [CrossRef] [PubMed]

cancers

MDPI

Review

Periprostatic Adipose Tissue as a Contributor to Prostate Cancer Pathogenesis: A Narrative Review

Julia Drewa [1,*], Katarzyna Lazar-Juszczak [2,3], Jan Adamowicz [1,4] and Kajetan Juszczak [1,*]

1 Department of Urology and Andrology, Collegium Medicum, Nicolaus Copernicus University, 85-094 Bydgoszcz, Poland
2 Primary Health Care Clinic of the Ujastek Medical Center, 31-752 Cracow, Poland
3 Krakow University of Health Promotion, 31-158 Cracow, Poland
4 Department of Regenerative Medicine, Collegium Medicum, Nicolaus Copernicus University, 85-094 Bydgoszcz, Poland
* Correspondence: drewajulia@wp.pl (J.D.); kaj.juszczak@gmail.com (K.J.)

Simple Summary: The role of periprostatic adipose tissue in the pathogenesis of prostate cancer seems to be unquestionable. Moreover, periprostatic adipose tissue is involved in the progression of prostate cancer. Our literature review provides detailed information on the involvement of periprostatic adipose tissue in the development of prostate cancer. The data so far indicate that periprostatic adipose tissue may become an attractive target for modern prostate cancer therapies, especially in patients with more aggressive and/or advanced stages of prostate cancer. Nevertheless, further research is necessary in this field.

Abstract: Periprostatic adipose tissue (PPAT) contributes to the pathogenesis of prostate cancer. The purpose of this study was to review and summarize the literature on the role of PPAT in prostate cancer pathogenesis. Moreover, we evaluated the clinical implication of PPAT in patients with prostate cancer. We performed a scoping literature review of PubMed from January 2002 to November 2024. Search terms included "periprostatic adipose tissue", "adipokines", and "prostate cancer". Secondary search involved reference lists of eligible articles. The key criterion was to identify studies that included PPAT, adipokines, and their role in prostate cancer biology and clinical features. In total 225 publications were selected for inclusion in this review. The studies contained in publications allowed us to summarize the data on the pathogenesis of PPAT as a contributor to prostate cancer biology and its aggressiveness. The review also presents new research directions for PPAT as a new target for the treatment of prostate cancer. Based on the current review, it can be stated that PPAT plays an important role in prostate cancer pathogenesis. Moreover, PPAT seems to be a promising target point when it comes to finding new therapies in patients with more aggressive and/or advanced stages of prostate cancer.

Keywords: periprostatic adipose tissue; prostate cancer; obesity; pathogenesis; adipokines

1. Introduction

Prostate cancer is the second most commonly diagnosed cancer in men [1]. In the European male population, prostate cancer remains the most frequently diagnosed cancer (excluding skin cancer) [2]. Prostate cancer is diagnosed on the basis of a prostate biopsy. Laboratory tests (assessment of the PSA level) and imaging tests (multiparametric magnetic resonance imaging) are helpful in diagnosis. Urine and serum biomarkers as well as tissue-based biomarkers have been proposed for improving detection and risk stratification of prostate cancer patients, potentially avoiding unnecessary biopsies. Most patients with prostate cancer require radical treatment (radical prostatectomy). However, taking into account the biology of prostate cancer and the clinical features of patients with prostate cancer (age, comorbidities, stage of the disease, etc.) in selected cases, we choose non-surgical methods (e.g., radical radiotherapy, hormonotherapy, chemotherapy, etc.). The pathogenesis of prostate cancer is multi-factorial but still incompletely understood [3]. Several etiological factors have been discussed as being associated with the risk of developing prostate cancer or as being etiologically important for the progression from latent to clinical prostate cancer [4]. The possible modifiable risk factors for the development of prostate cancer include metabolic syndrome, obesity, diet, and smoking [5].

A comprehensive meta-analysis provides epidemiological evidence supporting the association between body mass index (BMI) and cancer risk and reports an increased risk of aggressive prostate cancer in obese patients [6]. Despite advances in prostate cancer diagnosis and management, morbidity from prostate cancer still remains high. Despite hormonal therapy, patient with prostate cancer progress to castration-resistant prostate cancer (CRPC) approximately within 2–3 years of initiation of androgen deprivation therapy [7]. Bone metastases will occur in about 90% of patients with CRPC [8]. Therefore, there is a need for new therapeutic targets in patients witch prostate cancer, especially in CRPC clinical stage. Periprostatic adipose tissue (PPAT) contributes to the pathogenesis of prostate cancer development. Moreover, it is postulated that PPAT is involved in prostate cancer progression into metastatic disease.

The following review aims to discuss and provide information about the role of PPAT in prostate cancer pathogenesis and its clinical implication in patients with prostate cancer. The studies contained in publications allowed us to summarize the data on the pathogenesis of PPAT as a contributor to prostate cancer biology and its aggressiveness. The review also presents new research directions for PPAT as a new target for the treatment of prostate cancer, especially in patients with more aggressive and/or advanced stages of prostate cancer.

2. Obesity and Cancer

Obesity is strictly related to several chronic diseases, especially cardio-vascular illnesses, diabetes, sleep apnea, and osteoarthritis [9]. It is worth noting that there is growing evidence that overweight and obesity is a potential risk factor for cancer development [10]. Obesity attributes to about 4–8% of all cancers [11]. Previous studies showed the link between obesity and gastro-intestinal cancers (e.g., esophagus, stomach, colon, and rectum), gallbladder and pancreas cancer, genito-urinary cancers (e.g., prostate, uterus, and ovary), and breast cancer [11–14]. Aune et al.'s [15] study revealed that overweight and obesity is associated with increased risk of all-cause mortality. Additionally, obesity was associated with greater risk of recurrence and mortality overall in patients with cancer [16,17].

The potential pathomechanisms of obesity causing cancer are complex and multifactorial. This phenomenon remains incompletely explained. Obesity results from a chronic excessive accumulation of adipose tissue. In the literature, several potential cellular and molecular pathomechanisms linking cancer development, as well as cancer progression and metastasis development, to obesity were described [18]. These mechanisms include, among others, micro-environmental disturbances and extracellular matrix remodeling, altered fatty acid metabolism, hormonal disturbances (e.g., anabolic hormone), chronic inflammation, and immune instability [19]. Additionally, Renehan et al. [20] proposed several hormonal pathomechanisms attributed to cancer development, as follow: (1) adipokine-related pathways, (2) altered sex hormone metabolism, and (3) elevated insulin level and increased bioavailability of insulin-like growth factor 1 (IGF-1). Moreover, it is postulated that interstitial microbiota dysregulation is important in obesity, obesity-related diseases, and cancer development [21]. Roger et al. [22] draws attention to intestinal microbiome dysregulation affect proper bacterial metabolism, which may lead to production of potential procarcinogenic metabolites. Additionally, metabolic dysfunction due to boost energy extraction, nutrient availability, and induction of inflammation seems to contribute to tumor cells development and/or growth.

3. Obesity and Prostate Cancer

The relationship between obesity and the risk of prostate cancer is still unclear. Previous studies confirmed that obese men are at higher risk for dying of prostate cancer [23]. Moreover, men with obesity predispose to more aggressive form of prostate cancer [24,25]. Previous meta-analyses indicate a positive association between prostate cancer and obesity. In general, the relative risks (RRs) were from 1.01 (95% confidence interval [CI], 1.0–1.02) per 1 kg/m^2 increase in BMI [26] to 1.05 (95% CI, 1.01–1.08) [25] and 1.03 (95% CI, 1.0–1.07) [27] per 5 kg/m^2 increment in BMI [24].

There are two types of adipose tissue: white adipose tissue (WAT) and brown adipose tissue (BAT). Moreover, third type of adipose tissue can be distinguished: a "beige" adipose tissue due to the "browning" of WAT phenomenon. Many studies indicate the active participation of adipose tissue in the development and progression of prostate cancer via endocrine and paracrine signalling [28]. Hond et al. [29] study showed that that adipose tissue covered about 48% of the prostate gland surfaces.

Allott et al. [24] study described a close positive correlation among prostate cancer and other comorbidities (e.g., metabolic syndrome and obesity). There are currently several potential mechanisms explaining the relationship between obesity and the development of prostate cancer. First, generalized and local inflammatory response stimulated by immune system cells present in the adipose tissue, including that surrounding the prostate gland. Second, obesity and excess adipose tissue lead to the development of hyperinsulinemia. Third, excess adipose tissue predisposes to changes in the availability of a number of substances with para- and endocrine effects, including the so-called adipokines [30]. White adipose tissue surrounding the prostate gland forms the so-called PPAT and is one of the most important components of the prostate microenvironment, taking an active part in the physiological conditions as well as in the development of prostate cancer. Namely, the periprostatic adipose tissue is an active endocrine tissue, influencing the activity of prostate cells, but above all, by modulating the microenvironment, it promotes the processes of migration, invasion, and aggressiveness of prostate cancer cells [30,31].

In people with normal body weight, a proper balance between pro- and anti-inflammatory pathways is maintained in the adipose tissue. Thanks to the secretion of greater amounts of anti-inflammatory substances from the extracellular matrix and the adipose cells themselves [32]. As body weight increases, a predominance of pro-inflammatory activity is observed. This is due to increased production of adipokines associated with developing insulin resistance and increased inflammation. In addition, the cell death of some hypertrophic adipocytes and the release of intracellular substances are observed, which increase the already existing inflammation, intensifying the pro-inflammatory response [33].

Early childhood and puberty are important periods for the development of normal adipose tissue mass. After puberty, adipocyte number and size become static in lean individuals [34]. In obese subjects (in development and adulthood), the increment in adipose tissue mass is due to adipocyte size (hypertrophy) and increased adipocyte number (hyperplasia) [35]. In adults, a high-fat diet transiently induces adipocyte precursors to proliferate, which leads to the increased formation of adipocytes in diet-induced obesity. The development of PPAT appears to be parallel with the development of obesity, particularly of the visceral type. The increase in PPAT mass results mainly from the enlargement of adipocytes already present there. However, the coexistence of adipocyte proliferation cannot be ruled out. The extent of PPAT seems to be related to the degree of visceral obesity due to their morphological and functional similarities. Obesity is associated with changes in adipocyte gene expression spanning many pathways. These changes alter fuel partitioning between adipose tissue and other tissues. In addition, they alter the hormonal milieu by changing the relative expression of adipose hormones, adipokines. Finally, many metabolites act as signaling molecules; thus, their redistribution alters signaling pathways in adipose and other tissues [36].

4. PPAT and Prostate Cancer Biology

Adipocytes contained in PPAT are thought to influence cancer cell activity via pathological feedback loops dependent on paracrine secretion of adipokines. These adipokines influence cancer cell growth and survival. Park et al. [30] described the close interactions of cancer cell and adipocytes via endocrine and paracrine pathways. Several proposed pathophysiological mechanisms of prostate cancer tumorigenesis have been described at the cellular level, including: (1) the insulin and IGF axis, (2) deregulated adipokine signalling, and (3) the expansion of adipose/stromal stem cells population [37–39]. It is worth remembering, however, that the "adipocytes—prostate cancer cells" interaction is not one-way. Several studies have confirmed the observation that prostate cancer cells demonstrate the ability to induce genetic and phenotypic changes in neighbouring adipocytes, leading to their transformation into so-called "cancer-associated adipocytes" [40]. During tumour growth, epithelial cells leave the glandular niche and invade the microenvironment becoming exposed to huge concentrations of adipokines released by PPAT that boost their proliferation [28,41].

At the same time, remodelling of the extracellular matrix seems to be an inherent pathophysiological mechanism influencing tumour development and progression. Moreover, obesity predispose to infiltration of adipose tissues by inflammatory cells (e.g., macrophages and leukocytes) and in a consequence trigger the local and systemic inflammatory response and insulin resistance [42]. During local inflammatory process the reactive oxygen species are generated that act as tumour promoters at a low concentration [43]. Adipocytes, stromal cells, and infiltrating inflammatory cells in adipose tissue secrete several adipokines and other cytokines, which play a crucial role in the development of obesity-related cancer [42,44] (Figure 1).

5. PPAT and Adipokines

Adipose tissue releases a number of substances named adipokines. The adipokines include chemokines, cytokines (e.g., interleukin-1 (IL-1), interleukin-6 (IL-6) and tumour necrosis factor (TNF)-α), angiogenic factors (e.g., vascular endothelial growth factor (VEGF), and other substances (e.g., leptin, adiponectin, and insulin-like growth factor 1 (IGF1), etc.) [28,42] (Figure 2).

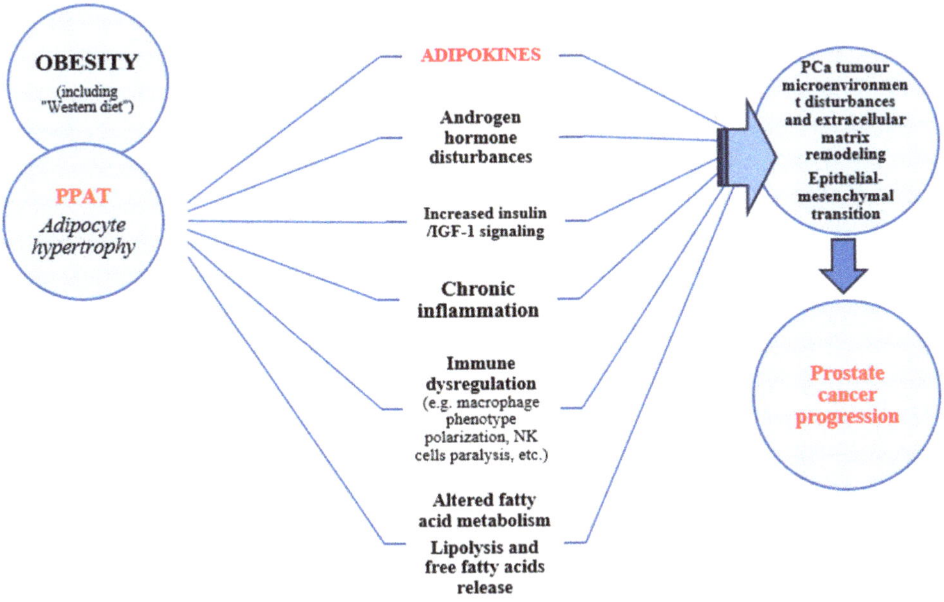

Figure 1. Obesity-associated pathomechanisms of prostate cancer development. PPAT—Periprostatic adipose tissue, IGF-1—Insulin-like growth factor-1, NK—Natural Killer, PCa—prostate cancer.

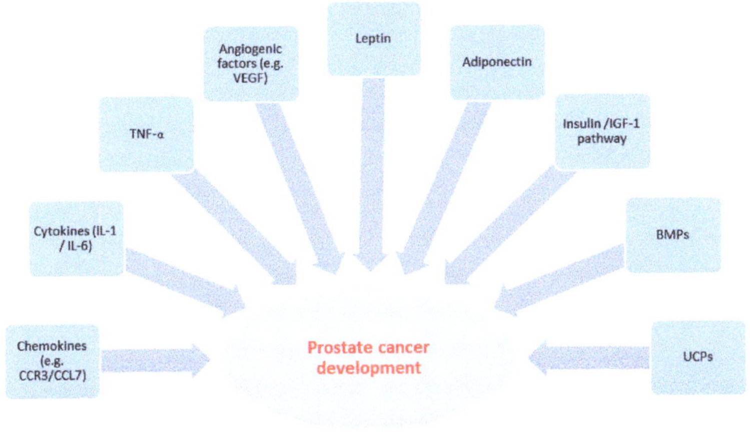

Figure 2. Adipokines released from PPAT affect prostate cancer development. CCR3—chemokine receptor 3, CCL7—chemokine ligand 7, IL-1—interleukin-1, IL-6—interleukin-6, TNF-α—tumor necrosis factor α, VEGF—vascular endothelial growth factor, IGF-1—Insulin-like growth factor-1, BMPs—Bone Morphogenetic Proteins, UCPs—mitochondrial uncoupling protein.

5.1. Chemokines

Chemokines are small molecules that function as chemotactic factors, which regulate the migration, infiltration, and accumulation of immune cells [45]. Laurent et al.'s [46] study showed that PPAT, especially its adipocytes, is directly involved in prostate cancer cell migration outside the prostate gland. Additionally, obesity promotes this migration. There are several adipokines involved in prostate cancer cell migration. The chemokine CCL7 secreted by adipocytes is pivotal in extensive migration. CCL7 diffuses through the prostatic capsule to the peripheral zone of the prostate gland and consequently stimulates the migration of the CCR3 = positive prostate cancer cells outside the prostate. Obesity predisposes to higher secretion of chemokines (e.g., CCL7) by hypertrophic adipocyte cells from PPAT and secondarily facilitates extraprostatic extension, leading to locally advanced disease. Additionally, CCR3/CCL7 axis blockade leads to inhibition of increased obesity-related cancer cell migration. The expression of the CCR3 receptor is associated with the occurrence of aggressive disease with extended local dissemination and a higher risk of biochemical recurrence of prostate cancer.

The adipocytes release the stromal cell derived factor 12 (CXCL12) through direct interaction with the chemokine receptor CXC type 4 (CXCR4) present in the membrane of tumour cells activates the intracellular cascade of gene transcription involved in cell survival, or migration and invasion, thus promoting EMT [28]. The process of epithelial–mesenchymal transition (EMT) plays a pivotal role in the development of metastatic castration resistant prostate cancer (m CRPC) [47]. The epithelial–mesenchymal transition (EMT) in important in prostate tumours growth and progression [48]. Moreover, the EMT phenomenon is promoted by obesity [49].

5.2. Leptin

Leptin is an obesity-associated adipokine. This molecule regulates energy metabolism and reproduction, as well as controls an appetite via the leptin receptor. Moreover, cancer cells and the tumour microenvironment expressing leptin and leptin receptors suggest that the potential leptin autocrine/paracrine signalling loop could affect tumour progression [50]. Gorrab et al. [51] demonstrated that high doses of leptin promote prostate cancer cell migration and EMT transition via stimulation of the STAT3 pathway. Moreover, the blockage of leptin receptors inhibits prostate cancer xenograft growth and progression in a mice model [52]. Cellular invasion and migration of androgen-resistant prostate cancer cells (PC-3 and DU-145 cell lines) are attenuated by leptin in a concentration-dependent manner in prostate cancer cell lines. Additionally, the proliferation of androgen-dependent and independent prostate cancer cell lines was observed in the presence of nanogram concentrations of leptin [53]. Serum levels of leptin positively correlate with prostate cancer development [54]. Chang et al. [55] study revealed that men with high-volume disease exhibited higher serum leptin concentrations overall and after stratification by age, testosterone level, height, and body mass index (BMI).

5.3. Adiponectin

Adiponectin interacts via ADIPOR1 and ADIPOR2 membrane receptors [56]. Adiponectin has significant anti-diabetic, anti-inflammatory, anti-atherosclerotic and anti-proliferative properties [54]. Patients with prostate cancer have lower serum adiponectin levels and decreased expression of adiponectin receptors in tumour tissues, which suggests that plasma adiponectin level is a risk factor for prostate cancer. Prostate cancer patients had significantly lower plasma adiponectin concentrations as compared to men with benign prostate hyperplasia and healthy controls. Men in the top two quartiles of adiponectin had a 71% to 73% reduced risk of prostate cancer as compared to men in the lowest quartile [57]. Li et al. [58] study showed that adiponectin concentrations were not associated with overall risk of prostate cancer. However, men with higher adiponectin concentrations had lower risk of developing high-grade or lethal cancer (metastatic or fatal disease). Endogenous adiponectin may function as a tumour suppressor gene through inhibiting the epithelial–mesenchymal transition of prostate cancer cells but is down-regulated in prostate cancer via promoter hypermethylation [59]. Contrarily, Tang et al.'s [60] study showed that adiponectin increased the migration and the expression of α5β1 integrin of human prostate cancer cells. One of the mechanisms underlying directed adiponectin migration was transcriptional up-regulation of α5β1 integrin and activation of AdipoR1 receptor, p38, AMPK, and NF-κB pathways. Previous studies revealed that that adiponectin presents anti-proliferative properties in prostate cancer cells and inhibits dihydrotestosterone-activated cell proliferation, IL-6, and IGF-I [61–63].

5.4. Insulin-like Growth Factor 1

Insulin-like growth factor (IGF)-1 is associated with a higher risk of prostate cancer [64]. Similarly, Qian et al. [65] revealed that the elevated serum IGF-1 levels increase the future risk of prostate cancer development in healthy men. Acromegaly patients with systemically high growth hormone (GH) and IGF-1 levels also have significantly higher incidence of prostate cancer and risk of prostate cancer-related mortality (HR = 1.33 and 1.44, respectively), suggesting that IGF-1 has a positive effect on prostate cancer development and progression [66]. IGF-1 is inhibited by IGF-binding protein (IGFBP)-1, which is defined as a marker for insulin activity. Insulin is responsible for proper carbohydrate and energy metabolism. It also has a strong mitogenic effect and stimulates prostate growth, which may contribute to the development of prostate cancer [67]. On the one hand, epidemiological studies to date clearly indicate the relationship between higher levels of circulating IGF-1 and an increased risk of prostate cancer development (especially low-grade cancer). On the other hand, the potential pathomechanisms related to insulin and IGF pathways remain unclear [68,69]. In patients with prostate cancer, the overexpression of IGF-1 receptor is observed. IGF-1 accelerated the growth of prostate cancer by activating phosphoinositide 3-kinase and mitogen-activated protein kinase or increasing sex hormone sensitivity [70]. Cao et al.'s [64] results showed that higher fasting IGF-binding protein (IGFBP-1) levels were associated with lower risk of prostate cancer, whereas higher IGF-1 levels were associated with increased prostate cancer risk. The associations were primarily driven by lower-grade and non-advanced prostate cancer. In patients with locally advanced and metastatic prostate cancer, androgen deprivation therapy remains very important therapeutical option. Experimental data confirmed the implication of IGF-1 axis in prostate cancer development. Moreover Ravi et al. [71] evaluate the association between IGF-1 and its binding proteins on outcomes in men with metastatic prostate cancer treated with androgen deprivation therapy, with or without docetaxel. The observations showed that a higher baseline and 6-month IGF-1:IGF-BP1 ratio was associated with better overall survival.

The normal function of white adipose tissue (WAT) is to store and release lipids. In obesity, WAT develops inflammation, fibrosis, and dysfunction and is sufficient to enhance cancer progression irrespective of diet. Periprostatic WAT, more abundant in obese patients, plays a particularly important role in prostate cancer [72]. Moreover, adipose tissue is considered to be more metabolically active than other tissues and to serve a prominent role in prostate cancer development. Visceral adipocyte tissue produces multiple molecules. PPAT is a type of visceral adipose tissue which serves an important role in prostate cancer biology. The ability of PPAT to secrete a number of molecules (cytokines, hormones, IGF-1, etc.) makes this tissue extremely similar to visceral adipose tissue [73].

In obesity pathogenesis, growth hormone (GH)/insulin-like growth factor (IGF)-dependent pathways remain crucial. Both GH and IGF-I have direct effects on adipocyte proliferation and differentiation. Insulin resistance, which is commonly associated with obesity, has been shown to promote prostate cancer by increasing circulating levels of bioactive IGF-1, a growth factor implicated in numerous types of cancer [74,75]. Yang et al.'s [76] study showed that metformin intake significantly increased IGF-1 level. On the other hand, Tosca et al.'s [77] study revealed that metformin reduces cell growth, protein synthesis, MAPK3/1, and P90RSK phosphorylation in response to IGF1 through an AMPK-dependent mechanism in cultured bovine granulosa cells. However, the influence of metformin on prostate cancer biology remains inconclusive [78]. Kim et al. [79] did not identify a significant positive correlation between metformin and prostate cancer. However, preoperational PSA and PSA velocity tended to be lower in the metformin cohort.

5.5. Interleukins

In obese patient the elevated level of IL-1 is observed [28]. It is postulated that IL-1 is a risk factor of cancer (e.g., colorectal and lung cancer) [80]. IL-1 is released by the activated macrophages present in the tumour microenvironment, but it is also produced by adipose tissue [81]. Proinflammatory cytokines can influence neuroendocrine differentiation in prostate cancer and be involved in disease progression [82]. Inflammation is known to promote tumour formation and progression. Fan et al. [83] found a natural anti-inflammatory factor, interleukin (IL)-1 receptor antagonist (IL1RN), in a mouse transgenic adenocarcinoma of the mouse prostate (TRAMP)-C1-derived tumour microenvironment.

Interleukin 6 (IL-6). IL-6 is also released by adipocytes in case of obesity. Interestingly, it has been found that although IL-6 is primarily considered a pro-inflammatory cytokine, it also has many regenerative or anti-inflammatory activities. Due to its modulatory effect on inflammation, IL-6 is associated with cancer development [28]. In patients with untreated metastatic or castration-resistant prostate cancer (CRPC), the serum level of IL-6 is increased and also correlates negatively with tumour survival and response to chemotherapy. In vitro and in vivo studies showed that IL-6 promote prostate cancer cell proliferation and inhibit apoptosis through several cellular pathways, such as (1) the Janus tyrosine family kinase (JAK-signal transducer and activator of transcription (STAT) pathway, (2) the extracellular signal-regulated kinase 1 and 2 (ERK1/2)-mitogen activated protein kinase (MAPK) pathway, (and 3) the phosphoinositide 3-kinase (PI3-K) pathway [84]. Additionally, IL-6 is associated with aggressive prostate cancer phenotype and may be involved in the metastatic process through regulation of the epithelial–mesenchymal transition (EMT) and homing of cancer cells to the bone [84]. Similarly, Okamoto et al.'s [85] in vitro experiments pointed that IL-6 acts as a paracrine growth factor for androgen-sensitive and slow-growing prostate cancer cell lines (LNCaP) and as an autocrine growth factor for androgen-insensitive and fast-growing prostate cancer cell lines (DU145 and PC3).

5.6. Tumor Necrosis Factor α (TNF-α)

TNF-α is an adipokine of multidirectional action [86]. Previous studies showed that TNF-α presents of different actions in prostate cancer (pro- and anti-carcinogenic) [87]. TNF-α expression levels correlate with disease progression. The highest expression of TNF-α was observed in prostate cancer as compared to benign prostate hyperplasia [88]. Maolake et al. [89] results showed that TNF-α acts as a regulator of increased tumour cell migration through the upregulation of C-C chemokine receptor 7 (CCR7). Moreover, TNF-α in involved in the initiation of castrate-resistant prostate cancer by inducing hypersensitivity to androgen (in vitro LNCaP cells). Contrarily, anti-cancer activities include, among other activities, the inhibition of angiogenesis at high doses of TNF-α in in vitro and in vivo studies [90]. TNF-α is chronically produced at low levels within the tumour microenvironment [91]. Additionally, stimulates antitumour immunity by enhancing the generation and proliferation of cytotoxic T cells [91]. Additionally, Lee et al.'s [92] results showed that TNF-α induces apoptosis of androgen-sensitive, non-metastatic prostate cancer cell lines (LNCaP).

5.7. Vascular Endothelial Growth Factor (VEGF)

The physiological activity of VEGF consists of angiogenesis, development, wound healing, and haematopoiesis. VEGF presents pro-tumour properties. The angiogenesis and expansive vascularization are a critical process which determine the growth and progression of tumour. The most potent pro-angiogenic factor is VEGF-A. Previous studies showed that the inhibition of VEGF-dependent pathways may lead to regression of vascular network and inhibition of a tumour growth [93]. Duque et al. [94] study indicates that patients with metastatic prostate cancer have higher plasma VEGF levels than patients with localized disease or healthy controls. Wang et al.'s [95] results showed that the Neuropilin-2 (NRP2), which functions as a VEGF receptor on tumour cells, is an attractive target to activate antitumor immunity in prostate cancer because VEGF-NRP2 signalling sustains PD-L1 expression. Moreover, the blockade of the binding of VEGF to NRP2 using a mouse-specific anti-NRP2 monoclonal antibody led to necrosis and tumour regression in mouse prostate cancer models. Adipose-derived mesenchymal stem cells (ADSCs) play a critical role in vascularization. ADSCs secrete a wide range of cytokines and growth, angiogenic, and antiapoptotic factors. The angiogenic and antiapoptotic properties are exacerbated under hypoxemic conditions [96,97]. Systemic insulin, IGF-1 and other biomolecules (e.g., HIF-1, VEGF, etc.) may modify ADSCs homeostasis within PPAT, with further effects on prostate cancer biology.

5.8. Bone Morphogenetic Proteins (BMPs)

BMPs belongs to multifunctional molecules which acts as a modulators of cell differentiation, proliferation, survival, and motility. BMPs play important roles in the development and progression of prostate cancer, breast cancer and lung cancer. Additionally, BMPs are involved in cancer-related angiogenesis. It is believed that BMP can either directly regulate the functions of vascular endothelial cells or indirectly influence the angiogenesis via regulation of angiogenic factors, such as VEGF [98]. The higher expression of BMP-6 is closely related to higher-grade primary tumours and metastatic prostate cancer. Moreover, BMP-6 plays a role in the progression of castration-resistant prostate cancer [99,100]. Contrarily, Kobayashi et al.'s [101] results showed that BMP-7 plays a critical role in tumour dormancy and recurrence. The elevated level of extracellular BMP-7 suppresses the migration and invasion of tumour cells. BMP-7 counteracts physiological epithelial-to-mesenchymal transition. The expression of BMP-7 in prostate cancer tissue was strongly down-regulated compared with normal prostate tissue [102]. Additionally, the BMP7 administration inhibited the growth of cancer cells in bone in mouse model [100].

BMPs are secretory proteins which are involved in morphogenetic activities and cell differentiation throughout the body, including the development of adipose tissue and adipogenic differentiation. BMP-4 and BMP-7 are related to white adipogenesis and brown adipogenesis, respectively, but other BMPs (e.g., BMP-2, BMP-6, and BMP-8b) have been shown to also affect adipogenesis [103]. BMPs induce various effects by regulating multiple types of cells and orchestrating them to remodel adipose tissue for adaptation [104]. Adipocyte turnover is relevant to the morphology and function of adipose tissue as well as the physiological and pathological states of adipose tissues [105]. The low adipocyte generation rates are associated with adipose tissue overgrowth without an increased number of cells (hypertrophy), whereas high generation rates are associated with adipose hyperplasia. Hypertrophic adipocytes resulting from lipid overload induce a series of adverse effects, such as hypoxia, lipotoxicity, inflammation, and metabolic impairment [104,105]. Differentiation generates new adipocytes, and cell death clears old or abnormal adipocytes. The undoubtable impact of BMPs on adipocytes may also have an impact on the activity of PPAT, in consequence leading to secretome profile changes.

5.9. Mitochondrial Uncoupling Protein (UCP)

Uncoupling proteins (UCPs) 1–3 are mitochondrial anion carrier proteins, which play a crucial function in diminishing reactive oxygen species production [106]. Mitochondrial uncoupling protein 2 (UCP2) uncouples electron transport from ATP production. UCP-2 play an important role in obesity and diabetes. In prostate cancer tissue the levels of UCP-2 were significantly higher than that in the adjacent normal tissues [107]. Sadehgi et al. [108] results showed that the increased UCP-2 expression was correlated with decreased survival in prostate cancer. UCP-2 reprograms the immune state of the tumour microenvironment by altering its cytokine milieu in an interferon-regulatory-factor-5-dependent manner [109]. Tumour-associated macrophages (TAMs), due to modulation of tumour microenvironmental features, promote tumour progression and metastasis development [110]. Macrophages present an expression of UPC-2 [111]. Macrophages have a very interesting property that allows them to adapt to hypoxemic conditions in conjunction with tumour growth and local ischemia. Despite hypoxia, macrophages can adapt to these conditions, reprogramming their metabolism and being still activated and promoting further tumour growth [112] (Figure 3).

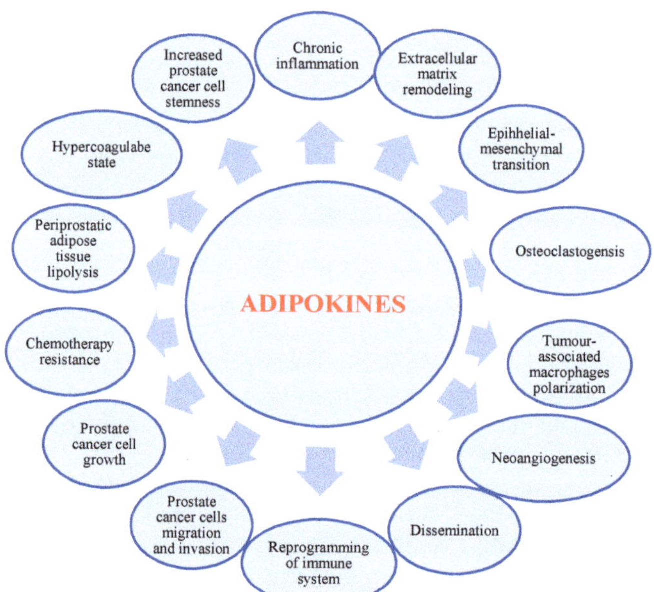

Figure 3. The multidirectional action of adipokines released by periprostatic adipose tissue (e.g., chemokines, cytokines, angiogenic factors, and other substances (e.g., leptin, adiponectin, IGF1, HIF-1α, etc.) in prostate cancer pathogenesis.

6. MicroRNAs

MicroRNAs (miRNAs) are single-stranded non-coding RNA molecules that play a regulatory role in gene expression and cancer cell signalling. The miR-628-5p (miR-628) was identified as a potential biomarker in serum samples from men with prostate cancer [113]. Srivastava et al.'s [114] results showed exposure to leptin, downregulated the expression of miR-628, and increased cell proliferation/migration in prostate cancer cells. miR-21 contributes to androgen-dependent and androgen-independent prostate cancer growth [115,116]. Dybos et al. [117] study showed that miR-148a-3p is upregulated in men with prostate cancer, and the miRNA is differentially expressed in patients with prostate cancer compared to healthy controls. miR-148a is an androgen-responsive microRNA that promotes LNCaP prostate cell (androgen-sensitive cells) [118]. He et al. [119] clinical study showed that serum miR-148a-3p level positively correlates while miR-485-5p level negatively correlates with prostate cancer's progressing and postoperative recurrence. Considering the impact of diet and dairy on the risk of developing prostate cancer, it is worth mentioning that cow milk contains large amounts of microRNAs (miRNAs) [120]. miR-17-5p, miR-25, miR-27b, and miR-9-5p were significantly reduced in ultra-high-temperature-treatment milk ($p < 0.05$) but not significantly affected in pasteurized milk (except miR-27b) [121]. Zhang et al. [121] described that the bioactive miRNA in raw milk was lost after ultra-high-temperature treatment but not in pasteurized treatment. miR-17-5p has been reported to increase cell proliferation and the risk of metastasis in prostate cancer. Additionally, a high cancer cell expression of miR-17-5p was an independent negative prognostic factor in prostate cancer [122].

7. PPAT and Extracellular Matrix Remodelling

The two-way interaction between PPAT and prostate cancer is predisposed to the modification of the cancer microenvironment in favour of cancer development. Each component of PPAT, which consists of adipocytes, an extracellular matrix (ECM) and immune cells plays a role in this process. ECM due to specific architecture plays role in cell adhesion, as well as tissue regeneration and repair. Moreover, ECM acts in cell proliferation, migration, and apoptosis. Obesity leads to adipocytes hypertrophy as a consequence of excessive lipid accumulation. It provokes further changes, such as (1) local infiltration by immune cells, (2) an increased accumulation of collagens, elastin, and fibronectin in ECM (fibrosis), and (3) inflammation response. These processes seem to be strictly related to local hypoxia and insulin resistance [123]. Cancer development is predisposed to dysregulation of the ECM architecture and its function. The most common component of ECM is collagen, which provides the basic mechanical and functional properties of ECM. Developing cancer cells release several molecules such as collagenases and metalloproteinases leading to significant changes in the deposition or degradation of collagen and in a consequence the loss of ECM homeostasis. Previously, it was believed that collagen, a component of ECM, was only a passive barrier protecting cancer cells from developing cancer. However, it is now known that it plays an active role in its development and progression [124,125]. A dynamic interplay between the microenvironment and cancer cells is observed, leading to structural changes of the surrounding ECM during cancer cell proliferation. Increased secretion of fibronectin and different types of collagens (I, III, and IV) indicates that tumour progression demand a continuous interaction between the ECM and tumour cells [126]. Additionally, Paszek et al. [127] revealed that increased deposition of matrix proteins promotes tumour progression by interfering with cell-to-cell adhesion, cell polarity, and ultimately amplifying growth factor signalling.

The tumour scaffold is based on collagen. ECM remodelling by collagen degradation and re-deposition affects tumour microenvironment, as well as promotes tumour infiltration, angiogenesis, invasion and migration [124]. Collagen changes in ECM release biomechanical signals, which are sensed by both tumour cells and stromal cells, trigger a cascade of biological events [124]. It is worth noting that a slight disturbance in tumour microenvironment homeostasis can have significant effects on the proliferation of cancer cells [93].

8. PPAT and Prostate Cancer Aggressiveness and Progression

In obesity, the normal balance of adipose tissue (including PPAT) secretory proteins is perturbed. This condition is associated with a greater risk of aggressive prostate cancer with increased local dissemination [24,128]. Su et al.'s [129] study establishes adipose stromal cells derived from white adipose tissue as the main source of CXCL12 driving prostate cancer aggressiveness by increasing the survival and proliferation of cancer cells. Through CXCR4-mediated signalling, the epithelial–mesenchymal transition (EMT) is also promoted, which intensifies the aggressiveness of prostate cancer. Another pathophysiological mechanism that enables the expansion of the prostate cancer tumour is the change in the structure of the extracellular matrix with the participation of PPAT. The adipocytes in PPAT through collagenases (CLG) and metalloproteinases (MMPs) leads to extracellular matrix remodelling, which, in conjunction with EMT, favours cancer cells migration out of the primary niche and their further dissemination [28]. Previous clinical studies showed that in comparison with normal weight patient, the obese individuals are at higher risk of prostate cancer progression after radical prostatectomy. Moreover, this cohort more likely develop metastatic prostate cancer and/or the cause of death will be prostate cancer [130]. These observations undoubtedly indicate that obesity is closely related to a more aggressive form of prostate cancer with a greater potential for clinical progression. Ribeiro et al.'s [130] study showed that the PPAT modulates extra-prostatic tumour cells' microenvironment through increased MMPs activity and to promote prostate cancer cell survival and migration. Matrix metalloproteinases are associated with cancer-cell invasion and metastasis due to its proteolytic features [131]. MMP9 elicit epithelial-to-mesenchymal transition in tumour cells, leading to more aggressive phenotype of cancer [132]. The extra-capsular extension of cancer cells into the periprostatic area is a factor of early disease recurrence and worse prognosis in patient with prostate cancer [133]. Sacca et al. [134] study showed that PPAT releases pro-MMP-9 which induces the invasive capacity of androgen dependent prostate cancer cell lines (LNCaP cells). Therefore, it is postulated that PPAT via MMP-dependent pathways may modulate prostate cancer progression even from the early stages of the disease. Previous studies showed that obesity is more related to the aggressiveness of the tumours and not directly related to the risk of development of prostate cancer. Moreover, prostate cancer progression depends on tumour activity as well as the active function of the microenvironment [135,136]. In obese patients with prostate cancer, the risk of cancer progression is more potent due to chronic inflammation, which is strictly related to increased secretion of pro-inflammatory adipokines and overproduction of reactive oxygen species. PPAT, which is a part of surrounding microenvironment for prostate cancer, participate in the bi-directional interplay with cancer cells via paracrine route. Moreover, the molecules excreted by cancer cells, stromal cells, adipocyte, and adipose stem cells into the tumour microenvironment play a critical function in cancer progression. Sacca et al.'s [137] study provides that in prostate cancer the metabolic dysfunction of PPAT occur. The prostate cancer microenvironment is altered by adipokines and fatty acids (FAs) secreted by PPAT. In locally advanced prostate cancer (T3 stage) the secretome of PPAT is enriched in several pathways related to energy production, indicating a greater energy requirement by the tumour, when compared to the organ-confined prostate cancer (T2 stage) [137]. Moreover, T3 stage prostate cancer presents enrichment in pathways related to hormone response, polyamine synthesis, and control of protein synthesis through amino acid, RNA, and nucleotide metabolism [137]. Balaban et al. [138]

results revealed interesting feature of prostate cancer cells. These cells use extracellular FAs as both fuel for oxidation and the primary substrates for complex lipid synthesis such as triacylglycerols, and that high extracellular lipid availability further enhances FA flux in these cells. Iordanescu et al. [139] clinical study showed the linear association between periprostatic adipose tissue fatty acid composition and extracapsular extension of prostate cancer and is marked by elevated monounsaturated and reduced saturated fatty acids in the PPAT relative to subcutaneous adipose tissue. The pathological stage of prostate cancer determines the different FA compositions of PPAT, leading to alteration in proper lipid metabolism [137]. It is postulated that PPAT remains an important reservoir of FAs for prostate cancer cells. In accordance with Yue at al.'s [140] observations, the expression of several genes related to lipid metabolism (e.g., CD36) was decreased when PPAT explants from patients with prostate cancer who underwent radical prostatectomy were co-cultured with prostate cancer cell lines. This strictly indicates a progressive decline in PPAT lipid production and utilization. Additionally, it is worth noting that increased lipid absorption and more potent lipid accumulation in prostate cancer cells, which secondarily leads to an increased number of intracellular lipid droplets (esterified cholesterol), was associated with more aggressive potential of prostate cancer (high-grade prostate cancer and metastases) [140]. In vitro study in prostate cancer cell lines showed that the loss of tumour suppressor PTEN and subsequent activation of the phosphatidylinositol 3-kinase (PI3K)/AKT pathway led to extensive cholesteryl ester accumulation. Contrarily, in a mouse animal model, the inhibition of cholesteryl ester storage significantly reduced cancer proliferation, impaired cancer invasion capability, and suppressed tumour growth [140]. FA uptake was increased in human prostate cancer via the CD36 fatty acid transporter. The modulation of fatty acid transporter CD36 activity ameliorates free FA uptake and consequently diminishes the prostate cancer progression [141,142].

Several pathomechanisms of prostate cancer progression (described as tumour growth, local invasion, and bone metastasis development) were defined as follows: (1) neovascularisation, (2) immunosuppression and macrophage phenotype modification, (3) dissemination growth, and (4) osteoclastogensis. PPAT secretes many molecules, which regulate all of the above mentioned processes. The neovascularisation is mediated via several adipokines, e.g., VEGF, basic-FGF and IL-8). Immunosuppression is regulated by IL-10 and TGF-β. Yunna et al. [143] described that macrophages may change their phenotypes (M1 and M2 populations) due to variety of factors. M1-typed macrophages are mostly involved in the pro-inflammatory response, contrary to the M2 type, which presents anti-inflammatory features. The polarisation of the tumour-associated macrophage (TAM) population is affected by IL-4 and IL-13. In cases of more advanced stages of prostate cancer, dissemination growth, and osteoclastogenesis in critical in-bone metastasis development. The former process is regulated by IL-6, IL-8, TNF-α and TGF-β. On the other hand, the latter process is influenced by parathyroid hormone-related protein (PTHrP), IL-1, IL-6, TNF-α and TGF-β.

It is worth nothing that a large group of patients diagnosed with prostate cancer were previously treated with 5α-reductase inhibitors, which may also affect the biology of prostate cancer. This appears to be consistent with Taussky et al.'s [144] results, which showed that 5α-reductase inhibitor treatment for at least 12 months reduces PPAT volume. Moreover, it points that 5α-reductase inhibitors may affect the prostate cancer biology through modulation of PPAT activity.

Prostate-specific antigen (PSA) expression level in prostate cancer cells is one of the strongest prognostic features in this tumour entity [145]. PSA is an insulin-like growth factor binding protein-3 protease. Thus, PSA may modulate IGF-dependent pathways function by altering IGF-IGFBP-3 [146]. There are no clear data on the occurrence of

PSA expression on the adipocytes that form PPAT. However, prostate cancer cells present a positive expression of PSA [145]. Additionally, such expression may lead to crosstalk between prostate cancer cells and PPAT by modulatory function on PPAT secretome through the IGF-1 dependent pathway.

The PPAT contributes through paracrine mechanisms to prostate cancer progression and affects its aggressiveness [147]. Detection of PPAT thickness above 3 mm was observed to be an independent risk factor for upstage in prostate cancer patients [148]. Jiang et al. study [149] showed that the PPAT thickness (PPATT)/subcutaneous adipose tissue (SAT) thickness (SATT) ratio is an independent risk factor for biochemical recurrence after radical prostatectomy. This indicates that patients with thicker PPATT and thinner SATT have a higher probability of biochemical recurrence. This clinical study strictly highlights the role of PPATT and overall fat distribution in predicting biochemical recurrence and overall survival in patients with prostate cancer. Moreover, patients with higher PPATT/SATT ratio had relatively higher Gleason scores (total score ≥ 9, 81.6% vs. 68.3%). The PPATT/SATT ratio > 0.22 is an independent risk factor for biochemical recurrence after radical prostatectomy. Additionally, van Roermund et al. [150] showed a significant association between periprostatic fat density and risk of having a high-risk disease in T1-3N0M0 prostate cancer patient qualified to radiotherapy. Similarly, Shao et al. [73] study showed that PPAT was significantly associated with extracapsular prostate cancer extension. Furthermore, in vitro experiments revealed that PPAT could inhibit prostate cancer cell proliferation by secreting factors that activated immune responses and could thereby promote cancer cell apoptosis. This mechanism may act as a first line of defence in the early stages of prostate cancer [73].

9. Thrombotic Cascade Activation via PPAT and Prostate Cancer Progression

In obesity, the insulin resistance and excessive caloric intake lead to adipose tissue expansion and adipocytes hypertrophy, and in consequence reduce adipose tissue oxygenation. Localised hypoxia increases the adipocyte cell death and stimulate the local adipocyte tissue inflammation which is corelated with extensive inflammatory cytokines and adipokines release. Previous studies showed that in obesity-related disorders (e.g., cardio-vascular diseases, diabetes, and cancer), a hypercoagulable state seems to be a contributor in their pathogenesis. In obesity, the inflammation within adipocyte tissue provides increased expression and activation of factor X (FXa) and thrombin as well as different isoforms of the protease-activated receptors (PARs), leading to a hypercoagulable state [151]. It is postulated that exacerbated inflammation process in PPAT predispose to prostate cancer phenotype progression including through thrombotic cascade activation. Ebrahimi et al. [152] described that inflammation induced via thrombin-dependent pathway facilitate tumour cells proliferation, angiogenesis, invasion, and metastasis. These processes are caused through increased expression of cytokines, adhesion molecules, angiogenic factors, and matrix-degrading proteases. The activation of coagulation cascade is boosted via tissue factor (TF) and factor VII. Moreover, adipocyte tissue is a major source of TF. The level of TF is increased in chronic inflammation [153]. Prostate (prostate epithelium and the stroma) is a rich reservoir of thrombin. Thrombin procoagulant activity is associated with more advanced disease and a worse prognosis in patients with prostate cancer [154]. It is worth noting that cellular effects of thrombin are mediated by PARs [155]. Additionally, improper expression of PARs provides increased angiogenesis, tumour growth, and metastasis of various cancers. Kaushal et al. [156] resulted revealed that PAR-1 expression is increased in advanced-stage of prostate cancer and is localized to endothelial cells in the vascular network of prostate tumour areas. Moreover, Black et al. [157] showed that

PAR mRNA expression in prostate specimens after radical prostatectomy was higher in cancer, and protein expression was increased in PAR-1 (45%), PAR-2 (42%), and PAR-4 (68%) compared to normal prostate glands. Moreover, increased expression of PAR-1 in periglandular stroma of the prostate was associated with higher rates of biochemical recurrence in prostate cancer.

Additionally, the thrombin-dependent pathway affects the macrophage population. Thrombin promoted the differentiation of macrophages into an M1-like phenotype polarization with an increased production of proinflammatory cytokines. The cellular actions of thrombin on macrophages were mediated in part by PAR-1 [158].

Additionally, the increased lipolysis in PPAT, evoked by thrombin, release free FAs, which participate in the development of oxidative stress in the prostatic tissue and exacerbation of inflammatory process [151]. Prostate cancer cells accumulate the released free FAs, which enhance the invasive potency of cancer cells. This triggers a further cascade consisting of the induction of an isoform of NADPH oxidase (NOX5) and intracellular ROS production. In the next stage, the HIF-1α/MMP-14 signalling pathway is launched via intracellular ROS [151,159]. In obesity, the tumour-surrounding adipocytes are more prone to activating the HIF-1α/MMP-14 signalling pathway. Additionally, the expression of NOX5 and MMP-14 is upregulated in areas of the tumour that are in the proximity of the PPAT [159].

10. Other PPAT Molecules and Prostate Cancer Pathogenesis

In addition to the previously discussed molecules that have an established role in the development of prostate cancer and obesity, there are many molecules in the literature that may influence the pathogenesis of prostate cancer and obesity (e.g., visfatin, omentin, resistin, LCN2, FABP4, osteopontin, etc.) [151]. The importance of these molecules in prostate cancer is outlined below.

10.1. Visfatin

Macrophages which infiltrate adipocyte tissue are characterized by increases level of visfatin. Previous studies showed that upregulation of visfatin in malignancies (e.g., in prostate cancer). Marked visfatin expression was detected in human locally advanced prostate cancer tissues (with extraprostatic extension) compared to minimal expression of organ-confined diseases. Visfatin plasma concentration was elevated in patients with prostate cancer. Additionally, the greater level of visfatin was observed in cases of prostate cancer with extraprostatic extension compared to organ-confined disease [160]. Moreover, the results of in vitro cell culture and in vivo preclinical mouse model studies performed by Sun et al. [160] confirmed visfatin-mediated enhancement of prostate cancer invasiveness into muscle tissues. The blockade of visfatin by polyclonal antibodies leads to the suppression of prostate cancer invasiveness.

10.2. Omentin

Omentin (intelectin-1) was identified at higher plasma concentration in patients with different malignancies, as well as is collated with insulin resistance. The visceral adipose tissue synthetizes intelectin-1. Uyeturk et al. [161] study showed elevated level of circulating omentin in patients with prostate cancer compared to patients with benign prostate hyperplasia. The role of omentin in prostate cancer still remains unclear.

10.3. Resistin

Resistin (ADSF–adipose-tissue-specific secretory factor) peptide hormone derived from adipose tissue which characterize proinflammatory properties. This adipokine links obesity and diabetes by prompting insulin resistance. Moreover, ADSF plays a role in inflammation, proliferation, angiogenesis, and metastasis and also affects the cancer cells' metabolism [151,162]. Kim et al. [163] revealed that human prostate cancer cell lines PC-3 and DU-145 express human resistin mRNA. Additionally, in comparison to benign prostate hyperplasia, the increased level of resistin was observed in high-grade prostate cancer tissue. Several potential ADSF-dependent mechanisms affecting cancer biology (by promotion of cancer progression and/or increasing its aggressiveness) have been proposed, as follow: (1) invasion and metastasis, (2) epithelial-to-mesenchymal transition (EMT) and stemness, (3) angiogenesis, and (4) chemoresistance [164].

10.4. Lipocalin-2 (LCN2)

LCN2 is characterized by multidirectional action. LCN2 participates in cell membrane transport, modulates immune responses, and promotes epithelial cell differentiation. Although LNC2 is expressed at low levels in most human tissues, it is abundant in aggressive subtypes of several cancer (e.g., breast, colon, pancreas, thyroid, etc.). LCN2 has been associated with increased cell proliferation, angiogenesis, cell invasion, and metastasis [165]. Moreover, LCN2 is elevated in obesity [151]. Ulusoy et al.'s [166] results indicate that high LCN2 expression was strictly correlated with higher prostate cancer grade (Gleason score). LCN2 knockdown in PC3 and DU145 prostate cancer cells decreased cell proliferation, colony formation, cell cycle arrest, migration, and invasion [167]. Additionally, Ding et al.'s [168] results showed that LCN2 could facilitate cell proliferation of castration-resistant prostate cancer (CRPC) via androgen receptor transcriptional activity. Moreover, LCN2 promotes cell migration and invasion of prostate cancer by inducing epithelial-to-mesenchymal transition via the extracellular signal-regulated kinase (ERK)/SLUG pathway. The positive correlation between higher concentration of LCN2 and prostate cancer invasiveness in in vivo and in vitro studies [169]. SLUG is a zinc-finger transcription factor that plays a role in migration and invasion of tumour cells. SLUG promotes prostate cancer cell migration and invasion via CXCR4/CXCL12 axis [170].

10.5. Fatty Acid Binding Protein 4 (FABP4)

FABP4, a member of the cytoplasmic fatty acid binding protein multigene family is secreted by adipocytes. The expression of FABP4 is increased in metabolic syndrome and in obesity [171]. Adipocytes release FABP4. Uehara et al. [171] showed that FABP4 treatment promoted serum-induced prostate cancer cell invasion in in vitro model. Moreover, in prostate cancer animal model the blockade of FABP4 diminished the tumour growth and metastasis, partly by inducing prostatic epithelial cell DNA damage and apoptosis. Elevated expression of FABP4 and secretion of FABP4 by prostate cancer cells trigger the invasiveness of the prostate cancer by stimulation of matrix metalloproteinases (MMPs) via phosphatidylinositol 3-kinase (PI3K) and mitogen-activated protein kinase (MAPK) signalling pathways [172]. Additionally, FABP4 facilitates prostate cancer aggressiveness through increased secretion of IL-6 and IL-8 [173].

10.6. Osteopontin (OPN)

OPN is an inflammatory cytokine, the expression of which is strongly upregulated in adipose tissue and liver upon obesity [173]. Prostate-cancer-afflicted individuals had higher plasma levels of OPN compared to patients with benign prostate hyperplasia [174].

Moreover, poor prognosis in prostate cancer was strictly associated with higher concentration of OPN [175]. OPN presents pro-tumorigenic effect through the activation of several signalling pathways after binding to integrin $\alpha v\beta 3$. Moreover, OPN upregulates CD44 and MMP-9 expression, providing a more potent ability for cancer cell invasion and metastasis development [176,177]. Khodavirdi et al.'s [178] results strictly indicated that OPN contributes to several steps in the process of prostate carcinogenesis and metastasis. Prostate cancer tumours with OPN overexpression seem to present an increased proliferative and invasive feature. It is postulated that prostate cancer progression is also mediated through OPNc, which activates androgen receptor signalling [179]. Prostate cancer cell culture (PC-3) with OPNc overexpression presents significantly induced endothelial cell adhesion, proliferation and migration [180]. As expected, decreased expression of OPN in PC-3 cell culture induced apoptosis of cell culture, leading to suppression of malignant potency of the cell colony [181].

11. PPAT, Chronic Hypoxemic State and Prostate Cancer

In obesity, the expression of HIF-1α in adipose tissue is increased. The HIF-1α activity is stimulated by several factors as follows: (1) adipogenesis, (2) insulin, and (3) hypoxia. Moreover, HIF-1α is a major transcriptional activator for the VEGF gene, but it is not sufficient for activation of VEGF gene expression in adipose tissue [182]. Additionally, García-Fuentes et al. [183] showed that morbidly obese subjects have a higher level of visceral adipose tissue HIF-1α. In comparison to other adipose tissue, PPAT has a sparse vascular network responsible for a chronic hypoxic state, leading to inflammation as well as fibrosis independent of obesity. Roumiguié et al. [184] study revealed an increase in expression of the oxygen-labile HIF-2α, but not of HIF-1α, in PPAT, indicating an adaptive response of this tissue to hypoxia. The higher level of VEGF secretion by PPAT when compared with adomino-pelvic adipose tissue may promote angiogenesis. Additionally, due to chronic hypoxia the PPAT exhibits hallmarks of chronic inflammation. Hypoxia-inducible factors (HIFs) play a pivotal role in cancer cell adaptation to hypoxic environments, contributing to treatment resistance. Peng et al.'s [185] in vitro studies showed that the marine-derived HIF-1α inhibitor reduces prostate cancer cell proliferation by targeting HIF-1 target genes.

12. PPAT, Diet and Prostate Cancer

PPAT is believed to be a so-called driving force for prostate cancer progression [186]. PPAT releases a wide range of molecules, which promotes tumour growth and the migration of cancer cells. However, some molecules released from PPAT, such as adiponectin and the n-6 or n-3 polyunsaturated fatty acids, have been shown to have anti-tumour properties. This fact points that the interplay between PPAT and prostate cancer biology depend on the balance between the pro- and anti-tumour components of PPAT [187]. Additionally, obesity and dietary factors seem to be involved in the risk and aggressiveness of prostate cancer through the modulatory impact on the interactions between PPAT and cancer cells and their consequences on the growth and the metastatic potential of prostate cancer.

The anti-inflammatory properties of vitamin D seem to be important in cancer prevention [188]. However, the results are conflicting and inconsistent [189]. Current data show an active role of vitamin D and its metabolites in physiological adipocyte and adipose tissue processes in adulthood. Vitamin D seems to affect the adipogenesis, energy metabolism, and inflammation process [190]. Insulin-like growth factor (IGF)-1 and its binding proteins are important in cancer growth, especially in prostate cancer [191]. The meta-analysis performed by Kord-Varkaneh et al. [192] indicates a non-significant increase in IGF-1 following vitamin D supplementation. Additionally, vitamin D dosages of <1000 IU/day and intervention durations of <12 weeks significantly raised IGF-1 levels. Additionally, Guzey et al. [193], in an animal model study, showed that vitamin D receptor deficiency in mice with prostate induces fat necrosis and individual cell apoptosis in PPAT, which regulates prostate cancer signalling pathways and affects prostate cancer progression.

Previous studies show that high-fat dairy, particularly whole milk, in healthy men may increase risk of aggressive prostate cancer. The potential impacts of a dairy diet on the risk of prostate cancer development are as follow: (1) high calcium intake decreasing vitamin D levels, (2) increased level of IGF-1 levels, (3) fluctuating phosphorus levels modifying vitamin D3 concentrations, and (4) elevated saturated fat intake modulating the immune response and inflammation [194]. Moreover, whole milk consumption after prostate cancer diagnosis was associated with increased risk of recurrence, particularly among very overweight or obese men [194]. Daily milk consumption in adolescence, but not in midlife or currently, was associated with a 3.2-fold risk of advanced prostate cancer [195]. Additionally, Song et al.'s study [196] showed that higher intake of skim/low-fat milk was associated with a greater risk of nonaggressive prostate cancer. Most importantly, only whole milk was consistently associated with higher incidence of fatal prostate cancer in the entire cohort and higher prostate cancer-specific mortality among cases. Similarly, men with higher intake of dairy foods, but not nondairy calcium, had a higher risk of prostate cancer compared with men having lower intakes [197]. Zhao et al.'s [197] meta-analysis showed an increased risk of prostate cancer with high intakes of total dairy products, milk, cheese, and butter. Dietary factors, especially cow milk consumption and dairy products, which raise systemic IGF-1 levels and donate abundant amounts of essential branched-chain amino acids of the leucine prototype may affect prostate cancer development. Increased insulin/IGF-1 signalling may promote tumour growth directly through insulin receptors or regulation of IGF and their binding proteins (IGFBP), which are involved in cell survival and proliferation [198]. Prostate cancer is dependent on androgen receptor signalling and aberrations of the PI3K-Akt-mTORC1 pathway mediating excessive and sustained growth signalling. The nutrient-sensitive kinase mTORC1 is upregulated in nearly 100% of advanced human prostate cancers, and this kinase is activated by leucine, insulin, IGF-1, and glucose. Oncogenic mTORC1 signalling activates key subsets of mRNAs that cooperate in distinct steps of prostate cancer initiation, cell growth, and progression [199]. Only milk proteins in comparison to meat and fish have the unique ability to preferentially increase both the insulin/IGF-1 and the leucine signalling pathways necessary for maximal mTORC1 activation [199]. mTORC1 activation is critically dependent on the availability of sufficient amounts of amino acids, especially of the branched-chain essential amino acid (BCAA) leucine [200]. Castration-resistant prostate cancer cells are addicted to leucine availability [201,202]. L-type amino acid transporters (LATs) uptake neutral amino acids, including L-leucine, into cells, stimulating mTORC1. LAT1 and LAT3 are overexpressed at different stages of prostate cancer, and they are responsible for increasing nutrients and stimulating cell growth. LAT inhibition suppressed M-phase cell cycle genes regulated by E2F family transcription factors including critical castration-resistant prostate cancer regulatory genes [203].

13. PPAT and Prostate Cancer Treatment (Radiotherapy, Androgen Deprivation Therapy, Chemotherapy)

Adipose tissue in the tumour microenvironment impacts the efficacy of chemotherapeutic agents and androgen deprivation treatments [204,205]. Androgen deprivation treatment (ADT) induces oxidative stress and inflammation in adipose tissue. This causes an increase in adipose tissue, cholesterol, oxidative stress, and inflammation, leading to tumour progression. Obesity-related proteins—thioesterase superfamily member 6 (THEM6) and yes-associated protein 1 (YAP1)—are associated with ADT resistance in prostate cancer by increasing cellular lipid content and activating the UPR [206,207]. THEM6, which is highly expressed in adipose tissue where it regulates intracellular fatty acid homeostasis, is upregulated in ADT-resistant prostate cancers, and activates the unfolded protein response (UPR) [208]. ADT affect the homeostasis of adipocyte tissue. Previous studies showed that ADT is a risk factor of insulin resistance and affect the adiponectin level [200,201]. Lam et al. [209] revealed that, in patients receiving ADT for 6 months, the PPAT presents a significant trend of pro-inflammatory, obesity-like adipose tissue. Obesity is a well-established risk factor for prostate cancer. Thus, ADT could potentially cause adverse effects on adipose tissue, linking it to tumour progression [206]. In case of radiotherapy, the irradiation to adipose tissue decreases lipogenic gene expression and increases reactive oxygen species and lipolysis. Both reactive oxygen species and lipolysis lead to the release of unsaturated fatty acids from the adipocytes, which cancer cells use to activate pro-cancer pathways. Additionally, radiation activates fat mass and obesity-associated (FTO) protein, which demethylates mRNA to promote radio-resistance [206]. Chemotherapy is often lipophilic and, therefore, easily sequestered and metabolized by adipocytes containing the aldo-keto reductase (AKR) protein, reducing the availability of the drug for prostate tumours [206,207]. Chemotherapy induces dysregulated cytokine secretion from adipose tissue, such as an increased release of IGF-1, causing the upregulation of TUBB2B, which is associated with chemo-resistance. PPAT secretes insulin-like growth factor-1 (IGF-1) leading to increased prostate cancer cell expression of TUBB2B, β-tubulin isoform 2B. TUBB2B is upregulated in metastatic prostate cancer and promotes docetaxel resistance by preventing drug-induced microtubule stabilization [206,210–212].

14. Exosome- and mTORC-Dependent Pathways and Prostate Cancer

Exosomes are extracellular vehicles (EVs) of endocytic and secretory exocytic origin that play a crucial role in cell-to-cell communication. Exosomes transport a wide range of cellular components (e.g., miRs, mRNAs, etc.) and are involved in different cancer development (e.g., breast, prostate, ovarian etc.) [213]. Primary human adipocytes shed EVs, specifically exosomes, that induced the expression of genes associated with epithelial-to-mesenchymal transition (EMT) and cancer-stem-like cell (CSC) traits in cocultured breast cancer cell lines [214,215]. Wang et al.'s [215] results showed that a mechanism of exosome-mediated cross-talk between metabolically abnormal adipocytes and breast cancer cells may promote tumour aggressiveness in patients with diabetes type 2. Exosomes regulate angiogenesis, immune suppression, metastasis, and drug and therapeutic resistance in prostate cancer [216]. Additionally, exosome release is stimulated by pH changes in prostate cancer microenvironment [216]. PPAT interplays with the tumour microenvironment via exosomes EVs. Sanchez-Martin et al.'s [217] study showed that the retinoic-acid-receptor-related orphan receptor alpha (RORA) gene was regulated by PPAT-EVs-derived miRNAs. The RORA gene has a role in prostate cancer cells proliferation and inflammation.

The mammalian target of rapamycin (mTOR) kinase is a master regulator of protein synthesis that couples nutrient sensing to cell growth and cancer. Several genes responsible for cancer cell metabolism, proliferation, and invasion regulated by mTOR signalling have been described [218]. Moreover, the complete mTOR inhibition by ATP site blockade reprograms this gene expression prevents prostate cancer invasion and metastasis [218]. Additionally, mTORC1 regulates polyamine dynamics, which are also important in carcinogenesis. In prostate cancer, alterations in the production of decarboxylated S-adenosylmethionine (dcSAM) and polyamine synthesis were observed. S-adenosylmethionine decarboxylase 1 (AMD1) was upregulated in prostate cancer specimens with activated mTORC1 [219]. Everolimus (the mTORC1 inhibitor) exhibited a predominant decrease in AMD1 immunoreactivity that was associated to a decrease in proliferation, in line with the requirement of dcSAM production for oncogenicity [220]. It is worth noting that in cases of prostate cancer, the activation of the phosphatidylinositol-3-kinase (PI3K), protein kinase B (PKB/AKT), and mTOR-dependent pathways facilitates tumour formation, disease progression, and therapeutic resistance. The complex crosstalk between the PI3K-AKT-mTOR pathway and multiple interacting cell signalling cascades can further promote prostate cancer progression and influence the sensitivity of prostate cancer cells to PI3K-AKT-mTOR-targeted therapies [221]. Regulation of the mTORC1 signalling pathway is performed by growth factors (through the insulin/IGF-1 pathway), energy (glucose level, AMP to ATP ratio changes, etc.) and oxygen levels [222]. In mouse models of prostate cancer, the signalling adaptor p62/Sqstm1 is selectively inactivated in adipocytes. p62 loss in adipocytes results in increased osteopontin secretion, which mediates tumour fatty acid oxidation and invasion, leading to aggressive metastatic prostate cancer in vivo. Furthermore, p62 deficiency triggers in adipocytes a general shutdown of energy-utilizing pathways through mTORC1 inhibition, which supports nutrient availability for cancer cells [223].

15. Tumour Microenvironment and Prostate Cancer

Several types of stromal cell support a tumorigenic primary niche. The immune system makes an attempt to eliminate tumour cells. Specific antigens of tumour cells play a role in this process and are recognized by cytotoxic immune cells, leading to their destruction. In the tumour microenvironment, macrophages and fibroblasts contribute to a growth-suppressive state; however, these cells may later become educated by the tumour to acquire pro-tumorigenic functions. On the other hand, tumour-associated macrophages (TAMs) support the primary tumour including growth, angiogenesis and invasion by secreting a wide range of pro-tumorigenic agents (e.g., proteases, cytokines and growth factors, etc.). Due to cytokine release during tumorigenesis the immune-suppressor cells are mobilized. Additionally, tumour cells release chemokines, which activate cancer-associated fibroblasts (CAFs). CAFs secrete extracellular matrix proteins and basement membrane components, as well as regulate differentiation, modulate immune responses, and contribute to deregulated homeostasis. Moreover, during the tumour growth the neo-angiogenesis is stimulated by VEGF released from CAFs. It is worth mentioning that parallelly to cellular alterations, the extracellular properties change (e.g., hypoxia, extracellular matrix components change) [224].

16. Conclusions

Current data strictly highlight the fundamental role of periprostatic adipose tissue (PPAT) and its active function in prostate cancer development and progression. The complexity of PPAT-related adipokines in prostate cancer pathogenesis points PPAT as a potential therapeutic target to modulate the interaction between the prostate cancer cells and microenvironment surrounding prostate gland. Considering the multipotential activity of PPAT and impact of prostate cancer biology, PPAT seems to become an interesting and promising avenue with potential therapeutic benefits in patients with prostate cancer.

17. Future Research Questions

The current epidemiological prognosis for the degree of obesity in the human population until 2050 is not optimistic [225]. This may have a huge impact on the incidence of prostate cancer. BMI > 25 kg/m^2 is associated with an increased risk of prostate cancer and mortality [226]. Recently, there has been an intensive increase in the use of novel drugs in the treatment of obesity, such a liraglutide (glucagon-like peptide-1 (GLP-1) agonist) and tirzepatide (a glucose-dependent insulinotropic polypeptide (GIP) and GLP-1 receptors agonist). Taking into account the fact that there is a close relationship between obesity, PPAT, and prostate cancer, a new field is opened for research aimed at explaining GIP as well as GLP-1 agonist and what effect the novel agents used in the treatment of obesity have on the biology of prostate cancer.

Author Contributions: Conceptualization, J.D., K.L.-J., J.A. and K.J.; methodology, J.D. and K.J.; formal analysis, J.D., K.L.-J. and K.J.; investigation, J.D., K.L.-J., J.A. and K.J.; data curation, J.D., K.L.-J. and K.J.; writing—original draft preparation, J.D., K.L.-J. and K.J.; writing—review and editing, J.D., K.L.-J., J.A. and K.J.; supervision, J.A. and K.J. All authors have read and agreed to the published version of the manuscript.

Funding: This research received no external funding.

Conflicts of Interest: The authors declare that the research was conducted in the absence of any commercial or financial relationships that could be construed as a potential conflict of interest.

List of Abbreviations

ADSCs	adipose-derived mesenchymal stem cells
ADSF	adipose-tissue-specific secretory factor
AKR	aldo-keto reductase
AMD1	S-adenosylmethionine decarboxylase 1
BAT	brown adipose tissue
BCAA	branched-chain essential amino acid
BMI	body mass index
BMPs	bone morphogenetic proteins
CAFs	cancer-associated fibroblasts
CLG	colagenase
CRPC	castration-resistant prostate cancer
CSC	cancer-stem-like cell
CXCR4	chemokine receptor CXC type 4
dcSAM	decarboxylated S-adenosylmethionine
ECM	extracellular matrix
EMT	epithelial–mesenchymal transition
ERK1/2	extracellular signal-regulated kinase 1 and 2
EVs	extracellular vehicles
FABP	fatty acid binding protein
GIP	glucose-dependent insulinotropic polypeptide
GLP-1	glucagon-like peptide-1
HIF	hypoxia-inducible factor
IFG-1	insulin-like growth factor 1
IGFBP-1	IGF-binding protein 1
IL-1	interleukin-1
IL-6	interleukin-6
JAK	the Janus tyrosine family kinase

LATs	L-type amino acid transporters
LCN	lipocalin
MAPK	mitogen activated protein kinase
MMPs	metalloproteinases
mTOR	mammalian target of rapamycin
NK	natural killer
OPN	osteopontin
PPAT	periprostatic adipose tissue
PPATT	periprostatic adipose tissue thickness
PAR	protease-activated receptors
PI3K	phosphatidylinositol-3-kinase
PSA	prostate-specific antigen
PTEN	tumour suppressor phosphatase and tensin homologue
PTHrP	parathyroid hormone-related protein
P90RSK	90 kDa ribosomal S6 kinases
RORA	retinoic acid-receptor-related orphan receptor alpha
ROS	reactive oxygen species
SATT	subcutaneous adipose tissue thickness
STAT	signal transducer and activator of transcription
TAMs	tumour-associated macrophages
TF	tissue factor
THEM6	thioesterase superfamily member 6
TNF-α	tumour necrosis factor
TUBB2B	tubulin beta 2B class IIb
UCP	mitochondrial uncoupling protein
WAT	white adipose tissue
VEGF	vascular endothelial growth factor

References

1. Culp, M.B.; Soerjomataram, I.; Efstathiou, J.A.; Bray, F.; Jemal, A. Recent Global Patterns in Prostate Cancer Incidence and Mortality Rates. *Eur. Urol.* **2020**, *77*, 38–52. [CrossRef] [PubMed]
2. Cornford, P.; van den Bergh, R.C.N.; Briers, E.; Van den Broeck, T.; Brunckhorst, O.; Darraugh, J.; Eberli, D.; De Meerleer, G.; De Santis, M.; Farolfi, A.; et al. EAU-EANM-ESTRO-ESUR-ISUP-SIOG Guidelines on Prostate Cancer-2024 Update. Part I: Screening, Diagnosis, and Local Treatment with Curative Intent. *Eur. Urol.* **2024**, *86*, 148–163. [CrossRef] [PubMed]
3. Murray, T.B.J. The Pathogenesis of Prostate Cancer. In *Prostate Cancer [Internet]*; Bott, S.R.J., Ng, K.L., Eds.; Exon Publications: Brisbane, QLD, Australia, 2021; Chapter 3. Available online: https://www.ncbi.nlm.nih.gov/books/NBK571321/ (accessed on 27 May 2021). [CrossRef]
4. Leitzmann, M.F.; Rohrmann, S. Risk factors for the onset of prostatic cancer: Age, location, and behavioral correlates. *Clin. Epidemiol.* **2012**, *4*, 1–11. [CrossRef] [PubMed] [PubMed Central]
5. Gandaglia, G.; Leni, R.; Bray, F.; Fleshner, N.; Freedland, S.J.; Kibel, A.; Stattin, P.; Van Poppel, H.; La Vecchia, C. Epidemiology and Prevention of Prostate Cancer. *Eur. Urol. Oncol.* **2021**, *4*, 877–892. [CrossRef] [PubMed]
6. Fang, X.; Wei, J.; He, X.; Lian, J.; Han, D.; An, P.; Zhou, T.; Liu, S.; Wang, F.; Min, J. Quantitative association between body mass index and the risk of cancer: A global Meta-analysis of prospective cohort studies. *Int. J. Cancer* **2018**, *143*, 1595–1603. [CrossRef] [PubMed]
7. Chandrasekar, T.; Yang, J.C.; Gao, A.C.; Evans, C.P. Mechanisms of resistance in castration-resistant prostate cancer (CRPC). *Transl. Androl. Urol.* **2015**, *4*, 365–380. [CrossRef] [PubMed] [PubMed Central]
8. Saad, F.; Aprikian, A.; Finelli, A.; Fleshner, N.E.; Gleave, M.; Kapoor, A.; Niazi, T.; North, S.A.; Pouliot, F.; Rendon, R.A.; et al. 2022 Canadian Urological Association (CUA)-Canadian Uro Oncology Group (CUOG) guideline: Management of castration-resistant prostate cancer (CRPC). *Can. Urol. Assoc. J.* **2022**, *16*, E506–E515. [CrossRef] [PubMed] [PubMed Central]

9. Kivimäki, M.; Strandberg, T.; Pentti, J.; Nyberg, S.T.; Frank, P.; Jokela, M.; Ervasti, J.; Suominen, S.B.; Vahtera, J.; Sipilä, P.N.; et al. Body-mass index and risk of obesity-related complex multimorbidity: An observational multicohort study. *Lancet Diabetes Endocrinol.* **2022**, *10*, 253–263. [CrossRef] [PubMed] [PubMed Central]
10. Sung, H.; Siegel, R.L.; Torre, L.A.; Pearson-Stuttard, J.; Islami, F.; Fedewa, S.A.; Goding Sauer, A.; Shuval, K.; Gapstur, S.M.; Jacobs, E.J.; et al. Global patterns in excess body weight and the associated cancer burden. *CA Cancer J. Clin.* **2019**, *69*, 88–112. [CrossRef] [PubMed]
11. Pati, S.; Irfan, W.; Jameel, A.; Ahmed, S.; Shahid, R.K. Obesity and Cancer: A Current Overview of Epidemiology, Pathogenesis, Outcomes, and Management. *Cancers* **2023**, *15*, 485. [CrossRef] [PubMed] [PubMed Central]
12. Jenabi, E.; Poorolajal, J. The effect of body mass index on endometrial cancer: A meta-analysis. *Public Health* **2015**, *129*, 872–880. [CrossRef] [PubMed]
13. Hoyo, C.; Cook, M.B.; Kamangar, F.; Freedman, N.D.; Whiteman, D.C.; Bernstein, L.; Brown, L.M.; Risch, H.A.; Ye, W.; Sharp, L.; et al. Body mass index in relation to oesophageal and oesophagogastric junction adenocarcinomas: A pooled analysis from the International BEACON Consortium. *Int. J. Epidemiol.* **2012**, *41*, 1706–1718. [CrossRef] [PubMed] [PubMed Central]
14. Wang, F.; Xu, Y. Body mass index and risk of renal cell cancer: A dose-response meta-analysis of published cohort studies. *Int. J. Cancer* **2014**, *135*, 1673–1686. [CrossRef] [PubMed]
15. Aune, D.; Sen, A.; Prasad, M.; Norat, T.; Janszky, I.; Tonstad, S.; Romundstad, P.; Vatten, L.J. BMI and all cause mortality: Systematic review and non-linear dose-response meta-analysis of 230 cohort studies with 3.74 million deaths among 30.3 million participants. *BMJ.* **2016**, *353*, i2156. [CrossRef] [PubMed] [PubMed Central]
16. Petrelli, F.; Cortellini, A.; Indini, A.; Tomasello, G.; Ghidini, M.; Nigro, O.; Salati, M.; Dottorini, L.; Iaculli, A.; Varricchio, A.; et al. Association of Obesity with Survival Outcomes in Patients with Cancer: A Systematic Review and Meta-analysis. *JAMA Netw. Open.* **2021**, *4*, e213520. [CrossRef] [PubMed] [PubMed Central]
17. Calle, E.E.; Rodriguez, C.; Walker-Thurmond, K.; Thun, M.J. Overweight, obesity, and mortality from cancer in a prospectively studied cohort of U.S. adults. *N. Engl. J. Med.* **2003**, *348*, 1625–1638. [CrossRef] [PubMed]
18. Liu, X.Z.; Pedersen, L.; Halberg, N. Cellular mechanisms linking cancers to obesity. *Cell Stress* **2021**, *5*, 55–72. [CrossRef] [PubMed] [PubMed Central]
19. Annett, S.; Moore, G.; Robson, T. Obesity and Cancer Metastasis: Molecular and Translational Perspectives. *Cancers* **2020**, *12*, 3798. [CrossRef] [PubMed] [PubMed Central]
20. Renehan, A.G.; Zwahlen, M.; Egger, M. Adiposity and cancer risk: New mechanistic insights from epidemiology. *Nat. Rev. Cancer* **2015**, *15*, 484–498. [CrossRef] [PubMed]
21. Islam, M.M.; Islam, M.M.; Rahman, M.A.; Ripon, M.A.R.; Hossain, M.S. Gut microbiota in obesity and related complications: Unveiling the complex interplay. *Life Sci.* **2023**, *334*, 122211. [CrossRef] [PubMed]
22. Rogers, C.J.; Prabhu, K.S.; Vijay-Kumar, M. The microbiome and obesity-an established risk for certain types of cancer. *Cancer J.* **2014**, *20*, 176–180. [CrossRef] [PubMed]
23. Freedland, S.J.; Aronson, W.J. Examining the relationship between obesity and prostate cancer. *Rev. Urol.* **2004**, *6*, 73–81. [PubMed] [PubMed Central]
24. Allott, E.H.; Masko, E.M.; Freedland, S.J. Obesity and prostate cancer: Weighing the evidence. *Eur. Urol.* **2013**, *63*, 800–809. [CrossRef] [PubMed] [PubMed Central]
25. MacInnis, R.J.; English, D.R. Body size and composition and prostate cancer risk: Systematic review and meta-regression analysis. *Cancer Causes Control.* **2006**, *17*, 989–1003. [CrossRef] [PubMed]
26. Bergström, A.; Pisani, P.; Tenet, V.; Wolk, A.; Adami, H.O. Overweight as an avoidable cause of cancer in Europe. *Int. J. Cancer* **2001**, *91*, 421–430; Erratum in *Int. J. Cancer* **2001**, *92*, 927. [CrossRef] [PubMed]
27. Renehan, A.G.; Tyson, M.; Egger, M.; Heller, R.F.; Zwahlen, M. Body-mass index and incidence of cancer: A systematic review and meta-analysis of prospective observational studies. *Lancet* **2008**, *371*, 569–578. [CrossRef] [PubMed]
28. Álvarez-Artime, A.; García-Soler, B.; Sainz, R.M.; Mayo, J.C. Emerging Roles for Browning of White Adipose Tissue in Prostate Cancer Malignant Behaviour. *Int. J. Mol. Sci.* **2021**, *22*, 5560. [CrossRef] [PubMed] [PubMed Central]
29. Hong, H.; Koch, M.O.; Foster, R.S.; Bihrle, R.; Gardner, T.A.; Fyffe, J.; Ulbright, T.M.; Eble, J.N.; Cheng, L. Anatomic distribution of periprostatic adipose tissue: A mapping study of 100 radical prostatectomy specimens. *Cancer* **2003**, *97*, 1639–1643. [CrossRef] [PubMed]
30. Park, J.; Euhus, D.M.; Scherer, P.E. Paracrine and endocrine effects of adipose tissue on cancer development and progression. *Endocr. Rev.* **2011**, *32*, 550–570. [CrossRef] [PubMed] [PubMed Central]
31. Hurwitz, A.A.; Foster, B.A.; Allison, J.P.; Greenberg, N.M.; Kwon, E.D. The TRAMP mouse as a model for prostate cancer. *Curr. Protoc. Immunol.* **2001**, *45*, 20.5.1–20.5.23. [CrossRef] [PubMed]

32. Brestoff, J.R.; Artis, D. Immune regulation of metabolic homeostasis in health and disease. *Cell* **2015**, *161*, 146–160. [CrossRef] [PubMed] [PubMed Central]
33. Howe, L.R.; Subbaramaiah, K.; Hudis, C.A.; Dannenberg, A.J. Molecular pathways: Adipose inflammation as a mediator of obesity-associated cancer. *Clin. Cancer Res.* **2013**, *9*, 6074–6083. [CrossRef] [PubMed] [PubMed Central]
34. Holtrup, B.; Church, C.D.; Berry, R.; Colman, L.; Jeffery, E.; Bober, J.; Rodeheffer, M.S. Puberty is an important developmental period for the establishment of adipose tissue mass and metabolic homeostasis. *Adipocyte* **2017**, *6*, 224–233. [CrossRef] [PubMed] [PubMed Central]
35. Wang, Q.A.; Tao, C.; Gupta, R.K.; Scherer, P.E. Tracking adipogenesis during white adipose tissue development, expansion and regeneration. *Nat. Med.* **2013**, *19*, 1338–1344. [CrossRef] [PubMed] [PubMed Central]
36. Attie, A.D.; Scherer, P.E. Adipocyte metabolism and obesity. *J. Lipid Res.* **2009**, *50*, S395–S399. [CrossRef] [PubMed] [PubMed Central]
37. Adesunloye, B.A. Mechanistic Insights into the Link between Obesity and Prostate Cancer. *Int. J. Mol. Sci.* **2021**, *22*, 3935. [CrossRef] [PubMed] [PubMed Central]
38. Prieto-Hontoria, P.L.; Pérez-Matute, P.; Fernández-Galilea, M.; Bustos, M.; Martínez, J.A.; Moreno-Aliaga, M.J. Role of obesity-associated dysfunctional adipose tissue in cancer: A molecular nutrition approach. *Biochim. Biophys. Acta* **2011**, *1807*, 664–678. [CrossRef] [PubMed]
39. Strong, A.L.; Burow, M.E.; Gimble, J.M.; Bunnell, B.A. Concise review: The obesity cancer paradigm: Exploration of the interactions and crosstalk with adipose stem cells. *Stem Cells* **2015**, *33*, 318–326. [CrossRef] [PubMed] [PubMed Central]
40. Wu, Q.; Li, B.; Li, Z.; Li, J.; Sun, S.; Sun, S. Cancer-associated adipocytes: Key players in breast cancer progression. *J. Hematol. Oncol.* **2019**, *12*, 95. [CrossRef] [PubMed] [PubMed Central]
41. Uehara, H.; Kobayashi, T.; Matsumoto, M.; Watanabe, S.; Yoneda, A.; Bando, Y. Adipose tissue: Critical contributor to the development of prostate cancer. *J. Med. Investig.* **2018**, *65*, 9–17. [CrossRef] [PubMed]
42. Kershaw, E.E.; Flier, J.S. Adipose tissue as an endocrine organ. *J. Clin. Endocrinol. Metab.* **2004**, *89*, 2548–2556. [CrossRef] [PubMed]
43. Ziech, D.; Franco, R.; Pappa, A.; Panayiotidis, M.I. Reactive oxygen species (ROS)–induced genetic and epigenetic alterations in human carcinogenesis. *Mutat. Res.* **2011**, *711*, 167–173. [CrossRef] [PubMed]
44. Roberts, D.L.; Dive, C.; Renehan, A.G. Biological mechanisms linking obesity and cancer risk: New perspectives. *Annu. Rev. Med.* **2010**, *61*, 301–316. [CrossRef] [PubMed]
45. Lekan, A.A.; Weiner, L.M. The Role of Chemokines in Orchestrating the Immune Response to Pancreatic Ductal Adenocarcinoma. *Cancers* **2024**, *16*, 559. [CrossRef] [PubMed] [PubMed Central]
46. Laurent, V.; Guérard, A.; Mazerolles, C.; Le Gonidec, S.; Toulet, A.; Nieto, L.; Zaidi, F.; Majed, B.; Garandeau, D.; Socrier, Y.; et al. Periprostatic adipocytes act as a driving force for prostate cancer progression in obesity. *Nat. Commun.* **2016**, *7*, 10230. [CrossRef] [PubMed] [PubMed Central]
47. Matuszak, E.A.; Kyprianou, N. Androgen regulation of epithelial-mesenchymal transition in prostate tumorigenesis. *Expert Rev. Endocrinol. Metab.* **2011**, *6*, 469–482. [CrossRef] [PubMed] [PubMed Central]
48. Grant, C.M.; Kyprianou, N. Epithelial mesenchymal transition (EMT) in prostate growth and tumor progression. *Transl. Androl. Urol.* **2013**, *2*, 202–211. [CrossRef] [PubMed] [PubMed Central]
49. Chavkin, N.W.; Vippa, T.; Jung, C.; McDonnell, S.; Hirschi, K.K.; Gokce, N.; Walsh, K. Obesity accelerates endothelial-to-mesenchymal transition in adipose tissues of mice and humans. *Front. Cardiovasc. Med.* **2023**, *10*, 1264479. [CrossRef] [PubMed] [PubMed Central]
50. Lin, T.C.; Hsiao, M. Leptin and Cancer: Updated Functional Roles in Carcinogenesis, Therapeutic Niches, and Developments. *Int. J. Mol. Sci.* **2021**, *22*, 2870. [CrossRef] [PubMed] [PubMed Central]
51. Gorrab, A.; Pagano, A.; Ayed, K.; Chebil, M.; Derouiche, A.; Kovacic, H.; Gati, A. Leptin Promotes Prostate Cancer Proliferation and Migration by Stimulating STAT3 Pathway. *Nutr. Cancer* **2021**, *73*, 1217–1227. [CrossRef] [PubMed]
52. Philp, L.K.; Rockstroh, A.; Sadowski, M.C.; Taherian Fard, A.; Lehman, M.; Tevz, G.; Libério, M.S.; Bidgood, C.L.; Gunter, J.H.; McPherson, S.; et al. Leptin antagonism inhibits prostate cancer xenograft growth and progression. *Endocr. Relat. Cancer* **2021**, *28*, 353–375. [CrossRef] [PubMed]
53. Deo, D.D.; Rao, A.P.; Bose, S.S.; Ouhtit, A.; Baliga, S.B.; Rao, S.A.; Trock, B.J.; Thouta, R.; Raj, M.H.; Rao, P.N. Differential effects of leptin on the invasive potential of androgen-dependent and -independent prostate carcinoma cells. *J. Biomed. Biotechnol.* **2008**, *2008*, 163902. [CrossRef] [PubMed] [PubMed Central]
54. Stattin, P.; Söderberg, S.; Hallmans, G.; Bylund, A.; Kaaks, R.; Stenman, U.H.; Bergh, A.; Olsson, T. Leptin is associated with increased prostate cancer risk: A nested case-referent study. *J. Clin. Endocrinol. Metab.* **2001**, *86*, 1341–1345. [CrossRef] [PubMed]
55. Chang, S.; Hursting, S.D.; Contois, J.H.; Strom, S.S.; Yamamura, Y.; Babaian, R.J.; Troncoso, P.; Scardino, P.S.; Wheeler, T.M.; Amos, C.I.; et al. Leptin and prostate cancer. *Prostate* **2001**, *46*, 62–67. [CrossRef] [PubMed]

56. Parker-Duffen, J.L.; Nakamura, K.; Silver, M.; Zuriaga, M.A.; MacLauchlan, S.; Aprahamian, T.R.; Walsh, K. Divergent roles for adiponectin receptor 1 (AdipoR1) and AdipoR2 in mediating revascularization and metabolic dysfunction in vivo. *J. Biol. Chem.* **2014**, *289*, 16200–16213. [CrossRef] [PubMed] [PubMed Central]
57. Michalakis, K.; Williams, C.J.; Mitsiades, N.; Blakeman, J.; Balafouta-Tselenis, S.; Giannopoulos, A.; Mantzoros, C.S. Serum adiponectin concentrations and tissue expression of adiponectin receptors are reduced in patients with prostate cancer: A case control study. *Cancer Epidemiol. Biomark. Prev.* **2007**, *16*, 308–313. [CrossRef] [PubMed]
58. Li, H.; Stampfer, M.J.; Mucci, L.; Rifai, N.; Qiu, W.; Kurth, T.; Ma, J. A 25-year prospective study of plasma adiponectin and leptin concentrations and prostate cancer risk and survival. *Clin. Chem.* **2010**, *56*, 34–43. [CrossRef] [PubMed] [PubMed Central]
59. Tan, W.; Wang, L.; Ma, Q.; Qi, M.; Lu, N.; Zhang, L.; Han, B. Adiponectin as a potential tumor suppressor inhibiting epithelial-to-mesenchymal transition but frequently silenced in prostate cancer by promoter methylation. *Prostate* **2015**, *75*, 1197–1205. [CrossRef] [PubMed]
60. Tang, C.H.; Lu, M.E. Adiponectin increases motility of human prostate cancer cells via adipoR, p38, AMPK, and NF-kappaB pathways. *Prostate* **2009**, *69*, 1781–1789. [CrossRef] [PubMed]
61. Bub, J.D.; Miyazaki, T.; Iwamoto, Y. Adiponectin as a growth inhibitor in prostate cancer cells. *Biochem. Biophys. Res. Commun.* **2006**, *340*, 1158–1166. [CrossRef] [PubMed]
62. Fenton, J.I.; Birmingham, J.M. Adipokine regulation of colon cancer: Adiponectin attenuates interleukin-6-induced colon carcinoma cell proliferation via STAT-3. *Mol. Carcinog.* **2010**, *49*, 700–709. [CrossRef] [PubMed] [PubMed Central]
63. Karnati, H.K.; Panigrahi, M.K.; Li, Y.; Tweedie, D.; Greig, N.H. Adiponectin as a Potential Therapeutic Target for Prostate Cancer. *Curr. Pharm. Des.* **2017**, *23*, 4170–4179. [CrossRef] [PubMed] [PubMed Central]
64. Cao, Y.; Nimptsch, K.; Shui, I.M.; Platz, E.A.; Wu, K.; Pollak, M.N.; Kenfield, S.A.; Stampfer, M.J.; Giovannucci, E.L. Prediagnostic plasma IGFBP-1, IGF-1 and risk of prostate cancer. *Int. J. Cancer* **2015**, *136*, 2418–2426. [CrossRef] [PubMed] [PubMed Central]
65. Qian, F.; Huo, D. Circulating Insulin-Like Growth Factor-1 and Risk of Total and 19 Site-Specific Cancers: Cohort Study Analyses from the UK Biobank. *Cancer Epidemiol. Biomarkers. Prev.* **2020**, *29*, 2332–2342. [CrossRef] [PubMed] [PubMed Central]
66. Watts, E.L.; Goldacre, R.; Key, T.J.; Allen, N.E.; Travis, R.C.; Perez-Cornago, A. Hormone-related diseases and prostate cancer: An English national record linkage study. *Int. J. Cancer* **2020**, *147*, 803–810. [CrossRef] [PubMed] [PubMed Central]
67. Argilés, J.M.; López-Soriano, F.J. Insulin and cancer (Review). *Int. J. Oncol.* **2001**, *18*, 683–687. [CrossRef] [PubMed]
68. Rowlands, M.A.; Gunnell, D.; Harris, R.; Vatten, L.J.; Holly, J.M.; Martin, R.M. Circulating insulin-like growth factor peptides and prostate cancer risk: A systematic review and meta-analysis. *Int. J. Cancer* **2009**, *124*, 2416–2429. [CrossRef] [PubMed] [PubMed Central]
69. Nimptsch, K.; Platz, E.A.; Pollak, M.N.; Kenfield, S.A.; Stampfer, M.J.; Willett, W.C.; Giovannucci, E. Plasma insulin-like growth factor 1 is positively associated with low-grade prostate cancer in the Health Professionals Follow-up Study 1993–2004. *Int. J. Cancer* **2011**, *128*, 660–667. [CrossRef] [PubMed] [PubMed Central]
70. Matsushita, M.; Fujita, K.; Hatano, K.; De Velasco, M.A.; Uemura, H.; Nonomura, N. Connecting the Dots between the Gut-IGF-1-Prostate Axis: A Role of IGF-1 in Prostate Carcinogenesis. *Front. Endocrinol.* **2022**, *13*, 852382. [CrossRef] [PubMed] [PubMed Central]
71. Ravi, P.; Wang, V.; Fichorova, R.N.; McGregor, B.; Wei, X.X.; Basaria, S.; Sweeney, C.J. IGF-1 axis changes with ADT and docetaxel in metastatic prostate cancer. *Endocr. Relat. Cancer* **2023**, *30*, e230241. [CrossRef] [PubMed] [PubMed Central]
72. Kolonin, M.G.; DiGiovanni, J. The role of adipose stroma in prostate cancer aggressiveness. *Transl. Androl. Urol.* **2019**, *8* (Suppl. S3), S348–S350. [CrossRef] [PubMed] [PubMed Central]
73. Shao, I.H.; Chang, T.H.; Chang, Y.H.; Hsieh, Y.H.; Sheng, T.W.; Wang, L.J.; Chien, Y.H.; Huang, L.K.; Chu, Y.C.; Kan, H.C.; et al. Periprostatic adipose tissue inhibits tumor progression by secreting apoptotic factors: A natural barrier induced by the immune response during the early stages of prostate cancer. *Oncol. Lett.* **2024**, *28*, 485. [CrossRef] [PubMed] [PubMed Central]
74. Lewitt, M.S. The Role of the Growth Hormone/Insulin-Like Growth Factor System in Visceral Adiposity. *Biochem. Insights* **2017**, *10*, 1178626417703995. [CrossRef] [PubMed] [PubMed Central]
75. Gallagher, E.J.; LeRoith, D. The proliferating role of insulin and insulin-like growth factors in cancer. *Trends Endocrinol. Metab.* **2010**, *21*, 610–618. [CrossRef] [PubMed] [PubMed Central]
76. Yang, X.; Kord-Varkaneh, H.; Talaei, S.; Clark, C.C.T.; Zanghelini, F.; Tan, S.C.; Zarezadeh, M.; Mousavi, S.M.; Rahmani, J.; Zhang, Y. The influence of metformin on IGF-1 levels in humans: A systematic review and meta-analysis. *Pharmacol. Res.* **2020**, *151*, 104588. [CrossRef] [PubMed]
77. Tosca, L.; Ramé, C.; Chabrolle, C.; Tesseraud, S.; Dupont, J. Metformin decreases IGF1-induced cell proliferation and protein synthesis through AMP-activated protein kinase in cultured bovine granulosa cells. *Reproduction* **2010**, *139*, 409–418. [CrossRef] [PubMed]

78. Galal, M.A.; Al-Rimawi, M.; Hajeer, A.; Dahman, H.; Alouch, S.; Aljada, A. Metformin: A Dual-Role Player in Cancer Treatment and Prevention. *Int. J. Mol. Sci.* **2024**, *25*, 4083. [CrossRef] [PubMed] [PubMed Central]
79. Kim, R.; Song, M.; Shinn, J.; Kim, H.S. Correlation between metformin intake and prostate cancer. Cardiovasc. *Prev. Pharmacother.* **2023**, *5*, 91–97.
80. Kim, S.; Keku, T.O.; Martin, C.; Galanko, J.; Woosley, J.T.; Schroeder, J.C.; Satia, J.A.; Halabi, S.; Sandler, R.S. Circulating levels of inflammatory cytokines and risk of colorectal adenomas. *Cancer Res.* **2008**, *68*, 323–328. [CrossRef] [PubMed] [PubMed Central]
81. Juge-Aubry, C.E.; Somm, E.; Giusti, V.; Pernin, A.; Chicheportiche, R.; Verdumo, C.; Rohner-Jeanrenaud, F.; Burger, D.; Dayer, J.M.; Meier, C.A. Adipose tissue is a major source of interleukin-1 receptor antagonist: Upregulation in obesity and inflammation. *Diabetes* **2003**, *52*, 1104–1110. [CrossRef] [PubMed]
82. Diaz, M.; Abdul, M.; Hoosein, N. Modulation of neuroendocrine differentiation in prostate cancer by interleukin-1 and -2. *Prostate Suppl.* **1998**, *8*, 32–36. [CrossRef] [PubMed]
83. Fan, Y.C.; Lee, K.D.; Tsai, Y.C. Roles of Interleukin-1 Receptor Antagonist in Prostate Cancer Progression. *Biomedicines* **2020**, *8*, 602. [CrossRef] [PubMed] [PubMed Central]
84. Nguyen, D.P.; Li, J.; Tewari, A.K. Inflammation and prostate cancer: The role of interleukin 6 (IL-6). *BJU Int.* **2014**, *113*, 986–992. [CrossRef] [PubMed]
85. Okamoto, M.; Lee, C.; Oyasu, R. Interleukin-6 as a paracrine and autocrine growth factor in human prostatic carcinoma cells in vitro. *Cancer Res.* **1997**, *57*, 141–146. [PubMed]
86. Sedger, L.M.; McDermott, M.F. TNF and TNF-receptors: From mediators of cell death and inflammation to therapeutic giants—Past, present and future. *Cytokine Growth Factor Rev.* **2014**, *25*, 453–472. [CrossRef] [PubMed]
87. Tse, B.W.; Scott, K.F.; Russell, P.J. Paradoxical roles of tumour necrosis factor-alpha in prostate cancer biology. *Prostate Cancer* **2012**, *2012*, 128965. [CrossRef] [PubMed] [PubMed Central]
88. Mizokami, A.; Gotoh, A.; Yamada, H.; Keller, E.T.; Matsumoto, T. Tumor necrosis factor-alpha represses androgen sensitivity in the LNCaP prostate cancer cell line. *J. Urol.* **2000**, *164 Pt 1*, 800–805. [CrossRef] [PubMed]
89. Maolake, A.; Izumi, K.; Natsagdorj, A.; Iwamoto, H.; Kadomoto, S.; Makino, T.; Naito, R.; Shigehara, K.; Kadono, Y.; Hiratsuka, K.; et al. Tumor necrosis factor-α induces prostate cancer cell migration in lymphatic metastasis through CCR7 upregulation. *Cancer Sci.* **2018**, *109*, 1524–1531. [CrossRef] [PubMed] [PubMed Central]
90. Lü, L.; Tang, D.; Wang, L.; Huang, L.Q.; Jiang, G.S.; Xiao, X.Y.; Zeng, F.Q. Gambogic acid inhibits TNF-α-induced invasion of human prostate cancer PC3 cells in vitro through PI3K/Akt and NF-κB signaling pathways. *Acta Pharmacol. Sin.* **2012**, *33*, 531–541. [CrossRef] [PubMed] [PubMed Central]
91. Gorelik, L.; Bar-Dagan, Y.; Mokyr, M.B. Insight into the mechanism(s) through which TNF promotes the generation of T cell-mediated antitumor cytotoxicity by tumor bearer splenic cells. *J. Immunol.* **1996**, *156*, 4298–4308. [CrossRef] [PubMed]
92. Lee, E.C.; Zhan, P.; Schallhom, R.; Packman, K.; Tenniswood, M. Antiandrogen-induced cell death in LNCaP human prostate cancer cells. *Cell Death Differ.* **2003**, *10*, 761–771. [CrossRef] [PubMed]
93. Chekhonin, V.P.; Shein, S.A.; Korchagina, A.A.; Gurina, O.I. VEGF in tumor progression and targeted therapy. *Curr. Cancer Drug Targets* **2013**, *13*, 423–443. [CrossRef] [PubMed]
94. Duque, J.L.; Loughlin, K.R.; Adam, R.M.; Kantoff, P.W.; Zurakowski, D.; Freeman, M.R. Plasma levels of vascular endothelial growth factor are increased in patients with metastatic prostate cancer. *Urology* **1999**, *54*, 523–527. [CrossRef] [PubMed]
95. Wang, M.; Wisniewski, C.A.; Xiong, C.; Chhoy, P.; Goel, H.L.; Kumar, A.; Zhu, L.J.; Li, R.; St Louis, P.A.; Ferreira, L.M.; et al. Therapeutic blocking of VEGF binding to neuropilin-2 diminishes PD-L1 expression to activate antitumor immunity in prostate cancer. *Sci. Transl. Med.* **2023**, *15*, eade5855. [CrossRef] [PubMed]
96. Rehman, J.; Traktuev, D.; Li, J.; Merfeld-Clauss, S.; Temm-Grove, C.J.; Bovenkerk, J.E.; Pell, C.L.; Johnstone, B.H.; Considine, R.V.; March, K.L. Secretion of angiogenic and antiapoptotic factors by human adipose stromal cells. *Circulation* **2004**, *109*, 1292–1298. [CrossRef] [PubMed]
97. Badimon, L.; Oñate, B.; Vilahur, G. Adipose-derived Mesenchymal Stem Cells and Their Reparative Potential in Ischemic Heart Disease. *Rev. Esp. Cardiol. (Engl. Ed.)* **2015**, *68*, 599–611. [CrossRef] [PubMed]
98. Ye, L.; Jiang, W.G. Bone morphogenetic proteins in tumour associated angiogenesis and implication in cancer therapies. *Cancer Lett.* **2016**, *380*, 586–597. [CrossRef] [PubMed]
99. Barnes, J.; Anthony, C.T.; Wall, N.; Steiner, M.S. Bone morphogenetic protein-6 expression in normal and malignant prostate. *World J. Urol.* **1995**, *13*, 337–343. [CrossRef] [PubMed]
100. Tamada, H.; Kitazawa, R.; Gohji, K.; Kitazawa, S. Epigenetic regulation of human bone morphogenetic protein 6 gene expression in prostate cancer. *J. Bone Miner. Res.* **2001**, *16*, 487–496. [CrossRef] [PubMed]

101. Kobayashi, A.; Okuda, H.; Xing, F.; Pandey, P.R.; Watabe, M.; Hirota, S.; Pai, S.K.; Liu, W.; Fukuda, K.; Chambers, C.; et al. Bone morphogenetic protein 7 in dormancy and metastasis of prostate cancer stem-like cells in bone. *J. Exp. Med.* **2011**, *208*, 2641–2655; Erratum in *J. Exp. Med.* **2012**, *209*, 639. [CrossRef] [PubMed] [PubMed Central]
102. Buijs, J.T.; Rentsch, C.A.; van der Horst, G.; van Overveld, P.G.; Wetterwald, A.; Schwaninger, R.; Henriquez, N.V.; Ten Dijke, P.; Borovecki, F.; Markwalder, R.; et al. BMP7, a putative regulator of epithelial homeostasis in the human prostate, is a potent inhibitor of prostate cancer bone metastasis in vivo. *Am. J. Pathol.* **2007**, *171*, 1047–1057. [CrossRef] [PubMed] [PubMed Central]
103. Blázquez-Medela, A.M.; Jumabay, M.; Boström, K.I. Beyond the bone: Bone morphogenetic protein signaling in adipose tissue. *Obes. Rev.* **2019**, *20*, 648–658. [CrossRef] [PubMed] [PubMed Central]
104. Qian, S.; Tang, Y.; Tang, Q.Q. Adipose tissue plasticity and the pleiotropic roles of BMP signaling. *J. Biol. Chem.* **2021**, *296*, 100678. [CrossRef] [PubMed] [PubMed Central]
105. Arner, E.; Westermark, P.O.; Spalding, K.L.; Britton, T.; Rydén, M.; Frisén, J.; Bernard, S.; Arner, P. Adipocyte turnover: Relevance to human adipose tissue morphology. *Diabetes* **2010**, *59*, 105–109. [CrossRef] [PubMed] [PubMed Central]
106. Mailloux, R.J.; Harper, M.E. Uncoupling proteins and the control of mitochondrial reactive oxygen species production. *Free Radic. Biol. Med.* **2011**, *51*, 1106–1115. [CrossRef] [PubMed]
107. Li, W.; Nichols, K.; Nathan, C.A.; Zhao, Y. Mitochondrial uncoupling protein 2 is up-regulated in human head and neck, skin, pancreatic, and prostate tumors. *Cancer Biomark.* **2013**, *13*, 377–383. [CrossRef] [PubMed]
108. Sadeghi, S.; Checchetto, V.; Varanita, T. A Comprehensive Pan-Cancer Analysis of the Mitochondrial Uncoupling Protein UCP2, with a Focus on Sex and Gender-Related Aspects. *Cell Physiol. Biochem.* **2024**, *58*, 630–653. [CrossRef] [PubMed]
109. Cheng, W.C.; Tsui, Y.C.; Ragusa, S.; Koelzer, V.H.; Mina, M.; Franco, F.; Läubli, H.; Tschumi, B.; Speiser, D.; Romero, P.; et al. Uncoupling protein 2 reprograms the tumor microenvironment to support the anti-tumor immune cycle. *Nat. Immunol.* **2019**, *20*, 206–217; Erratum in *Nat. Immunol.* **2019**, *20*, 515–516. [CrossRef] [PubMed]
110. Han, C.; Deng, Y.; Xu, W.; Liu, Z.; Wang, T.; Wang, S.; Liu, J.; Liu, X. The Roles of Tumor-Associated Macrophages in Prostate Cancer. *J. Oncol.* **2022**, *2022*, 8580043. [CrossRef] [PubMed] [PubMed Central]
111. van Dierendonck, X.A.M.H.; Sancerni, T.; Alves-Guerra, M.C.; Stienstra, R. The role of uncoupling protein 2 in macrophages and its impact on obesity-induced adipose tissue inflammation and insulin resistance. *J. Biol. Chem.* **2020**, *295*, 17535–17548. [CrossRef] [PubMed] [PubMed Central]
112. Monnier, M.; Paolini, L.; Vinatier, E.; Mantovani, A.; Delneste, Y.; Jeannin, P. Antitumor strategies targeting macrophages: The importance of considering the differences in differentiation/polarization processes between human and mouse macrophages. *J. Immunother. Cancer* **2022**, *10*, e005560; Erratum in *J. Immunother. Cancer* **2023**, *11*, e005560corr1. [CrossRef] [PubMed] [PubMed Central]
113. Srivastava, A.; Goldberger, H.; Dimtchev, A.; Marian, C.; Soldin, O.; Li, X.; Collins, S.P.; Suy, S.; Kumar, D. Circulatory miR-628-5p is downregulated in prostate cancer patients. *Tumour Biol.* **2014**, *35*, 4867–4873. [CrossRef] [PubMed] [PubMed Central]
114. Hu, X.; Hu, C.; Zhang, C.; Zhang, M.; Long, S.; Cao, Z. Role of Adiponectin in prostate cancer. *Int. Braz. J. Urol.* **2019**, *45*, 220–228. [CrossRef] [PubMed] [PubMed Central]
115. Ribas, J.; Lupold, S.E. The transcriptional regulation of miR-21, its multiple transcripts, and their implication in prostate cancer. *Cell Cycle* **2010**, *9*, 923–929. [CrossRef] [PubMed] [PubMed Central]
116. Ribas, J.; Ni, X.; Haffner, M.; Wentzel, E.A.; Salmasi, A.H.; Chowdhury, W.H.; Kudrolli, T.A.; Yegnasubramanian, S.; Luo, J.; Rodriguez, R.; et al. miR-21: An androgen receptor-regulated microRNA that promotes hormone-dependent and hormone-independent prostate cancer growth. *Cancer Res.* **2009**, *69*, 7165–7169. [CrossRef] [PubMed] [PubMed Central]
117. Dybos, S.A.; Flatberg, A.; Halgunset, J.; Viset, T.; Rolfseng, T.; Kvam, S.; Skogseth, H. Increased levels of serum miR-148a-3p are associated with prostate cancer. *APMIS* **2018**, *126*, 722–731. [CrossRef] [PubMed]
118. Murata, T.; Takayama, K.; Katayama, S.; Urano, T.; Horie-Inoue, K.; Ikeda, K.; Takahashi, S.; Kawazu, C.; Hasegawa, A.; Ouchi, Y.; et al. miR-148a is an androgen-responsive microRNA that promotes LNCaP prostate cell growth by repressing its target CAND1 expression. *Prostate Cancer Prostatic Dis.* **2010**, *13*, 356–361. [CrossRef] [PubMed]
119. He, W.; Zhang, F.; Jiang, F.; Liu, H.; Wang, G. Correlations between serum levels of microRNA-148a-3p and microRNA-485-5p and the progression and recurrence of prostate cancer. *BMC Urol.* **2022**, *22*, 195. [CrossRef] [PubMed] [PubMed Central]
120. Chen, X.; Gao, C.; Li, H.; Huang, L.; Sun, Q.; Dong, Y.; Tian, C.; Gao, S.; Dong, H.; Guan, D.; et al. Identification and characterization of microRNAs in raw milk during different periods of lactation, commercial fluid, and powdered milk products. *Cell Res.* **2010**, *20*, 1128–1137. [CrossRef] [PubMed]
121. Zhang, Y.; Xu, Q.; Hou, J.; Huang, G.; Zhao, S.; Zheng, N.; Wang, J. Loss of bioactive microRNAs in cow's milk by ultra-high-temperature treatment but not by pasteurization treatment. *J. Sci. Food. Agric.* **2022**, *102*, 2676–2685. [CrossRef] [PubMed]

122. Stoen, M.J.; Andersen, S.; Rakaee, M.; Pedersen, M.I.; Ingebriktsen, L.M.; Bremnes, R.M.; Donnem, T.; Lombardi, A.P.G.; Kilvaer, T.K.; Busund, L.T.; et al. High expression of miR-17-5p in tumor epithelium is a predictor for poor prognosis for prostate cancer patients. *Sci. Rep.* **2021**, *11*, 13864. [CrossRef] [PubMed] [PubMed Central]
123. Ruiz-Ojeda, F.J.; Méndez-Gutiérrez, A.; Aguilera, C.M.; Plaza-Díaz, J. Extracellular Matrix Remodeling of Adipose Tissue in Obesity and Metabolic Diseases. *Int. J. Mol. Sci.* **2019**, *20*, 4888. [CrossRef] [PubMed] [PubMed Central]
124. Fang, M.; Yuan, J.; Peng, C.; Li, Y. Collagen as a double-edged sword in tumor progression. *Tumour Biol.* **2014**, *35*, 2871–2882. [CrossRef] [PubMed] [PubMed Central]
125. Walker, C.; Mojares, E.; Del Río Hernández, A. Role of Extracellular Matrix in Development and Cancer Progression. *Int. J. Mol. Sci.* **2018**, *19*, 3028. [CrossRef] [PubMed] [PubMed Central]
126. Malik, R.; Lelkes, P.I.; Cukierman, E. Biomechanical and biochemical remodeling of stromal extracellular matrix in cancer. *Trends Biotechnol.* **2015**, *33*, 230–236. [CrossRef] [PubMed] [PubMed Central]
127. Paszek, M.J.; Zahir, N.; Johnson, K.R.; Lakins, J.N.; Rozenberg, G.I.; Gefen, A.; Reinhart-King, C.A.; Margulies, S.S.; Dembo, M.; Boettiger, D.; et al. Tensional homeostasis and the malignant phenotype. *Cancer Cell* **2005**, *8*, 241–254. [CrossRef] [PubMed]
128. Parker, A.S.; Thiel, D.D.; Bergstralh, E.; Carlson, R.E.; Rangel, L.J.; Joseph, R.W.; Diehl, N.; Karnes, R.J. Obese men have more advanced and more aggressive prostate cancer at time of surgery than non-obese men after adjusting for screening PSA level and age: Results from two independent nested case-control studies. *Prostate Cancer Prostatic Dis.* **2013**, *16*, 352–356. [CrossRef] [PubMed] [PubMed Central]
129. Su, F.; Daquinag, A.C.; Ahn, S.; Saha, A.; Dai, Y.; Zhao, Z.; DiGiovanni, J.; Kolonin, M.G. Progression of prostate carcinoma is promoted by adipose stromal cell-secreted CXCL12 signaling in prostate epithelium. *NPJ Precis. Oncol.* **2021**, *5*, 26. [CrossRef] [PubMed] [PubMed Central]
130. Ribeiro, R.; Monteiro, C.; Cunha, V.; Oliveira, M.J.; Freitas, M.; Fraga, A.; Príncipe, P.; Lobato, C.; Lobo, F.; Morais, A.; et al. Human periprostatic adipose tissue promotes prostate cancer aggressiveness in vitro. *J. Exp. Clin. Cancer Res.* **2012**, *31*, 32. [CrossRef] [PubMed] [PubMed Central]
131. Egeblad, M.; Werb, Z. New functions for the matrix metalloproteinases in cancer progression. *Nat. Rev. Cancer* **2002**, *2*, 161–174. [CrossRef] [PubMed]
132. Lin, C.Y.; Tsai, P.H.; Kandaswami, C.C.; Lee, P.P.; Huang, C.J.; Hwang, J.J.; Lee, M.T. Matrix metalloproteinase-9 cooperates with transcription factor Snail to induce epithelial-mesenchymal transition. *Cancer Sci.* **2011**, *102*, 815–827. [CrossRef] [PubMed]
133. Cheng, L.; Darson, M.F.; Bergstralh, E.J.; Slezak, J.; Myers, R.P.; Bostwick, D.G. Correlation of margin status and extraprostatic extension with progression of prostate carcinoma. *Cancer* **1999**, *86*, 1775–1782. [CrossRef] [PubMed]
134. Sacca, P.A.; Creydt, V.P.; Choi, H.; Mazza, O.N.; Fletcher, S.J.; Vallone, V.B.; Scorticati, C.; Chasseing, N.A.; Calvo, J.C. Human periprostatic adipose tissue: Its influence on prostate cancer cells. *Cell. Physiol. Biochem.* **2012**, *30*, 113–122. [CrossRef] [PubMed]
135. Moreira, Â.; Pereira, S.S.; Costa, M.; Morais, T.; Pinto, A.; Fernandes, R.; Monteiro, M.P. Adipocyte secreted factors enhance aggressiveness of prostate carcinoma cells. *PLoS ONE* **2015**, *10*, e0123217. [CrossRef] [PubMed] [PubMed Central]
136. Asmar, R.; Beebe-Dimmer, J.L.; Korgavkar, K.; Keele, G.R.; Cooney, K.A. Hypertension, obesity and prostate cancer biochemical recurrence after radical prostatectomy. *Prostate Cancer Prostatic Dis.* **2013**, *16*, 62–66. [CrossRef] [PubMed] [PubMed Central]
137. Sacca, P.A.; Calvo, J.C. Periprostatic Adipose Tissue Microenvironment: Metabolic and Hormonal Pathways during Prostate Cancer Progression. *Front. Endocrinol.* **2022**, *13*, 863027. [CrossRef] [PubMed] [PubMed Central]
138. Balaban, S.; Nassar, Z.D.; Zhang, A.Y.; Hosseini-Beheshti, E.; Centenera, M.M.; Schreuder, M.; Lin, H.M.; Aishah, A.; Varney, B.; Liu-Fu, F.; et al. Extracellular Fatty Acids Are the Major Contributor to Lipid Synthesis in Prostate Cancer. *Mol. Cancer Res.* **2019**, *17*, 949–962. [CrossRef] [PubMed]
139. Iordanescu, G.; Brendler, C.; Crawford, S.E.; Wyrwicz, A.M.; Venkatasubramanian, P.N.; Doll, J.A. MRS measured fatty acid composition of periprostatic adipose tissue correlates with pathological measures of prostate cancer aggressiveness. *J. Magn. Reson. Imaging* **2015**, *42*, 651–657. [CrossRef] [PubMed]
140. Yue, S.; Li, J.; Lee, S.Y.; Lee, H.J.; Shao, T.; Song, B.; Cheng, L.; Masterson, T.A.; Liu, X.; Ratliff, T.L.; et al. Cholesteryl ester accumulation induced by PTEN loss and PI3K/AKT activation underlies human prostate cancer aggressiveness. *Cell Metab.* **2014**, *19*, 393–406. [CrossRef] [PubMed] [PubMed Central]
141. Watt, M.J.; Clark, A.K.; Selth, L.A.; Haynes, V.R.; Lister, N.; Rebello, R.; Porter, L.H.; Niranjan, B.; Whitby, S.T.; Lo, J.; et al. Suppressing fatty acid uptake has therapeutic effects in preclinical models of prostate cancer. *Sci. Transl. Med.* **2019**, *11*, eaau5758. [CrossRef] [PubMed]
142. Cao, H.; Wang, Y.; Zhang, D.; Liu, B.; Zhou, H.; Wang, S. Periprostatic Adipose Tissue: A New Perspective for Diagnosing and Treating Prostate Cancer. *J. Cancer* **2024**, *15*, 204–217. [CrossRef] [PubMed] [PubMed Central]
143. Yunna, C.; Mengru, H.; Lei, W.; Weidong, C. Macrophage M1/M2 polarization. *Eur. J. Pharmacol.* **2020**, *877*, 173090. [CrossRef] [PubMed]

144. Taussky, D.; Barkati, M.; Campeau, S.; Zerouali, K.; Nadiri, A.; Saad, F.; Delouya, G. Changes in periprostatic adipose tissue induced by 5α-reductase inhibitors. *Andrology* **2017**, *5*, 511–515. [CrossRef] [PubMed]
145. Bonk, S.; Kluth, M.; Hube-Magg, C.; Polonski, A.; Soekeland, G.; Makropidi-Fraune, G.; Möller-Koop, C.; Witt, M.; Luebke, A.M.; Hinsch, A.; et al. Prognostic and diagnostic role of PSA immunohistochemistry: A tissue microarray study on 21,000 normal and cancerous tissues. *Oncotarget* **2019**, *10*, 5439–5453. [CrossRef] [PubMed] [PubMed Central]
146. Cohen, P.; Graves, H.C.; Peehl, D.M.; Kamarei, M.; Giudice, L.C.; Rosenfeld, R.G. Prostate-specific antigen (PSA) is an insulin-like growth factor binding protein-3 protease found in seminal plasma. *J. Clin. Endocrinol. Metab.* **1992**, *75*, 1046–1053. [CrossRef] [PubMed]
147. Estève, D.; Roumiguié, M.; Manceau, C.; Milhas, D.; Muller, C. Periprostatic adipose tissue: A heavy player in prostate cancer progression. *Curr. Opin. Endocr. Metab. Res.* **2020**, *10*, 29–35. [CrossRef]
148. Uzun, E.; Polat, M.E.; Ceviz, K.; Olcucuoglu, E.; Tastemur, S.; Kasap, Y.; Senel, S.; Ozdemir, O. The importance of periprostatic fat tissue thickness measured by preoperative multiparametric magnetic resonance imaging in upstage prediction after robot-assisted radical prostatectomy. *Investig. Clin. Urol.* **2024**, *65*, 53–61. [CrossRef] [PubMed] [PubMed Central]
149. Jiang, S.; Li, Y.; Guo, Y.; Gong, B.; Wei, C.; Liu, W.; Chen, C.; Pan, F.; Song, J.; He, Q.; et al. MRI-measured periprostatic to subcutaneous adipose tissue thickness ratio as an independent risk factor in prostate cancer patients undergoing radical prostatectomy. *Sci. Rep.* **2024**, *14*, 20896. [CrossRef] [PubMed] [PubMed Central]
150. van Roermund, J.G.; Hinnen, K.A.; Tolman, C.J.; Bol, G.H.; Witjes, J.A.; Bosch, J.L.; Kiemeney, L.A.; van Vulpen, M. Periprostatic fat correlates with tumour aggressiveness in prostate cancer patients. *BJU Int.* **2011**, *107*, 1775–1779. [CrossRef] [PubMed]
151. AlZaim, I.; Al-Saidi, A.; Hammoud, S.H.; Darwiche, N.; Al-Dhaheri, Y.; Eid, A.H.; El-Yazbi, A.F. Thromboinflammatory Processes at the Nexus of Metabolic Dysfunction and Prostate Cancer: The Emerging Role of Periprostatic Adipose Tissue. *Cancers* **2022**, *14*, 1679. [CrossRef] [PubMed]
152. Ebrahimi, S.; Rahmani, F.; Behnam-Rassouli, R.; Hoseinkhani, F.; Parizadeh, M.R.; Keramati, M.R.; Khazaie, M.; Avan, A.; Hassanian, S.M. Proinflammatory signaling functions of thrombin in cancer. *J. Cell. Physiol.* **2017**, *232*, 2323–2329. [CrossRef] [PubMed]
153. Samad, F.; Pandey, M.; Loskutoff, D.J. Regulation of tissue factor gene expression in obesity. *Blood* **2001**, *98*, 3353–3358. [CrossRef] [PubMed]
154. Kohli, M.; Williams, K.; Yao, J.L.; Dennis, R.A.; Huang, J.; Reeder, J.; Ricke, W.A. Thrombin expression in prostate: A novel finding. *Cancer Investig.* **2011**, *29*, 62–67. [CrossRef] [PubMed] [PubMed Central]
155. Martorell, L.; Martínez-González, J.; Rodríguez, C.; Gentile, M.; Calvayrac, O.; Badimon, L. Thrombin and protease-activated receptors (PARs) in atherothrombosis. *Thromb. Haemost.* **2008**, *99*, 305–315. [CrossRef] [PubMed]
156. Kaushal, V.; Kohli, M.; Dennis, R.A.; Siegel, E.R.; Chiles, W.W.; Mukunyadzi, P. Thrombin receptor expression is upregulated in prostate cancer. *Prostate* **2006**, *66*, 273–282. [CrossRef] [PubMed]
157. Black, P.C.; Mize, G.J.; Karlin, P.; Greenberg, D.L.; Hawley, S.J.; True, L.D.; Vessella, R.L.; Takayama, T.K. Overexpression of protease-activated receptors-1,-2, and-4 (PAR-1, -2, and -4) in prostate cancer. *Prostate* **2007**, *67*, 743–756. [CrossRef] [PubMed]
158. López-Zambrano, M.; Rodriguez-Montesinos, J.; Crespo-Avilan, G.E.; Muñoz-Vega, M.; Preissner, K.T. Thrombin Promotes Macrophage Polarization into M1-Like Phenotype to Induce Inflammatory Responses. *Thromb. Haemost.* **2020**, *120*, 658–670. [CrossRef] [PubMed]
159. Laurent, V.; Toulet, A.; Attané, C.; Milhas, D.; Dauvillier, S.; Zaidi, F.; Clement, E.; Cinato, M.; Le Gonidec, S.; Guérard, A.; et al. Periprostatic Adipose Tissue Favors Prostate Cancer Cell Invasion in an Obesity-Dependent Manner: Role of Oxidative Stress. *Mol. Cancer Res.* **2019**, *17*, 821–835. [CrossRef] [PubMed]
160. Sun, B.L.; Sun, X.; Casanova, N.; Garcia, A.N.; Oita, R.; Algotar, A.M.; Camp, S.M.; Hernon, V.R.; Gregory, T.; Cress, A.E.; et al. Role of secreted extracellular nicotinamide phosphoribosyltransferase (eNAMPT) in prostate cancer progression: Novel biomarker and therapeutic target. *EBioMedicine* **2020**, *61*, 103059. [CrossRef] [PubMed] [PubMed Central]
161. Uyeturk, U.; Sarıcı, H.; Kın Tekce, B.; Eroglu, M.; Kemahlı, E.; Uyeturk, U.; Gucuk, A. Serum omentin level in patients with prostate cancer. *Med. Oncol.* **2014**, *31*, 923. [CrossRef] [PubMed]
162. Deb, A.; Deshmukh, B.; Ramteke, P.; Bhati, F.K.; Bhat, M.K. Resistin: A journey from metabolism to cancer. *Transl. Oncol.* **2021**, *14*, 101178. [CrossRef] [PubMed] [PubMed Central]
163. Kim, H.J.; Lee, Y.S.; Won, E.H.; Chang, I.H.; Kim, T.H.; Park, E.S.; Kim, M.K.; Kim, W.; Myung, S.C. Expression of resistin in the prostate and its stimulatory effect on prostate cancer cell proliferation. *BJU Int.* **2011**, *108 Pt 2*, E77–E83. [CrossRef] [PubMed]
164. Sudan, S.K.; Deshmukh, S.K.; Poosarla, T.; Holliday, N.P.; Dyess, D.L.; Singh, A.P.; Singh, S. Resistin: An inflammatory cytokine with multi-faceted roles in cancer. *Biochim. Biophys. Acta Rev. Cancer* **2020**, *1874*, 188419. [CrossRef] [PubMed] [PubMed Central]
165. Santiago-Sánchez, G.S.; Pita-Grisanti, V.; Quiñones-Díaz, B.; Gumpper, K.; Cruz-Monserrate, Z.; Vivas-Mejía, P.E. Biological Functions and Therapeutic Potential of Lipocalin 2 in Cancer. *Int. J. Mol. Sci.* **2020**, *21*, 4365. [CrossRef] [PubMed] [PubMed Central]

166. Ulusoy, M.H.; Cirak, Y.; Adali, Y. Predictive and Prognostic Role of Lipocalin-2 Expression in Prostate Cancer and Its Association with Gleason Score. *Prostate Cancer* **2021**, *2021*, 8836043. [CrossRef] [PubMed] [PubMed Central]
167. Tung, M.C.; Hsieh, S.C.; Yang, S.F.; Cheng, C.W.; Tsai, R.T.; Wang, S.C.; Huang, M.H.; Hsieh, Y.H. Knockdown of lipocalin-2 suppresses the growth and invasion of prostate cancer cells. *Prostate* **2013**, *73*, 1281–1290. [CrossRef] [PubMed]
168. Ding, G.; Wang, J.; Feng, C.; Jiang, H.; Xu, J.; Ding, Q. Lipocalin 2 over-expression facilitates progress of castration-resistant prostate cancer via improving androgen receptor transcriptional activity. *Oncotarget* **2016**, *7*, 64309–64317. [CrossRef] [PubMed] [PubMed Central]
169. Ding, G.; Fang, J.; Tong, S.; Qu, L.; Jiang, H.; Ding, Q.; Liu, J. Over-expression of lipocalin 2 promotes cell migration and invasion through activating ERK signaling to increase SLUG expression in prostate cancer. *Prostate* **2015**, *75*, 957–968. [CrossRef] [PubMed]
170. Uygur, B.; Wu, W.S. SLUG promotes prostate cancer cell migration and invasion via CXCR4/CXCL12 axis. *Mol. Cancer* **2011**, *10*, 139. [CrossRef] [PubMed] [PubMed Central]
171. Uehara, H.; Takahashi, T.; Oha, M.; Ogawa, H.; Izumi, K. Exogenous fatty acid binding protein 4 promotes human prostate cancer cell progression. *Int. J. Cancer* **2014**, *135*, 2558–2568. [CrossRef] [PubMed]
172. Huang, M.; Narita, S.; Inoue, T.; Koizumi, A.; Saito, M.; Tsuruta, H.; Numakura, K.; Satoh, S.; Nanjo, H.; Sasaki, T.; et al. Fatty acid binding protein 4 enhances prostate cancer progression by upregulating matrix metalloproteinases and stromal cell cytokine production. *Oncotarget* **2017**, *8*, 111780–111794. [CrossRef] [PubMed] [PubMed Central]
173. Kiefer, F.W.; Zeyda, M.; Gollinger, K.; Pfau, B.; Neuhofer, A.; Weichhart, T.; Säemann, M.D.; Geyeregger, R.; Schlederer, M.; Kenner, L.; et al. Neutralization of osteopontin inhibits obesity-induced inflammation and insulin resistance. *Diabetes* **2010**, *59*, 935–946. [CrossRef] [PubMed] [PubMed Central]
174. Castellano, G.; Malaponte, G.; Mazzarino, M.C.; Figini, M.; Marchese, F.; Gangemi, P.; Travali, S.; Stivala, F.; Canevari, S.; Libra, M. Activation of the osteopontin/matrix metalloproteinase-9 pathway correlates with prostate cancer progression. *Clin. Cancer Res.* **2008**, *14*, 7470–7480. [CrossRef] [PubMed]
175. Ramankulov, A.; Lein, M.; Kristiansen, G.; Loening, S.A.; Jung, K. Plasma osteopontin in comparison with bone markers as indicator of bone metastasis and survival outcome in patients with prostate cancer. *Prostate* **2007**, *67*, 330–340. [CrossRef] [PubMed]
176. Zhao, H.; Chen, Q.; Alam, A.; Cui, J.; Suen, K.C.; Soo, A.P.; Eguchi, S.; Gu, J.; Ma, D. The role of osteopontin in the progression of solid organ tumour. *Cell Death Dis.* **2018**, *9*, 356. [CrossRef] [PubMed] [PubMed Central]
177. Desai, B.; Rogers, M.J.; Chellaiah, M.A. Mechanisms of osteopontin and CD44 as metastatic principles in prostate cancer cells. *Mol. Cancer* **2007**, *6*, 18. [CrossRef] [PubMed] [PubMed Central]
178. Khodavirdi, A.C.; Song, Z.; Yang, S.; Zhong, C.; Wang, S.; Wu, H.; Pritchard, C.; Nelson, P.S.; Roy-Burman, P. Increased expression of osteopontin contributes to the progression of prostate cancer. *Cancer Res.* **2006**, *66*, 883–888. [CrossRef] [PubMed]
179. Tilli, T.M.; Ferreira, L.B.; Gimba, E.R. Osteopontin-c mediates the upregulation of androgen responsive genes in LNCaP cells through PI3K/Akt and androgen receptor signaling. *Oncol. Lett.* **2015**, *9*, 1845–1850. [CrossRef] [PubMed] [PubMed Central]
180. Tilli, T.M.; Bellahcène, A.; Castronovo, V.; Gimba, E.R. Changes in the transcriptional profile in response to overexpression of the osteopontin-c splice isoform in ovarian (OvCar-3) and prostate (PC-3) cancer cell lines. *BMC Cancer* **2014**, *14*, 433. [CrossRef] [PubMed] [PubMed Central]
181. Zheng, J.; Hou, Z.B.; Jiao, N.L. Effects of osteopontin downregulation on the growth of prostate cancer PC-3 cells. *Mol. Med. Rep.* **2011**, *4*, 1225–1231. [CrossRef] [PubMed]
182. He, Q.; Gao, Z.; Yin, J.; Zhang, J.; Yun, Z.; Ye, J. Regulation of HIF-1{alpha} activity in adipose tissue by obesity-associated factors: Adipogenesis, insulin, and hypoxia. *Am. J. Physiol. Endocrinol. Metab.* **2011**, *300*, E877–E885. [CrossRef] [PubMed] [PubMed Central]
183. García-Fuentes, E.; Santiago-Fernández, C.; Gutiérrez-Repiso, C.; Mayas, M.D.; Oliva-Olivera, W.; Coín-Aragüez, L.; Alcaide, J.; Ocaña-Wilhelmi, L.; Vendrell, J.; Tinahones, F.J.; et al. Hypoxia is associated with a lower expression of genes involved in lipogenesis in visceral adipose tissue. *J. Transl. Med.* **2015**, *13*, 373. [CrossRef] [PubMed] [PubMed Central]
184. Roumiguié, M.; Estève, D.; Manceau, C.; Toulet, A.; Gilleron, J.; Belles, C.; Jia, Y.; Houël, C.; Pericart, S.; LeGonidec, S.; et al. Periprostatic Adipose Tissue Displays a Chronic Hypoxic State that Limits Its Expandability. *Am. J. Pathol.* **2022**, *192*, 926–942. [CrossRef] [PubMed]
185. Peng, S.; Guo, Y.; Irondelle, M.; Mazzu, A.; Kahi, M.; Ferreira Montenegro, P.; Bost, F.; Mazure, N.M. The marine-derived HIF-1α inhibitor, Yardenone 2, reduces prostate cancer cell proliferation by targeting HIF-1 target genes. *Cell. Mol. Biol. Lett.* **2024**, *9*, 101. [CrossRef] [PubMed] [PubMed Central]
186. La Civita, E.; Carbone, G.; Sicignano, E.; Crocetto, F.; Terracciano, D. Investigating periprostatic adipose tissue as a driving force of prostate cancer progression: A new source of information for the advancement of targeted therapy in metastatic prostate cancer. *J. Basic Clin. Physiol. Pharmacol.* **2023**, *34*, 245–247. [CrossRef] [PubMed]

187. Cancel, M.; Pouillot, W.; Mahéo, K.; Fontaine, A.; Crottès, D.; Fromont, G. Interplay between Prostate Cancer and Adipose Microenvironment: A Complex and Flexible Scenario. *Int. J. Mol. Sci.* **2022**, *23*, 10762. [CrossRef] [PubMed] [PubMed Central]
188. Fenercioglu, A.K. The Anti-Inflammatory Roles of Vitamin D for Improving Human Health. *Curr. Issues Mol. Biol.* **2024**, *46*, 13514–13525. [CrossRef] [PubMed] [PubMed Central]
189. Krumina, E.; Ocanto, A.; Couñago, F. Vitamin D and prostate cancer prevention. *World J. Clin. Oncol.* **2024**, *15*, 691–694. [CrossRef] [PubMed] [PubMed Central]
190. Bennour, I.; Haroun, N.; Sicard, F.; Mounien, L.; Landrier, J.F. Recent insights into vitamin D, adipocyte, and adipose tissue biology. *Obes. Rev.* **2022**, *23*, e13453. [CrossRef] [PubMed]
191. Cagigas, M.L.; Fiorito, G.; Bertozzi, B.; Masedunskas, A.; Cava, E.; Spelta, F.; Veronese, N.; Tosti, V.; Rajakumar, G.; Pelaia, T.; et al. Effects of protein restriction on insulin-like growth factor (IGF)-1 in men with prostate cancer: Results from a randomized clinical trial. *Biomark. Res.* **2024**, *12*, 68. [CrossRef] [PubMed] [PubMed Central]
192. Kord-Varkaneh, H.; Rinaldi, G.; Hekmatdoost, A.; Fatahi, S.; Tan, S.C.; Shadnoush, M.; Khani, V.; Mousavi, S.M.; Zarezadeh, M.; Salamat, S.; et al. The influence of vitamin D supplementation on IGF-1 levels in humans: A systematic review and meta-analysis. *Ageing Res. Rev.* **2020**, *57*, 100996. [CrossRef] [PubMed]
193. Guzey, M.; Jukic, D.; Arlotti, J.; Acquafondata, M.; Dhir, R.; Getzenberg, R.H. Increased apoptosis of periprostatic adipose tissue in VDR null mice. *J. Cell. Biochem.* **2004**, *93*, 133–141. [CrossRef] [PubMed]
194. Tat, D.; Kenfield, S.A.; Cowan, J.E.; Broering, J.M.; Carroll, P.R.; Van Blarigan, E.L.; Chan, J.M. Milk and other dairy foods in relation to prostate cancer recurrence: Data from the cancer of the prostate strategic urologic research endeavor (CaPSURE™). *Prostate* **2018**, *78*, 32–39. [CrossRef] [PubMed] [PubMed Central]
195. Torfadottir, J.E.; Steingrimsdottir, L.; Mucci, L.; Aspelund, T.; Kasperzyk, J.L.; Olafsson, O.; Fall, K.; Tryggvadottir, L.; Harris, T.B.; Launer, L.; et al. Milk intake in early life and risk of advanced prostate cancer. *Am. J. Epidemiol.* **2012**, *175*, 144–153. [CrossRef] [PubMed] [PubMed Central]
196. Song, Y.; Chavarro, J.E.; Cao, Y.; Qiu, W.; Mucci, L.; Sesso, H.D.; Stampfer, M.J.; Giovannucci, E.; Pollak, M.; Liu, S.; et al. Whole milk intake is associated with prostate cancer-specific mortality among U.S. male physicians. *J. Nutr.* **2013**, *143*, 189–196. [CrossRef] [PubMed] [PubMed Central]
197. Orlich, M.J.; Mashchak, A.D.; Jaceldo-Siegl, K.; Utt, J.T.; Knutsen, S.F.; Sveen, L.E.; Fraser, G.E. Dairy foods, calcium intakes, and risk of incident prostate cancer in Adventist Health Study-2. *Am. J. Clin. Nutr.* **2022**, *116*, 314–324. [CrossRef] [PubMed] [PubMed Central]
198. Zhao, Z.; Wu, D.; Gao, S.; Zhou, D.; Zeng, X.; Yao, Y.; Xu, Y.; Zeng, G. The association between dairy products consumption and prostate cancer risk: A systematic review and meta-analysis. *Br. J. Nutr.* **2023**, *129*, 1714–1731. [CrossRef] [PubMed]
199. Melnik, B.C.; John, S.M.; Carrera-Bastos, P.; Cordain, L. The impact of cow's milk-mediated mTORC1-signaling in the initiation and progression of prostate cancer. *Nutr. Metab.* **2012**, *9*, 74. [CrossRef] [PubMed] [PubMed Central]
200. Dodd, K.M.; Tee, A.R. Leucine and mTORC1: A complex relationship. *Am. J. Physiol. Endocrinol. Metab.* **2012**, *302*, E1329–E1342. [CrossRef] [PubMed]
201. Tee, A.R. Metastatic castration-resistant prostate cancer hungers for leucine. *J. Natl. Cancer Inst.* **2013**, *105*, 1427–1428. [CrossRef] [PubMed]
202. Wang, Q.; Bailey, C.G.; Ng, C.; Tiffen, J.; Thoeng, A.; Minhas, V.; Lehman, M.L.; Hendy, S.C.; Buchanan, G.; Nelson, C.C.; et al. Androgen receptor and nutrient signaling pathways coordinate the demand for increased amino acid transport during prostate cancer progression. *Cancer Res.* **2011**, *71*, 7525–7536. [CrossRef] [PubMed]
203. Wang, Q.; Tiffen, J.; Bailey, C.G.; Lehman, M.L.; Ritchie, W.; Fazli, L.; Metierre, C.; Feng, Y.J.; Li, E.; Gleave, M.; et al. Targeting amino acid transport in metastatic castration-resistant prostate cancer: Effects on cell cycle, cell growth, and tumor development. *J. Natl. Cancer Inst.* **2013**, *105*, 1463–1473. [CrossRef] [PubMed]
204. Mentoor, I.; Engelbrecht, A.M.; van Jaarsveld, P.J.; Nell, T. Chemoresistance: Intricate Interplay between Breast Tumor Cells and Adipocytes in the Tumor Microenvironment. *Front. Endocrinol.* **2018**, *9*, 758. [CrossRef] [PubMed] [PubMed Central]
205. Wade, C.A.; Kyprianou, N. Adipose tissue: Enabler of prostate cancer aggressive behavior. *Transl. Androl. Urol.* **2019**, *8* (Suppl. S3), S242–S245. [CrossRef] [PubMed] [PubMed Central]
206. Liermann-Wooldrik, K.T.; Kosmacek, E.A.; Oberley-Deegan, R.E. Adipose Tissues Have Been Overlooked as Players in Prostate Cancer Progression. *Int. J. Mol. Sci.* **2024**, *25*, 12137. [CrossRef] [PubMed] [PubMed Central]
207. Blomme, A.; Peter, C.; Mui, E.; Rodriguez Blanco, G.; An, N.; Mason, L.M.; Jamieson, L.E.; McGregor, G.H.; Lilla, S.; Ntala, C.; et al. THEM6-mediated reprogramming of lipid metabolism supports treatment resistance in prostate cancer. *EMBO Mol. Med.* **2022**, *14*, e14764. [CrossRef] [PubMed] [PubMed Central]
208. Choi, S.M.; Kam, S.C. Metabolic effects of androgen deprivation therapy. *Korean J. Urol.* **2015**, *56*, 12–18. [CrossRef] [PubMed] [PubMed Central]

209. Lam, T.; Birzniece, V.; McLean, M.; Gurney, H.; Hayden, A.; Cheema, B.S. The Adverse Effects of Androgen Deprivation Therapy in Prostate Cancer and the Benefits and Potential Anti-oncogenic Mechanisms of Progressive Resistance Training. *Sports Med. Open.* **2020**, *6*, 13. [CrossRef] [PubMed] [PubMed Central]
210. Sheng, X.; Parmentier, J.H.; Tucci, J.; Pei, H.; Cortez-Toledo, O.; Dieli-Conwright, C.M.; Oberley, M.J.; Neely, M.; Orgel, E.; Louie, S.G.; et al. Adipocytes Sequester and Metabolize the Chemotherapeutic Daunorubicin. *Mol. Cancer Res.* **2017**, *15*, 1704–1713. [CrossRef] [PubMed] [PubMed Central]
211. Liotti, A.; La Civita, E.; Cennamo, M.; Crocetto, F.; Ferro, M.; Guadagno, E.; Insabato, L.; Imbimbo, C.; Palmieri, A.; Mirone, V.; et al. Periprostatic adipose tissue promotes prostate cancer resistance to docetaxel by paracrine IGF-1 upregulation of TUBB2B beta-tubulin isoform. *Prostate* **2021**, *81*, 407–417. [CrossRef]
212. Nami, B.; Wang, Z. Genetics and Expression Profile of the Tubulin Gene Superfamily in Breast Cancer Subtypes and Its Relation to Taxane Resistance. *Cancers* **2018**, *10*, 274. [CrossRef]
213. Melnik, B.C.; John, S.M.; Carrera-Bastos, P.; Schmitz, G. MicroRNA-21-Enriched Exosomes as Epigenetic Regulators in Melanomagenesis and Melanoma Progression: The Impact of Western Lifestyle Factors. *Cancers* **2020**, *12*, 2111. [CrossRef] [PubMed] [PubMed Central]
214. Wang, Y.Y.; Attané, C.; Milhas, D.; Dirat, B.; Dauvillier, S.; Guerard, A.; Gilhodes, J.; Lazar, I.; Alet, N.; Laurent, V.; et al. Mammary adipocytes stimulate breast cancer invasion through metabolic remodeling of tumor cells. *JCI Insight* **2017**, *2*, e87489. [CrossRef] [PubMed] [PubMed Central]
215. Jafari, N.; Kolla, M.; Meshulam, T.; Shafran, J.S.; Qiu, Y.; Casey, A.N.; Pompa, I.R.; Ennis, C.S.; Mazzeo, C.S.; Rabhi, N.; et al. Adipocyte-derived exosomes may promote breast cancer progression in type 2 diabetes. *Sci. Signal.* **2021**, *14*, eabj2807. [CrossRef] [PubMed] [PubMed Central]
216. Dey, D.; Ghosh, S.; Mirgh, D.; Panda, S.P.; Jha, N.K.; Jha, S.K. Role of exosomes in prostate cancer and male fertility. *Drug Discov. Today* **2023**, *28*, 103791. [CrossRef] [PubMed]
217. Sánchez-Martin, S.; Altuna-Coy, A.; Arreaza-Gil, V.; Bernal-Escoté, X.; Fontgivell, J.F.G.; Ascaso-Til, H.; Segarra-Tomás, J.; Ruiz-Plazas, X.; Chacón, M.R. Tumoral periprostatic adipose tissue exovesicles-derived miR-20a-5p regulates prostate cancer cell proliferation and inflammation through the RORA gene. *J. Transl. Med.* **2024**, *22*, 661. [CrossRef] [PubMed] [PubMed Central]
218. Hsieh, A.C.; Liu, Y.; Edlind, M.P.; Ingolia, N.T.; Janes, M.R.; Sher, A.; Shi, E.Y.; Stumpf, C.R.; Christensen, C.; Bonham, M.J.; et al. The translational landscape of mTOR signalling steers cancer initiation and metastasis. *Nature* **2012**, *485*, 55–61. [CrossRef] [PubMed] [PubMed Central]
219. Zabala-Letona, A.; Arruabarrena-Aristorena, A.; Martín-Martín, N.; Fernandez-Ruiz, S.; Sutherland, J.D.; Clasquin, M.; Tomas-Cortazar, J.; Jimenez, J.; Torres, I.; Quang, P.; et al. mTORC1-dependent AMD1 regulation sustains polyamine metabolism in prostate cancer. *Nature* **2017**, *547*, 109–113; Erratum in *Nature* **2018**, *554*, 554. [CrossRef] [PubMed] [PubMed Central]
220. Tabernero, J.; Rojo, F.; Calvo, E.; Burris, H.; Judson, I.; Hazell, K.; Martinelli, E.; Ramon y Cajal, S.; Jones, S.; Vidal, L.; et al. Dose- and schedule-dependent inhibition of the mammalian target of rapamycin pathway with everolimus: A phase I tumor pharmacodynamic study in patients with advanced solid tumors. *J. Clin. Oncol.* **2008**, *26*, 1603–1610; Erratum in *J. Clin. Oncol.* **2010**, *28*, 5350. [CrossRef] [PubMed]
221. Shorning, B.Y.; Dass, M.S.; Smalley, M.J.; Pearson, H.B. The PI3K-AKT-mTOR Pathway and Prostate Cancer: At the Crossroads of AR, MAPK, and WNT Signaling. *Int. J. Mol. Sci.* **2020**, *21*, 4507. [CrossRef] [PubMed] [PubMed Central]
222. Zhang, S.; Lin, X.; Hou, Q.; Hu, Z.; Wang, Y.; Wang, Z. Regulation of mTORC1 by amino acids in mammalian cells: A general picture of recent advances. *Anim. Nutr.* **2021**, *7*, 1009–1023. [CrossRef] [PubMed] [PubMed Central]
223. Huang, J.; Duran, A.; Reina-Campos, M.; Valencia, T.; Castilla, E.A.; Müller, T.D.; Tschöp, M.H.; Moscat, J.; Diaz-Meco, M.T. Adipocyte p62/SQSTM1 Suppresses Tumorigenesis through Opposite Regulations of Metabolism in Adipose Tissue and Tumor. *Cancer Cell* **2018**, *33*, 770–784.e6. [CrossRef] [PubMed] [PubMed Central]
224. Quail, D.F.; Joyce, J.A. Microenvironmental regulation of tumor progression and metastasis. *Nat. Med.* **2013**, *19*, 1423–1437. [CrossRef] [PubMed] [PubMed Central]
225. GBD 2021 US Obesity Forecasting Collaborators. National-level and state-level prevalence of overweight and obesity among children, adolescents, and adults in the USA, 1990–2021, and forecasts up to 2050. *Lancet* **2024**, *404*, 2278–2298. [CrossRef] [PubMed]
226. Ramadani, F.G.; Perdana, N.R.; Ringoringo, D.R.L. Body mass index, obesity and risk of prostate cancer: A systematic review and meta-analysis. *Cent. Eur. J. Urol.* **2024**, *77*, 176–188.

cancers

MDPI

Review

Role of Lutetium Radioligand Therapy in Prostate Cancer

Ignacy Książek [1], Artur Ligęza [1], Franciszek Drzymała [1], Adam Borek [1], Marcin Miszczyk [2,3,*], Marcin Radosław Francuz [1], Akihiro Matsukawa [2,4], Takafumi Yanagisawa [4], Tamás Fazekas [5,6], Łukasz Zapała [7] and Paweł Rajwa [1,2,*]

1 Department of Urology, Medical University of Silesia, 41-800 Zabrze, Poland; ignacyk98@gmail.com (I.K.); adam_b1998@interia.pl (A.B.)
2 Department of Urology, Medical University of Vienna, 1090 Vienna, Austria
3 Collegium Medicum—Faculty of Medicine, WSB University, 41-300 Dąbrowa Górnicza, Poland
4 Department of Urology, Jikei University School of Medicine, Tokyo 105-8461, Japan
5 Department of Urology, Semmelweis University, 1085 Budapest, Hungary
6 Centre for Translational Medicine, Semmelweis University, 1085 Budapest, Hungary
7 Clinic of General, Oncological and Functional Urology, Medical University of Warsaw, 02-091 Warsaw, Poland
* Correspondence: marcinmmiszczyk@gmail.com (M.M.); pawelgrajwa@gmail.com (P.R.)

Simple Summary: Lutetium-177-PSMA—a radiopharmaceutical composed of a radionuclide lutetium-177 and a PSMA-binding ligand—is a theranostic medicine for prostate cancer. In this review, a summary of the impact of this drug on castration-resistant prostate cancer, hormone-sensitive prostate cancer, and localized prostate cancer is provided. Available data demonstrate that ^{177}Lu-PSMA could be a successful therapy in those types of prostate cancers, but it is not without adverse effects. Conclusions revealed the need for further well-designed high-quality controlled trials to evaluate long-term outcomes and effectiveness.

Abstract: Theranostics utilize ligands that chelate radionuclides and selectively bind with cancer-specific membrane antigens. In the case of prostate cancer (PCa), the state-of-the-art lutetium-177-PSMA combines the radioactive β-emitter ^{177}Lu with Vipivotide Tetraxetan, a prostate-specific membrane antigen (PSMA)-binding ligand. Several studies have been conducted, and the therapy is not without adverse effects (e.g., xerostomia, nausea, and fatigue); however, few events are reported as severe. The available evidence supports the use of ^{177}Lu-PSMA in selected metastatic castration-resistant prostate cancer patients, and the treatment is considered a standard of care in several clinical scenarios. Emerging research shows promising results in the setting of hormone-sensitive prostate cancer; however, evidence from high-quality controlled trials is still missing. In this review, we discuss the available evidence for the application of ^{177}Lu-PSMA in the management of PCa patients.

Keywords: prostate cancer; Lutetium-177-PSMA; radioactive isotopes; radiation therapy

1. Introduction

The treatment of prostate cancer (PC) has evolved significantly over the years—surgical techniques, chemotherapy, abundant forms of radiotherapy, androgen receptor signaling inhibitors (ARSIs), agonists and antagonists of luteinizing hormone-releasing hormone (LHRH), and poly (ADP-ribose) polymerase inhibitors (PARPi) represent the treatment landscape of PC. However, there are many effects associated with these treatments [1–3]. Despite a favorable prognosis in the localized and regional stages, patients with distant cancer still have a poor prognosis [4,5]. Therefore, novel agents are being investigated to elevate both the life expectancy and quality of life (QoL) of patients with advanced PC. One promising group of anti-cancer agents is based on theranostics, which describes a technique that, depending on the radionuclide and ligand, can be used for both therapeutic and diagnostic purposes. Molecularly-targeted radioligand therapies include the alpha and beta-emitters actinium-225 and lutetium-177.

Lutetium-177-PSMA is a radiopharmaceutical composed of a radionuclide lutetium-177 attached to a transmembrane glycoprotein known as prostate-specific membrane antigen (PSMA), also referred to as glutamate carboxypeptidase II or folate hydrolase. Conceptually, this should lead to highly selective delivery of radiation to the metastatic lesions, similar to radiotherapy-based metastasis-directed therapy (MDT) [6–8]. Lutetium-177 is an unstable isotope ($T_{1/2}$ = 6.65 days) produced in a particle accelerator called a cyclotron through the irradiation of ^{176}Lu or ^{176}Yb. The use of ^{176}Lu is considered the direct route, as its primary product is ^{177}Lu. Conversely, the utilization of ^{176}Yb is termed the indirect route due to the short-lived intermediate ^{177}Yb. Vipivotide tetraxetan chelates the radionuclide ^{177}Lu and binds to human prostate-specific membrane antigens. Once administered intravenously, ^{177}Lu-PSMA is distributed to targeted tissues within 2.5 h. There are no identified enzymes or transporters that interact with vipivotide tetraxetan ^{177}Lu. Approximately 60–70% of ^{177}Lu vipivotide tetraxetan binds to human plasma proteins and is primarily eliminated through the kidneys in its unchanged form. A decrease in creatinine clearance may extend exposure time, though the drug itself does not appear to be nephrotoxic. However, in the VISION trial, several cases of renal disorders were observed [9]. A portion of the drug can bind to the salivary glands, leading to a dry mouth. Higher tumor burden correlates with lower doses observed in other organs [10–12]. Post-administration, ^{177}Lu decays to stable hafnium-177, emitting beta particles with a maximum energy of 0.497 MeV and maximal tissue penetration of 2 mm. This helps minimize damage to non-tumor tissues [13–15]. Moreover, gamma particles are emitted too, which is used in prostate cancer imaging [16].

The most studied theranostic PSMA ligands (PSMA-617 and PSMA Imaging and Therapy) are appropriate for therapeutic usage and have similar in vivo behavior, toxicity profiles, and efficacy in metastatic castration-resistant prostate cancer (mCRPC) patients [17]. Unlike normal tissues, prostate cancer cells express PSMA at levels substantially higher than those found in the kidney, gut, and salivary gland tissues. Therefore, these agents accumulate specifically in prostate cancer cells, causing DNA damage and signaling cell death while sparing healthy tissue [17,18]. Emerging prospective data suggests these agents' efficacy is similar to that of cabazitaxel and beneficial for heavily pretreated patients with mCRPC [9,19]. In numerous early-phase investigations, radioligand therapy exhibits encouraging biochemical and radiographic response rates, reduced pain, and tolerable toxicity [9]. These studies are summarized in Tables 1 and 2. The objective of this narrative review is to evaluate the existing evidence on the use of ^{177}Lu-PSMA radioligand therapy in managing PC.

Table 1. The basic characteristics of the studies on the use of ^{177}Lu-PSMA in the treatment of prostate cancer (original work).

Study	Phase	Type of Study	Origin (Country)	Patients Total S Arm (Study) C Arm (Control)	Median Age	Primary mCRPC or Pre-Treated	PSA Response	Recruitment Years	Follow up Period	Drugs Used
					mCRPC					
VISION trial, Sartor et al. [9]	3	Open-label, randomized prospective	International	S 551 C 280	S 70.0 C 71.5	Pre-treated	S 71.5% C 35.5%	2018–2019	20.9 months	^{177}Lu-PSMA-617
TheraP Hofman et al. [19]	2	Prospective randomized, open-label	Australia	S 99 C 101	S 72.1 C 71.8	Pre-treated	S 66% C 37%	2018–2019	Mean 18.4 months	S ^{177}Lu-PSMA-617 C Cabazitaxel
Satapathy et al. [20]	2	Parallel group	India	S 20 C 20	68	no chemotherapy, only novel androgen-axis drugs	S 50% C 40%	2019–2021	20 months	^{177}LuPSM-617, docetaxel
Barber et al. [21]	-	Retrospective	Australia	S1 83 S2 84	S1 69,3 S2 70.8	Pre-treated and naïve.	S1 40% S2 57%	2013–2016	10.6 months	^{177}Lu-PSMA-617 and ^{177}Lu-PSMA-I&T
Baum et al. [22]	2	Single-center prospective	Germany	S 56	72	Pre-treated	S 80.4%	2013–2015	Median 15 months, total 28 months	^{177}Lu-PSMA
LuPSMA trial Hofman et al. [23]	2	Prospective single-arm	Australia	S 30	71	Pre-treated	S 97%	2015–2016	12 weeks	^{177}Lu-PSMA-617
Violet et al. [24]	2	Prospective	Australia	S 50	71	Pre-treated	S 64%	2015–2016, 2017	Mean 31.4 months	^{177}Lu-PSMA-617
Rahbar et al. [25]	-	Retrospective	Germany	S 104	70	Pre-treated	Any—67% decline $\geq$50% −33%	2014–2016	Overall survival	^{177}Lu-PSMA-617
					Localized PC					
Golan et al. [26]	1	Single-arm clinical trial	Israel	S 14	67	Primary	after 2 doses, 64% after 3 doses, 75%	2019–2021	12 months	^{177}Lu-PSMA
LuTectomy Dhiantravan et al. [27]	1/2	Single-arm Study open-label nonrandomised	Australia	S 20	66	Primary	45%	2020–2022	36 months	^{177}Lu-PSMA (later prostatectomy + pelvic nodes dissection)
					mHSPC					
Privé et al. [28]	1	Prospective Pilot Study	Netherlands	S 10	67.2	Primary	No Data	2018–2019	10.6 months	^{177}Lu-PSMA
BULLSEYE trial Prive et al. [29]	2	Two-arm randomized open-label	Netherlands	S 29 C 29	No data	only local therapy, no hormonal or chemotherapy	No data	2020–2023	6 months	^{177}Lu-PSMA-I&T

Table 2. Information summary of 12 studies on the use of ^{177}Lu-PSMA in the treatment of prostate cancer (original work).

Study	Inclusion Criteria	Exclusion Criteria	HR, OR	Adverse Events	Notable Findings	Overall Effect
			mCRPC			
VISION trial, Sartor et al. [9]	Adults with CRPC with at least one metastatic lesion Disease progression after anti-androgen treatment (abiraterone and enzalutamide)	Any PSMA-negative lesions Eastern Cooperative Oncology Group performance score of—through 2 (0–5 scale) Life expectancy of at least 6 months Adequate organ/bone marrow function	HR for progression or death: 0.40 (CI 99.2%) HR for overall survival: 0.62 (CI 95%)	Fatigue Dry mouth Nausea Anemia Back pain Arthralgia Decreased appetite Constipation Diarrhea Vomiting Thrombocytopenia Lymphopenia Leukopenia	Low rate of adverse events Extended overall survival in a population with androgen-receptor pathway inhibitor-resistant disease	Overall survival versus standard care alone-: 4 months Progression-free versus standard care alone: 5.3 months
TheraP Hofman et al. [19]	PSMA-positive disease no sites of metastatic disease with discordant FDG-positive and PSMA-negative findings	Low uptake on [68Ga]Ga-PSMA-11 PET-CT discordant	HR for delayed progression: 0.63 (CI 95%)	Fatigue Pain Dry mouth Diarrhea Nausea Thrombocytopenia Dry eyes Anaemia Neuropathy Dysgeusia Haematuria Neutropenia Insomnia Vomiting Dizziness Leukopenia		Outcomes were better for cabazitaxel than for [^{177}Lu]Lu-PSMA-617
Satapathy et al. [20]	Metastatic disease on 68 Ga-PSMA-11 PET/CT with significant PSMA expression Chemotherapy-naive, however, patients with prior treatment of NAADs were included. ECOG 0-2 adequate hematological, renal, and liver function	Histological evidence of sarcomatous, spindle-cell or small-cell differentiation, and Sjogren syndrome	No data	Nausea/vomiting Constipation Fatigue Dryness of the mouth or eyes Abdominal pain Generalized pain Loss of weight or appetite Hematological toxicity Nephrotoxicity Hepatotoxicity	The outcomes are not significantly different between the two arms; one possible explanation for this could be the relatively higher tumor burden in the ^{177}Lu-PSMA-617 arm. This is evident from the higher median baseline PSA.	^{177}Lu-PSMA-617 was demonstrated to be non-inferior to docetaxel. Moreover, ^{177}Lu-PSMA-617 was tolerated well vis-à-vis docetaxel, with less frequent grade 3/4 adverse events.

Table 2. *Cont.*

Study	Inclusion Criteria	Exclusion Criteria	HR, OR	Adverse Events	Notable Findings	Overall Effect
Barber et al. [21]	Selection for ^{177}Lu-PRLT was based on PSMA-avid metastatic disease confirmed on pretherapy 68Ga-PSMA PET/CT imaging. In this study, patients were classified as either taxane che-motherapy pretreated (T-pretreated) or naïve (T-naïve) depending on whether they had received taxane-based chemotherapy (first- or second-line) prior to ^{177}Lu-PRLT	T-naive patients who had been previously treated with non-taxane-based cytotoxic chemotherapy before ^{177}Lu-PRLT were excluded from this analysis.	No data	Hematologic toxicity Anemia Leukocytopenia Thrombocytopenia Renal toxicity Creatinine Hepatic toxicity	^{177}Lu-PRLT is a promising therapy in mCRPC, with encouraging outcomes and minimal associated toxicity seen in both our T-naive and heavily pretreated patient cohorts.	^{177}Lu-PRLT was safe, with minimal adverse effects evident during follow-up in both T-pretreated and T-naive patients.
Baum et al. [22]	PSMA expression, progressive mCRPC, rising prostate-specific antigen (PSA) levels, 68Ga-PSMA PET/CT before therapy, renal function, hematologic status, previous treatments, and Karnofsky Performance Status score	No data	No data	Mild reversible xerostomia, reduction in erythrocyte and leukocyte counts, leukocytopenia	Safe and effective, objective responses with minimal toxicity in patients whose prostate cancer had progressed despite all standard treatments	PSMA RLT with ^{177}Lu-PSMA is feasible, safe, and effective in end-stage progressive mCRPC with appropriate selection and follow-up of patients by 68Ga-PSMA PET/CT through application of the concept of theranostics.
LuPSMA trial Hofman et al. [23]	Pathologically (adenocarcinoma) confirmed metastatic castration-resistant prostate cancer with progressive disease after standard treatments, including taxane-based chemotherapy and second-generation anti-androgen treatment (abiraterone, enzalutamide, or both).	Low PSMA-avidity or FDG-discordant disease	No data	Dry mouth Lymphocytopenia Thrombocytopenia Fatigue Nausea Anaemia Neutropenia Pain Vomiting Anorexia Dry eyes Weight loss Disseminated intravascular coagulation Oculomotor nerve disorder Spinal fracture Hip fracture	Improved cognitive functioning and insomnia	^{177}Lu-PSMA was well tolerated and could be a useful therapeutic option for mCRPC.

Table 2. *Cont.*

Study	Inclusion Criteria	Exclusion Criteria	HR, OR	Adverse Events	Notable Findings	Overall Effect
Violet et al. [24]	Pathologically confirmed mCRPC with progressive disease after taxane-based chemotherapy and second-generation antiandrogen therapy (abiraterone, enzalutamide, or both). Radiographic progression or new pain in an area of radiographically evident disease and an ECOG Performance Status of 2 or less must have occurred within 12 months. Tumor SUVmax (standardized uptake value) had to be at least 1.5 times the liver SUVmean to indicate PSMA intensity at disease sites.	Significant hematologic abnormalities, renal or liver insufficiency Prior to radiotherapy within 6 weeks, or uncontrolled disease. PET showed major discordant disease sites: 18F-FDG-positive and PSMA-negative.	No data	Dry mouth Lymphocytopenia Thrombocytopenia Fatigue Nausea Anemia Neutropenia Bone pain Vomiting Anorexia Dry eyes Renal injury	Long-term outcomes (after LuPSMA trial) high therapeutic efficacy and low toxicity, improvement in QoL in multiple domains. high response rates but less durable responses in patients rechallenged with ^{177}Lu-PSMA on progression	High response rates, low toxicity, and improved QoL with ^{177}Lu-PSMA radioligand therapy. On progression, rechallenge ^{177}Lu-PSMA demonstrated higher response rates than other systemic therapies.
Rakhbar et al. [25]	Interdisciplinary tumor board, lacking other therapeutic options and disease progression despite established therapies according to mCRPC management guidelines, treated with ^{177}Lu-PSMA-617, received at least one line of chemotherapy (docetaxel and/or cabazitaxel) and at least one next-generation antihormonal therapy (enzalutamide and/or abiraterone), and PSMA imaging was performed in all patients using 68Ga-PSMA-11 PET-CT or PET-MRI.	Bone marrow depression, Abnormal renal or liver function, upper urinary tract obstruction	HR 0.38 (CI 95%) (any PSA response vs. PSA progression) HR 0.28 (CI 95%) (PSA decline ≥20.87% as cutpoint)	No data	PSA decline ≥20.87% as the most noticeable cut-off prognosticating longer survival, which remained an independent prognosticator of improved OS in the multivariate analysis.	^{177}Lu-PSMA-617 RLT is a new effective therapeutic and seems to prolong survival in patients with advanced mCRPC pretreated with chemotherapy, abiraterone, and/or enzalutamide.

Table 2. *Cont.*

Study	Inclusion criteria	Exclusion Criteria	HR, OR	Adverse Events	Notable Findings	Overall Effect
			Localized PC			
Golan et al. [26]	Adult with high-risk localized prostate cancer (cT3/4, Gleason score $\geq$ 8, prostate biopsy, PSA $\geq$ 20 ng/dL) or loco-regional prostate cancer (pelvic lymphadenopathy $\geq$ 2 cm on axial imaging). PET/CT PSMA showed higher PSMA expression than the liver. There were no PET FDG-positive sites without high PSMA expression. Patients should have an ECOG performance status score of 1 or lower. Life expectancy is >10 years.	Radiotherapy within two months. Combining nephrotoxic drugs. Distal lymphadenopathy, visceral, or bone metastases. Renal or liver insufficiency, hematologic abnormalities	No data	Nausea, Fatigue, Xerostomia	^{177}Lu-PSMA, followed by RARP, seems to be tolerated similarly to RARP alone and has a high safety profile.	Absence of serious systemic adverse effects. Histological examination shows typical radiation-induced changes.
LuTectomy Dhiantravan et al. [27]	An adult with histologically verified adenocarcinoma of the prostate, planned for radical prostatectomy and pelvic lymph node dissection with the objective to cure. Classified as having high- or intermediate risk localized or loco-regional prostate cancer, in accordance with the European Association of Urology's criteria. Significant PSMA avidity on 68 Ga-PSMA PET/CT—SUVmax of 20 or greater. Hematological and serum biochemistry parameters fall within normal ranges.	Rare prostate cancer with neuroendocrine or other pathology. Past prostate cancer treatment with radiotherapy or androgen deprivation. Any metastasis or lymph nodes above the common iliac artery bifurcation. Renal impairment Sjogren syndrome Any conditions, treatments, or laboratory abnormalities that could confound the trial results	No data	No data	No data	The first results will be known in June 2023.

Table 2. *Cont.*

Study	Inclusion Criteria	Exclusion Criteria	HR, OR	Adverse Events	Notable Findings	Overall Effect
			mHSPC			
Privé et al. [28]	Prostate histological adenocarcinoma, Over 50 years old Prior local therapy with biochemical recurrence or clinical progression PSA doubling time: <6 months Local treatment is no longer viable 68Ga-PSMA-11-PET/CT positive metastases in bones and/or lymph nodes: ≥1 to 10 metastases (at least 1 lesion ≥1 cm for dosimetry studies) Free of visceral metastases. Normal liver function and blood count	68Ga-PSMA-11-PET/CT showed no lesions below the liver uptake. An alternative to prostate adenocarcinoma. Any medical condition that the investigator believes will affect patients' clinical status in this trial. Prior hip replacement surgery Contraindications for MRI, Glucagon, or Buscopan	No data	Fatigue Nausea Xerostomia Rash Pain	Findings regarding both toxicity and efficacy are performed in a small cohort of selected patients.	^{177}Lu-PSMA appeared to be a feasible and safe treatment modality in ten patients with low-volume mHSPC. Although the patients were treated with a relatively low dose of ^{177}Lu-PSMA, the majority of patients showed a promising response to this therapy. This supports the need for the following trials to further evaluate the efficacy of ^{177}Lu-PSMA in low-volume metastatic disease as well as in HSPC.
BULLSEYE trial Privé et al. [29]	Histologically proven prostate adenocarcinoma Biochemical recurrence and PSA-doubling time < 6 months. Positive 18F-PSMA-PET/CT metastases in bones and/or lymph nodes (N1/M1ab): ≥1 to 5 metastases. Local treatment is no longer possible. No prior hormonal, docetaxel or cabazitaxel therapy Lesion with an SUVmax > 15 ECOG Performance Status: 0–1. Life expectancy is >6 months. Normal liver and renal function, along with blood count	Known subtypes other than prostate adenocarcinoma, PSMA-based radioligand treatment, visceral or brain metastases, Any medical condition the investigator believes will affect patients' clinical status in this trial. Prior hip replacement. Sjogren's Syndrome Another active cancer is prostate cancer. Sexually active patients who cannot use medically acceptable barrier contraception.	No data	The study is not finished.	Patients in the SOC arm are eligible to receive ^{177}Lu-PSMA-I&T after meeting the primary study objective, which is the fraction of patients who show disease progression during the study follow-up.	The study is not finished.

2. mCRPC

The mCRPC represents an advanced stage of PC with a notably poor prognosis due to resistance to androgen deprivation therapy (ADT). In this terminal disease phase, the treatment often comprises docetaxel, abiraterone/prednisolone (AAP), enzalutamide, cabazitaxel, olaparib, niraparib/AAP, and talazoparib/enzalutamide [30]. However, these therapeutic strategies often come with numerous adverse effects and limited efficacy. Patients with mCRPC are first-choice candidates for enrollment in clinical trials that evaluate novel, promising molecules for PC treatment. Notable studies conducted on a large patient cohort include the Phase 3 VISION trial by Sartor et al. [9]. However, despite the high number of patients included, the study provides a limited understanding of the role of ^{177}Lu due to sub-standard treatment methods in the control arm and highly unbalanced dropout rates between arms [31]. It is possible that a considerable number of patients discontinue participation due to the availability of more efficient standard-of-care (SoC) therapeutic options than those allowed in the control arm, such as taxane-based chemotherapy.

Noteworthy is that ^{177}Lu-PSMA efficacy was evaluated in heavily pretreated mCRPC patients and compared against a few SoC therapies [9,19]. Several moderators of ^{177}Lu-PSMA-617 efficacy were identified, including the clinical stage at ^{177}Lu-PSMA-617 treatment initiation, prior taxane-based chemotherapy, or prostate-specific antigen (PSA) decline following drug administration. In two studies, ^{177}Lu-PSMA was compared to chemotherapy in chemotherapy-naive patients [20,21], and two studies compared ^{177}Lu-PSMA against chemotherapy, suggesting non-inferiority of the treatment [19,20]. However, both studies used intermediate clinical endpoints, such as progression-free survival (PFS) and PSA response, that were recently shown to be insufficient for overall survival (OS) surrogacy, and survival outcomes need to be analyzed to verify the non-inferiority of the treatment [32,33].

In the TheraP study, there was no statistically significant difference in PFS between patients treated with ^{177}Lu-PSMA and cabazitaxel [19]. Sartor et al. demonstrated an improvement in both OS (HR 0.62) (95% CI; 0.52 to 0.74; p < 0,001) and PFS (HR 0.4) (99.2% CI; 0.29 to 0.57; p < 0.001) in the study group. However, it is important to note that the trial included restrictive criteria for SoC therapy in the control group, which led to many patients being offered possibly sub-standard therapy, and unbalanced dropout rates between arms [9]. For example, the median PFS duration varied depending on whether the patient had prior taxane treatment (6 vs. 8.8 months; pre-treated vs. taxane-naïve) [21]. In a retrospective analysis by Barber et al., the median overall survival was higher in taxane-naive patients, lasting up to 27.1 months [21]. Sartor et al. prove that patients who underwent SoC and chemotherapy experienced a median overall survival between 11.3 and 15.3 months [9].

Although the objective responses achieved in this single-center prospective clinical trial showed promising results with minimal toxicity, it is important to note that the study had certain limitations. There were no specific initial criteria for selecting patients, and the patients were a diverse group. The individuals seeking medical treatment varied widely. PSMA RLT was considered a logical therapeutic choice, and the decision to pursue this treatment was made by oncologists and urologists after exploring all other available options [22]. It is recommended to implement lutetium treatment and include it in clinical trials at earlier disease stages, using the same criteria for inclusion and exclusion as in other studies, to facilitate comparison [9,19–25].

2.1. Long-Term Response

Several authors reported that reaching a given PSA reduction threshold is an indicator of a long-term response. An association between longer median PFS and PSA declines of over 50% was found by Hoffman et al. [23]. While ^{177}Lu-PSMA appeared to induce a greater PSA decline than Cabazitaxel and Ra-223 [19,23], Violet et al. found that patients with a PSA decline of over 50% exhibited significantly longer median overall survival compared to those with less than 50% (18.4 months vs. 8.7 months) [24]. Rahbar et al. suggested that a PSA decline of approximately 20% is the most significant prognostic predictor for longer survival (HR 0.28) [25]. While these findings show that the concept of biochemical response is a promising predictor of survival in patients treated with ^{177}Lu, it must also be noted that a posteriori analyses introduce a significant immortal-time bias and that biochemical endpoints were shown to be insufficient surrogates of survival in both metastatic hormone-sensitive prostate cancer (mHSPC) and mCRPC patients [32,33].

Furthermore, attention should be drawn to PSMA-based radioligand treatment in homologous recombination repair (HRR)-deficient PC patients. HRR deficiency is a phenotype defined by a cell's incapacity to use the HRR pathway to efficiently repair double-strand DNA breaks. Privé et al. reported that DNA damage repair defects are not significantly associated with exceptional responsiveness to PSMA therapy [33,34]. However, further studies in larger prospective cohorts are necessary to verify the association between DNA damage repair gene defects and differential responses to PSMA-RLT.

2.2. *Quality of Life*

When assessing treatment options, the impact on a patient's QoL should be carefully considered, with special emphasis on pain relief, as it can significantly enhance a patient's life quality. For individuals with mCRPC, it is crucial to focus on improving their QoL and minimizing harmful treatment side effects, considering that many are already burdened with disease symptoms. ^{177}Lu-PSMA seems especially adept at relieving pain, with a considerable number of patients reporting rapid relief following the initial treatment cycle. Among 27 patients who had initial pain, 37% noted improvement after their first treatment round. This amount of pain reduction is promising and is comparable to that obtained with other medications, such as cabazitaxel. However, particular attention should be paid to the level of pain that patients enroll in the trial with, as this may affect the test results and interpretation of the efficacy of lutetium [23]. The therapy also showed greater improvements in fatigue, social functioning, and insomnia compared to cabazitaxel. Therefore, ^{177}Lu-PSMA-617 may be appropriate for individuals who are ineligible for other forms of therapy owing to age or comorbidities [19]. Another study indicated that ^{177}Lu-PSMA-617 had improved health-related QoL compared to docetaxel. More extensive studies should be conducted with larger groups of participants to assess how ^{177}Lu-PSMA-617 performs against other interventions in the initial treatment of mCRPC [20]. According to all the studies conducted, the treatment has exhibited minimal toxicity and high tolerability, with rare occurrences of dose reduction or discontinuation of the medication [9,19–25].

2.3. *Take Home Message*

Further research is required to investigate correlations between the effectiveness of ^{177}Lu-PSMA at different dosages, as well as to evaluate long-term outcomes in a larger patient cohort, building upon studies such as Satapathy et al. Currently, the available evidence suggests that ^{177}Lu-PSMA is a successful therapy with tolerable toxicity rates for heavily pretreated mCRPC patients expressing PSMA who have progressed after other lines of therapy. The results of mCRPC research serve as a foundation for further studies in other patient groups, such as localized PCa and mHSPC [20,21,24,25].

3. Localized

The unequivocal role of neoadjuvant therapies, such as chemohormonal or androgen deprivation therapy, for unfavorable localized prostate cancer is yet to be determined. Despite the absence of concrete evidence demonstrating improvement in oncological outcomes from neoadjuvant therapy preceding radical prostatectomy [35,36], nearly 65% of patients require supplemental therapy post-surgery, and a third will ultimately experience progression [37,38]. In such cases, ^{177}Lu-PSMA emerges as a promising agent due to its direct targeting of cancer cells, inclusive of micrometastases, potentially preventing disease progression.

Golan et al. conducted a clinical trial with 14 patients with high-risk localized prostate cancer [26]. Before robot-assisted radical prostatectomy (RARP), patients were treated with

2–3 doses of ^{177}Lu-PSMA administered at two-week intervals. The median PSA reduction registered was 3.45 ng/mL (IQR 0.4–5.2) after two, and 4.3 ng/mL (IQR 0.92–6.8) after three ^{177}Lu-PSMA doses. The salivary gland damage was reduced by applying ice packs 10 min before and 30 min post-administration. All prostatic specimens showed adenocarcinoma upon histological examination, with a positive surgical margin observed in seven patients (53%). Radiation-induced changes, such as clear vacuolated cytoplasm and pyknotic nuclei, were evident. The authors did not observe anatomical alterations in the prostate area, and no significant intraoperative complications were recorded. Most patients required one or fewer pads three months post-surgery, and 50% retained erections. Overall, the treatment was well-tolerated [26]. In the LuTectomy clinical trial, 20 patients received ^{177}Lu-PSMA intravenously before a planned radical prostatectomy and pelvic lymph node dissection. Almost half of the patients achieved a 50% PSA reduction at 6 weeks after administrating ^{177}Lu-PSMA, and the treatment was well tolerated. In conclusion, ^{177}Lu-PSMA shows initial efficacy as a neoadjuvant treatment before radical prostatectomy, and the treatment appears to be safe and feasible. Certain estimates suggest that ^{177}Lu-PSMA could not only augment surgery but even possibly replace it as the first line setting in selected patients in the future [27,39].

Take Home Message

^{177}Lu-PSMA appears to hold promise as a therapeutic option in the context of localized disease, in particular as a neo-adjuvant treatment. However, the preliminary results should be verified in prospective, controlled studies.

4. mHSPC

Currently, there is a wide range of approved agents for the treatment of mHSPC. Still, the backbone of the therapy involves combining ADT with ARSIs (abiraterone, apalutamide, or enzalutamide) and the option to add docetaxel. The treatment protocol also encompasses the combination of ADT, darolutamide, and docetaxel. Additionally, patients with low metastatic burden may benefit from prostate radiotherapy, cytoreductive prostatectomy, or MDT [8,40–42]. The selection of therapy should be individualized, taking into account various factors such as expected therapy results, the patient's condition, disease burden, patient preferences, and treatment toxicity. Prive et al. conducted a prospective pilot study assessing the efficacy of ^{177}Lu-PSMA in 10 patients with low-volume mHSPC [28]. Half of the patients experienced a PSA reduction of >50%, with one patient achieving an undetectable PSA. At 24 weeks after the second cycle, five patients displayed at least a partial response, with one patient revealing a complete response, and the disease progressed in four patients. The most common symptoms reported were fatigue that subsided after 2–4 weeks. Other complaints included nausea, xerostomia, rash, and pain. In laboratory tests, no signs of kidney, liver, or bone marrow damage were observed. Moderate side effects may result from using a low dose and low cycle number; hence, there is a need for further research to evaluate the safety of higher dose and cycle numbers. Currently, a third-phase clinical trial of PSMAddition is ongoing to assess the effectiveness and safety of ADT and ARSI in combination with ^{177}Lu-PSMA-617 therapy compared to androgen deprivation therapy and ARSI alone. In this study, about 1126 patients will be randomized in a 1:1 ratio and receive up to 6 cycles of ^{177}Lu-PSMA-617 (7.4 GBq) every 6 weeks [43]. BULLSEYE is an ongoing prospective randomized multicenter II phase study that compares ^{177}Lu-PSMA-617 to the current standard of care in oligometastatic HSPC. It is also being investigated whether ^{177}Lu-PSMA-617 can delay ADT [29].

Take Home Message

Preliminary results suggest that ^{177}Lu-PSMA is a promising therapy for mHSPC, but further investigation is necessary to confirm these conjectures.

5. Adverse Effects of Lutetium Therapy

Among the adverse effects of ^{177}Lu-PSMA, mild and moderate ones were predominant, with only a few incidents reported as severe or life-threatening. A significant retrospective analysis at various centers showed that xerostomia, nausea, and fatigue were experienced by 8%, 6%, and 13% of patients, respectively. Grade 3–4 hematologic adverse events were recorded in just 12% of patients, where anemia was found to occur in 10% of instances [44]. As this research was retrospective, underreporting of adverse events is a common issue and might be the case here. Prospective trials are therefore more dependable for monitoring adverse events [45]. An international phase III open-label prospective study found that the most common complications were fatigue (43.1%), dry mouth (38.8%), and nausea (35.3%), most of which were Grade 1 or 2 according to the CTCAE (Common Terminology Criteria for Adverse Events) [9]. Concerns have been raised regarding disorders of the blood and lymphatic system, with anemia being the most common. Symptoms classified as Grade 3 or higher occurred in 12.9% of patients, and overall, 31.8% of patients had anemia. Careful consideration should also be given to other conditions such as thrombocytopenia (17.2%), lymphopenia (14.2%), and leukopenia (12.5%). These hematological complications are more likely to present as grade 3 or above than non-hematological complications [9]. However, information on potential long-term adverse effects, which may be of great importance, is missing from the present study. Despite the documented side effects, just a small percentage of patients (11.9%) withdrew from treatment or needed to lower their dosage (5.7%). These findings highlight the overall safety of this therapy [9]. While previous studies have mainly focused on the immediate post-treatment period, future research should investigate the long-term effects associated with the use of ^{177}Lu-PSMA [46].

6. The Future of Lutetium Therapy

Beta emitters such as ^{177}Lu have demonstrated therapeutic efficacy in treating large tumor masses due to their long radiation range and ability to induce a cross-fire effect [47,48]. Targeted alpha-radiation therapy (TAT) using ^{225}Ac may be even more effective in treating patients with disseminated metastatic disease due to the shorter radiation range coupled with high-linear-energy transfer that induces targeted tumor cell killing by causing a higher number of double-strand DNA breaks in tumor cells, resulting in their destruction, while minimizing damage to surrounding tissues for instance red bone marrow. This treatment shows promise and requires further research with larger cohort studies. These studies should include ^{177}Lu and ^{225}Ac, as well as immunohistochemical analysis and genomic profiling of patients with mCRPC [49].

7. Conclusions

The treatment of prostate cancer is still evolving. Collected evidence supports lutetium-177-PSMA as a standard-of-care treatment for castration-resistant prostate cancer. Other research shows promising results in the management of hormone-sensitive prostate cancer and localized prostate cancer. However, therapy has its drawbacks, such as nausea, xerostomia, and fatigue. Despite optimistic results, further research is required with a larger cohort to assess long-term outcomes and efficiency with various patient groups.

Author Contributions: Conceptualization, P.R.; writing—original draft preparation, I.K., A.L., F.D. and A.B.; writing—review and editing, M.M., M.R.F., A.M., T.Y., T.F., Ł.Z. and P.R.; all authors; supervision. All authors have read and agreed to the published version of the manuscript.

Funding: This research received no external funding.

Conflicts of Interest: The authors declare no conflicts of interest.

References

1. Cao, B.; Kim, M.; Reizine, N.M.; Moreira, D.M. Adverse Events and Androgen Receptor Signaling Inhibitors in the Treatment of Prostate Cancer: A Systematic Review and Multivariate Network Meta-analysis. *Eur. Urol. Oncol.* **2023**, *6*, 237–250. [CrossRef] [PubMed]
2. Oing, C.; Bristow, R.G. Systemic treatment of metastatic hormone-sensitive prostate cancer-upfront triplet versus doublet combination therapy. *ESMO Open* **2023**, *8*, 101194. [CrossRef] [PubMed]
3. Rosario, E.; Rosario, D.J. *Localized Prostate Cancer*; StatPearls: Treasure Island, FL, USA, 2023.
4. Saad, F.; Clarke, N.W.; Oya, M.; Shore, N.; Procopio, G.; Guedes, J.D.; Arslan, C.; Mehra, N.; Parnis, F.; Brown, E.; et al. Olaparib plus abiraterone versus placebo plus abiraterone in metastatic castration-resistant prostate cancer (PROpel): Final prespecified overall survival results of a randomised, double-blind, phase 3 trial. *Lancet. Oncol.* **2023**, *24*, 1094–1108. [CrossRef] [PubMed]
5. Siegel, D.A.; O'Neil, E.M.; Richards, T.B.; Dowling, N.F.; Weir, H.K. Prostate Cancer Incidence and Survival, by Stage and Race/Ethnicity—United States, 2001–2017. *MMWR Morb. Mortal. Wkly. Rep.* **2020**, *69*, 1473–1480. [CrossRef] [PubMed]
6. Di Iorio, V.; Boschi, S.; Cuni, C.; Monti, M.; Severi, S.; Paganelli, G.; Masini, C. Production and Quality Control of [^{177}Lu]Lu-PSMA-I&T: Development of an Investigational Medicinal Product Dossier for Clinical Trials. *Molecules* **2022**, *27*, 4143. [CrossRef] [PubMed]
7. Ghosh, A.; Heston, W.D.W. Tumor target prostate specific membrane antigen (PSMA) and its regulation in prostate cancer. *J. Cell. Biochem.* **2004**, *91*, 528–539. [CrossRef] [PubMed]
8. Miszczyk, M.; Rajwa, P.; Yanagisawa, T.; Nowicka, Z.; Shim, S.R.; Laukhtina, E.; Kawada, T.; von Deimling, M.; Pradere, B.; Rivas, J.G.; et al. The Efficacy and Safety of Metastasis-directed Therapy in Patients with Prostate Cancer: A Systematic Review and Meta-analysis of Prospective Studies. *Eur. Urol.* **2024**, *85*, 125–138. [CrossRef] [PubMed]
9. Sartor, O.; De Bono, J.; Chi, K.N.; Fizazi, K.; Herrmann, K.; Rahbar, K.; Tagawa, S.T.; Nordquist, L.T.; Vaishampayan, N.; Haddad, G.E.; et al. Lutetium-177–PSMA-617 for Metastatic Castration-Resistant Prostate Cancer. *N. Engl. J. Med.* **2022**, *385*, 1091–1103. [CrossRef] [PubMed]
10. Keam, S.J. Lutetium Lu 177 Vipivotide Tetraxetan: First Approval. *Mol. Diagn. Ther.* **2022**, *26*, 467–475. [CrossRef]
11. Rosar, F.; Kochems, N.; Bartholomä, M.; Maus, S.; Stemler, T.; Linxweiler, J.; Khreish, F.; Ezziddin, S. Renal Safety of [^{177}Lu]Lu-PSMA-617 Radioligand Therapy in Patients with Compromised Baseline Kidney Function. *Cancers* **2021**, *13*, 3095. [CrossRef]
12. Violet, J.; Jackson, P.; Ferdinandus, J.; Sandhu, S.; Akhurst, T.; Iravani, A.; Kong, G.; Kumar, A.R.; Thang, S.P.; Eu, P.; et al. Dosimetry of ^{177} Lu-PSMA-617 in Metastatic Castration-Resistant Prostate Cancer: Correlations Between Pretherapeutic Imaging and Whole-Body Tumor Dosimetry with Treatment Outcomes. *J. Nucl. Med.* **2019**, *60*, 517–523. [CrossRef]
13. Vogel, W.V.; Van der Marck, S.C.; Versleijen, M.W.J. Challenges and future options for the production of lutetium-177. *Eur. J. Nucl. Med. Mol. Imaging* **2021**, *48*, 2329–2335. [CrossRef] [PubMed]
14. Dash, A.; Pillai, M.R.A.; Knapp, F.F. Production of ^{177}Lu for Targeted Radionuclide Therapy: Available Options. *Nucl. Med. Mol. Imaging* **2015**, *49*, 85–107. [CrossRef]
15. Krebs, S.; Dunphy, M. Role of nuclear medicine in diagnosis and management of hepatopancreatobiliary disease. In *Blumgart's Surgery of the Liver, Biliary Tract and Pancreas, 2-Volume Set*; Elsevier: Amsterdam, The Netherlands, 2017; pp. 285–315.e3.
16. Ghodsirad, M.A.; Pirayesh, E.; Akbarian, R.; Javanmard, B.; Kaghazchi, F.; Tavakoli, M.; Fattahi, K. Diagnostic Utility of Lutetium-177 (Lu 177) Prostate-Specific Membrane Antigen (PSMA) Scintigraphy in Prostate Cancer Patients with PSA Rise And Negative Conventional Imaging. *Urol. J.* **2020**, *17*, 374–378. [CrossRef]
17. Ling, S.W.; De Blois, E.; Hooijman, E.; Van der Veldt, A.; Brabander, T. Advances in ^{177}Lu-PSMA and 225Ac-PSMA Radionuclide Therapy for Metastatic Castration-Resistant Prostate Cancer. *Pharmaceutics* **2022**, *14*, 2166. [CrossRef]
18. Van Kalmthout, L.W.M.; Van der Sar, E.C.A.; Braat, A.J.A.T.; de Keizer, B.; Lam, M.G.E.H. Lutetium-177-PSMA therapy for prostate cancer patients—A brief overview of the literature. *Tijdschr. Voor Urol.* **2020**, *10*, 141–146. [CrossRef]
19. Hofman, M.S.; Emmett, L.; Sandhu, S.; Iravani, A.; Joshua, A.M.; Goh, J.C.; Pattison, D.A.; Tan, T.H.; Kirkwood, I.D.; Ng, S.; et al. [^{177}Lu] Lu-PSMA-617 versus cabazitaxel in patients with metastatic castration-resistant prostate cancer (TheraP): A randomised, open-label, phase 2 trial. *Lancet* **2021**, *397*, 797–804. [CrossRef] [PubMed]
20. Satapathy, S.; Mittal, B.R.; Sood, A.; Das, C.K.; Mavuduru, R.S.; Goyal, S.; Shukla, J.; Singh, S.K. ^{177}Lu-PSMA-617 versus docetaxel in chemotherapy-naïve metastatic castration-resistant prostate cancer: A randomized, controlled, phase 2 non-inferiority trial. *Eur. J. Nucl. Med. Mol. Imaging* **2022**, *49*, 1754–1764. [CrossRef] [PubMed]
21. Barber, T.W.; Singh, A.; Kulkarni, H.R.; Niepsch, K.; Billah, B.; Baum, R.P. Clinical outcomes of ^{177}Lu-PSMA radioligand therapy in earlier and later phases of metastatic castration-resistant prostate cancer grouped by previous taxane chemotherapy. *J. Nucl. Med.* **2019**, *60*, 955–962. [CrossRef]
22. Baum, R.P.; Kulkarni, H.R.; Schuchardt, C.; Singh, A.; Wirtz, M.; Wiessalla, S.; Schottelius, M.; Mueller, D.; Klette, I.; Wester, H.J. ^{177}Lu-labeled prostate-specific membrane antigen radioligand therapy of metastatic castration-resistant prostate cancer: Safety and efficacy. *J. Nucl. Med.* **2016**, *57*, 1006–1013. [CrossRef]
23. Hofman, M.S.; Violet, J.; Hicks, R.J.; Ferdinandus, J.; Ping Thang, S.; Akhurst, T.; Iravani, A.; Kong, G.; Ravi Kumar, A.; Murphy, D.G.; et al. [^{177}Lu]-PSMA-617 radionuclide treatment in patients with metastatic castration-resistant prostate cancer (LuPSMA trial): A single-centre, single-arm, phase 2 study. *Lancet Oncol.* **2018**, *19*, 825–833. [CrossRef] [PubMed]

24. Violet, J.; Sandhu, S.; Iravani, A.; Ferdinandus, J.; Thang, S.P.; Kong, G.; Kumar, A.R.; Akhurst, T.; Pattison, D.; Beaulieu, A.; et al. Long-term follow-up and outcomes of retreatment in an expanded 50-patient single-center Phase II prospective trial of ^{177}Lu-PSMA-617 theranostics in metastatic castration-resistant prostate cancer. *J. Nucl. Med.* **2020**, *61*, 857–865. [CrossRef]
25. Rahbar, K.; Boegemann, M.; Yordanova, A.; Eveslage, M.; Schäfers, M.; Essler, M.; Ahmadzadehfar, H. PSMA targeted radioligandtherapy in metastatic castration resistant prostate cancer after chemotherapy, abiraterone and/or enzalutamide. A retrospective analysis of overall survival. *Eur. J. Nucl. Med. Mol. Imaging* **2018**, *45*, 12–19. [CrossRef]
26. Golan, S.; Frumer, M.; Zohar, Y.; Rosenbaum, E.; Yakimov, M.; Kedar, D.; Margel, D.; Baniel, J.; Steinmetz, A.P.; Groshar, D.; et al. Neoadjuvant ^{177}Lu-PSMA-I&T Radionuclide Treatment in Patients with High-risk Prostate Cancer Before Radical Prostatectomy: A Single-arm Phase 1 Trial. *Eur. Urol. Oncol.* **2022**, *6*, 151–159. [CrossRef] [PubMed]
27. Dhiantravan, N.; Violet, J.; Eapen, R.; Alghazo, O.; Scalzo, M.; Jackson, P.; Keam, S.P.; Mitchell, C.; Neeson, P.J.; Sandhu, S.; et al. Clinical Trial Protocol for LuTectomy: A Single-arm Study of the Dosimetry, Safety, and Potential Benefit of ^{177}Lu-PSMA-617 Prior to Prostatectomy. *Eur. Urol. Focus* **2021**, *7*, 234–237. [CrossRef]
28. Privé, B.M.; Peters, S.M.B.; Muselaers, C.H.J.; van Oort, I.M.; Janssen, M.J.R.; Michiel Sedelaar, J.P.; Konijnenberg, M.W.; Zámecnik, P.; Uijen, M.J.M.; Schilham, M.G.M.; et al. Lutetium-177-PSMA-617 in low-volume hormone-sensitive metastatic prostate cancer: A prospective pilot study. *Clin. Cancer Res.* **2021**, *27*, 3595–3601. [CrossRef] [PubMed]
29. Privé, B.M.; Janssen, M.J.R.; van Oort, I.M.; Muselaers, C.H.J.; Jonker, M.A.; van Gemert, W.A.; de Groot, M.; Westdorp, H.; Mehra, N.; Verzijlbergen, J.F.; et al. Update to a randomized controlled trial of lutetium-177-PSMA in Oligo-metastatic hormone-sensitive prostate cancer: The BULLSEYE trial. *Trials* **2021**, *22*, 768. [CrossRef] [PubMed]
30. EAU Guidelines. *Edition Presented at the EAU Annual Congress Paris*; EAU: Arnhem, The Netherlands, 2024; ISBN 978-94-92671-23-3.
31. Prasad, V. Lutetium 177 PSMA—Problems with the Vision Trial, YouTube. 2021. Available online: https://www.youtube.com/watch?v=pAsPzPt2avc (accessed on 1 June 2023).
32. Miszczyk, M.; Rajwa, P.; Fazekas, T.; Briganti, A.; Karakiewicz, P.I.; Rouprêt, M.; Shariat, S.F. The State of Intermediate Clinical Endpoints as Surrogates for Overall Survival in Prostate Cancer in 2024. *Eur. Urol. Oncol.* 2024. [CrossRef]
33. Fazekas, T.; Széles, Á.D.; Teutsch, B.; Csizmarik, A.; Vékony, B.; Kói, T.; Ács, N.; Hegyi, P.; Hadaschik, B.; Nyirády, P.; et al. Poly (ADP-ribose) Polymerase Inhibitors Have Comparable Efficacy with Platinum Chemotherapy in Patients with BRCA-positive Metastatic Castration-resistant Prostate Cancer. A Systematic Review and Meta-analysis. *Eur. Urol. Oncol.* **2024**, *7*, 365–375. [CrossRef]
34. Privé, B.M.; Slootbeek, P.H.J.; Laarhuis, B.I.; Naga, S.P.; van der Doelen, M.J.; van Kalmthout, L.W.M.; de Keizer, B.; Ezziddin, S.; Kratochwil, C.; Morgenstern, A.; et al. Impact of DNA damage repair defects on response to PSMA radioligand therapy in metastatic castration-resistant prostate cancer. *Prostate Cancer Prostatic Dis.* **2022**, *25*, 71–78. [CrossRef]
35. Tosco, L.; Briganti, A.; D'amico, A.V.; Eastham, J.; Eisenberger, M.; Gleave, M.; Haustermans, K.; Logothetis, C.J.; Saad, F.; Sweeney, C.; et al. Systematic Review of Systemic Therapies and Therapeutic Combinations with Local Treatments for High-risk Localized Prostate Cancer. *Eur. Urol.* **2019**, *75*, 44–60. [CrossRef]
36. Eastham, J.A.; Heller, G.; Halabi, S.; Monk, J.P.; Beltran, H.; Gleave, M.; Evans, C.P.; Clinton, S.K.; Szmulewitz, R.Z.; Coleman, J.; et al. Cancer and leukemia group B 90203 (Alliance): Radical prostatectomy with or without neoadjuvant chemohormonal therapy in localized, high-risk prostate cancer. *J. Clin. Oncol.* **2020**, *38*, 3042–3050. [CrossRef] [PubMed]
37. Yossepowitch, O.; Eastham, J.A. Radical prostatectomy for high-risk prostate cancer. *World J. Urol.* **2008**, *26*, 219–224. [CrossRef] [PubMed]
38. Stephenson, A.J.; Kattan, M.W.; Eastham, J.A.; Bianco, F.J.; Yossepowitch, O.; Vickers, A.J.; Klein, E.A.; Wood, D.P.; Scardino, P.T. Prostate cancer-specific mortality after radical prostatectomy for patients treated in the prostate-specific antigen era. *J. Clin. Oncol.* **2009**, *27*, 4300–4305. [CrossRef]
39. Eapen, R.S.; Buteau, J.P.; Jackson, P.; Mitchell, C.; Oon, S.F.; Alghazo, O.; McIntosh, L.; Dhiantravan, N.; Scalzo, M.J.; O'Brien, J.; et al. Administering [(177)Lu]Lu-PSMA-617 Prior to Radical Prostatectomy in Men with High-risk Localised Prostate Cancer (LuTectomy): A Single-centre, Single-arm, Phase 1/2 Study. *Eur. Urol.* **2024**, *85*, 217–226. [CrossRef] [PubMed]
40. Parker, C.; Castro, E.; Fizazi, K.; Heidenreich, A.; Ost, P.; Procopio, G.; Tombal, B.; Gillessen, S. Prostate cancer: ESMO Clinical Practice Guidelines for diagnosis, treatment and follow-up†. *Ann. Oncol.* **2020**, *31*, 1119–1134. [CrossRef]
41. Burdett, S.; Boevé, L.M.; Ingleby, F.C.; Fisher, D.J.; Rydzewska, L.H.; Vale, C.L.; van Andel, G.; Clarke, N.W.; Hulshof, M.C.; James, N.D.; et al. Prostate Radiotherapy for Metastatic Hormone-sensitive Prostate Cancer: A STOPCAP Systematic Review and Meta-analysis. *Eur. Urol.* **2019**, *76*, 115–124. [CrossRef]
42. Rajwa, P.; Robesti, D.; Chaloupka, M.; Zattoni, F.; Giesen, A.; Huebner, N.A.; Krzywon, A.; Miszczyk, M.; Moll, M.; Stando, R.; et al. Outcomes of Cytoreductive Radical Prostatectomy for Oligometastatic Prostate Cancer on Prostate-specific Membrane Antigen Positron Emission Tomography: Results of a Multicenter European Study. *Eur. Urol. Oncol.* 2023. [CrossRef]
43. Sartor, A.O.; Tagawa, S.T.; Saad, F.; De Bono, J.S.; Feng, F.Y.; Fizazi, K.; Sakharova, O.V.; Morris, M.J. PSMAddition: A phase 3 trial to compare treatment with ^{177}Lu-PSMA-617 plus standard of care (SOC) versus SOC alone in patients with metastatic hormone-sensitive prostate cancer. *J. Clin. Oncol.* **2022**, 40. [CrossRef]
44. Rahbar, K.; Ahmadzadehfar, H.; Kratochwil, C.; Haberkorn, U.; Schafers, M.; Essler, M.; Baum, R.P.; Kulkarni, H.R.; Schmidt, M.; Drzezga, A.; et al. German multicenter study investigating ^{177}Lu-PSMA-617 Radioligand therapy in advanced prostate cancer patients. *J. Nucl. Med.* **2017**, *58*, 85–90. [CrossRef]

45. Seitzer, K.E.; Seifert, R.; Kessel, K.; Roll, W.; Schlack, K.; Boegemann, M.; Rahbar, K. Lutetium-177 labelled PSMA targeted therapy in advanced prostate cancer: Current status and future perspectives. *Cancers* **2021**, *13*, 3715. [CrossRef] [PubMed]
46. Rahbar, K.; Afshar-Oromieh, A.; Jadvar, H.; Ahmadzadehfar, H. PSMA Theranostics: Current Status and Future Directions. *Mol. Imaging* **2018**, *17*, 1–9. [CrossRef] [PubMed]
47. Rathke, H.; Giesel, F.L.; Flechsig, P.; Kopka, K.; Mier, W.; Hohenfellner, M.; Haberkorn, U.; Kratochwil, C. Repeated ^{177}Lu-Labeled PSMA-617 Radioligand Therapy Using Treatment Activities of Up to 9.3 GBq. *J. Nucl. Med.* **2018**, *59*, 459–465. [CrossRef] [PubMed]
48. Haberkorn, U.; Giesel, F.; Morgenstern, A.; Kratochwil, C. The Future of Radioligand Therapy: α, β, or Both? *J. Nucl. Med.* **2017**, *58*, 1017–1018. [CrossRef]
49. Van der Doelen, M.J.; Mehra, N.; Van Oort, I.M.; Looijen-Salamon, M.G.; Janssen, M.J.R.; Custers, J.A.E.; Slootbeek, P.H.J.; Kroeze, L.I.; Bruchertseifer, F.; Morgenstern, A.; et al. Clinical outcomes and molecular profiling of advanced metastatic castration-resistant prostate cancer patients treated with (225)Ac-PSMA-617 targeted alpha-radiation therapy. *Urol. Oncol.* **2021**, *39*, 729.e7–729.e16. [CrossRef]

cancers

MDPI

Review

Role of Receptor for Advanced Glycation End-Products in Endometrial Cancer: A Review

Kamila Zglejc-Waszak [1,*], Marcin Jozwik [2], Michael Thoene [3] and Joanna Wojtkiewicz [4,*,†]

1 Department of Anatomy, Faculty of Medicine, Collegium Medicum, University of Warmia and Mazury in Olsztyn, 10-082 Olsztyn, Poland

2 Department of Gynecology and Obstetrics, Collegium Medicum, University of Warmia and Mazury in Olsztyn, 10-045 Olsztyn, Poland

3 Department of Medical Biology, Faculty of Health Sciences, University of Warmia and Mazury in Olsztyn, Żołnierska 14C Str., 10-561 Olsztyn, Poland; michael.thoene@uwm.edu.pl

4 Department of Human Physiology and Pathophysiology, Faculty of Medicine, Collegium Medicum, University of Warmia and Mazury in Olsztyn, 10-082 Olsztyn, Poland

* Correspondence: kamila.zglejc@uwm.edu.pl or kamilazglejc@gmail.com (K.Z.-W.); joanna.wojtkiewicz@uwm.edu.pl (J.W.); Tel.: +48-(089)-524-53-01 (K.Z.-W. & J.W.)

† Senior author.

Simple Summary: The RAGE signaling pathway is associated with many chronic disorders. One of them may be endometrial cancer (EC). EC is one of the most common gynecologic cancers among women. The aim of our considerations was to decipher the role of RAGE and its ligands in the progression of EC. We confirmed that disruptions in the RAGE signaling pathways may be a reason for EC progression. The cross-talk between RAGE and Diaph1 plays a crucial role in downstream signaling pathways during EC progression. However, we assume that DNA methylation may regulate the activity of the RAGE signaling pathways in the endometrium. Thus, DNA methylation may create an epigenetic memory that may trigger perturbations in the endometrium.

Abstract: Endometrial cancer (EC) is the most common gynecological malignancy. EC is associated with metabolic disorders that may promote non-enzymatic glycation and activate the receptor for advanced glycation end-products (RAGE) signaling pathways. Thus, we assumed that RAGE and its ligands may contribute to EC. Of particular interest is the interaction between diaphanous-related formin 1 (Diaph1) and RAGE during the progression of human cancers. Diaph1 is engaged in the proper organization of actin cytoskeletal dynamics, which is crucial in cancer invasion, metastasis, angiogenesis, and axonogenesis. However, the detailed molecular role of RAGE in EC remains uncertain. In this review, we discuss epigenetic factors that may play a key role in the RAGE-dependent endometrial pathology. We propose that DNA methylation may regulate the activity of the RAGE pathway in the uterus. The accumulation of negative external factors, such as hyperglycemia, inflammation, and oxidative stress, may interfere with the DNA methylation process. Therefore, further research should take into account the role of epigenetic mechanisms in EC progression.

Keywords: endometrial cancer; glycation; RAGE; Diaph1; DNA methylation

1. Introduction

Endometrium is an important tissue in pregnancy development, essential for reproductive success [1,2]. Yet, endometrium is also a site of the most common malignancy of the female reproductive system, endometrial cancer (EC) [3–5]. Many novel aspects of the physiology and pathology of the endometrium are currently under study [6,7].

The inspiration to write a review were the results of NGS studies, which revealed the association of metabolic changes with the development of EC in women [4]. In this review, we aimed to summarize the current knowledge on the role of the receptor for advanced glycation end-products (RAGE) in EC. Our previous studies have indicated that RAGE and its ligands are involved in diabetic/metabolic complications, as well as in neurodegenerative diseases [8–14]. We demonstrated that the RAGE signaling pathway may be activated in uterine tissues during the estrous cycle [6]. Zheng et al. [5] showed a stimulative effect of RAGE on the formation of microvessels in EC. This can be seen as an analogy to diabetic disorders, like retinopathy [15]. Previous studies have indicated that RAGE signaling may be associated with renal cell carcinoma, as well as prostate, lung, breast, and colorectal cancers [5,16–18]. Therefore, we analyzed the role of RAGE as a potential prognostic protein of uterine carcinogenesis. We assumed that the RAGE signaling pathway may be involved in EC development.

The insights on the role of RAGE signaling in EC provided in this review have been based on the literature as well as on the results of our previous studies. We describe recent advances and current theories on the etiology of EC, highlighting the function of the RAGE signaling system in endometrial pathology. As EC is a broad topic with new information coming out almost every week, we, therefore, focused our review on aberrant RAGE-mediated signaling in EC to formulate a new hypothesis. We believe that limiting the scope has allowed us to focus on how the interaction between RAGE and its ligand may play a pivotal role in endometrial complications in animal models and human patients and if understanding this pathway can uncover targets for safe and effective therapeutic intervention for EC.

2. Molecular Dialogue between the RAGE Signaling Pathway and Endometrial Pathology

RAGE is a multi-ligand receptor widely expressed in good health and in embryogenesis, as well as in health disorders [8–14,19,20]. The consequential discovery that RAGE was a multi-ligand receptor set the stage for a better understanding of the biology of RAGE in homeostasis and in disease. We observed that the expression of RAGE was elevated during neurodegenerative diseases and in diabetes [8–14,20,21]. We noted that the RAGE signaling pathway is activated in the uterus during the estrous cycle [6]. It has, therefore, been difficult to separate the physiological role of RAGE from its pathological influence on the development of EC. Nowadays, EC is the most common cancer of female reproductive organs, and new insights into the RAGE signaling pathway may find novel indications for the early detection and treatment of EC.

Approximately 40% of EC cases are associated with acquired metabolic disorders, such as obesity and diabetes [4,22,23]. Nevertheless, Sidorkiewicz and co-workers [4] identified genes associated with metabolic status in EC. Transcriptomic studies showed that *solute carrier family 7 member 11* (*SLC7A11*), *solute carrier family 7 member 5* (*SLC7A5*), *Runt-related transcription factor 1* (*RUNX1*), *laminin subunit alpha 4* (*LAMA4*), *collagen type VI alpha 3 chain* (*COL6A3*), *phosphoinositide-dependent kinase-1* (*PDK1*), *cyclin A1* (*CCNA1*), *enolase 1* (*ENO1*), *pyruvate kinase muscle isozyme* (*PKM*), *nuclear receptor subfamily 2 group F member 1* (*NR2F1*), and *N-acetylated alpha-linked acidic dipeptidase 2* (*NAALAD2*) are directly associated with the KEGG signaling pathway, the central carbon metabolism in cancer (hsa05230) [4].

The GeneMANIA [24] analysis of selected genes, including *SLC7A11*, *SLC7A5*, *RUNX1*, *LAMA4*, *COL6A3*, *PDK1*, *CCNA1*, *ENO1*, *PKM*, *NR2F1*, *NAALAD2* [4], and *AGER* (the gene encoding RAGE), revealed that only *NAALAD2* was not connected to one network (Figure 1). The GeneMANIA network comprises 32 genes (20 related genes) and consists of genes related to multiple biological functions (Table S1). The analysis revealed that the selected genes were mainly involved in metabolic functions (Table 1). Moreover, we observed that *AGER* directly interacts with *PKM* and *SLC7A8* (a co-expression interaction) and *RUNX1* (a co-localization interaction, Figure 1).

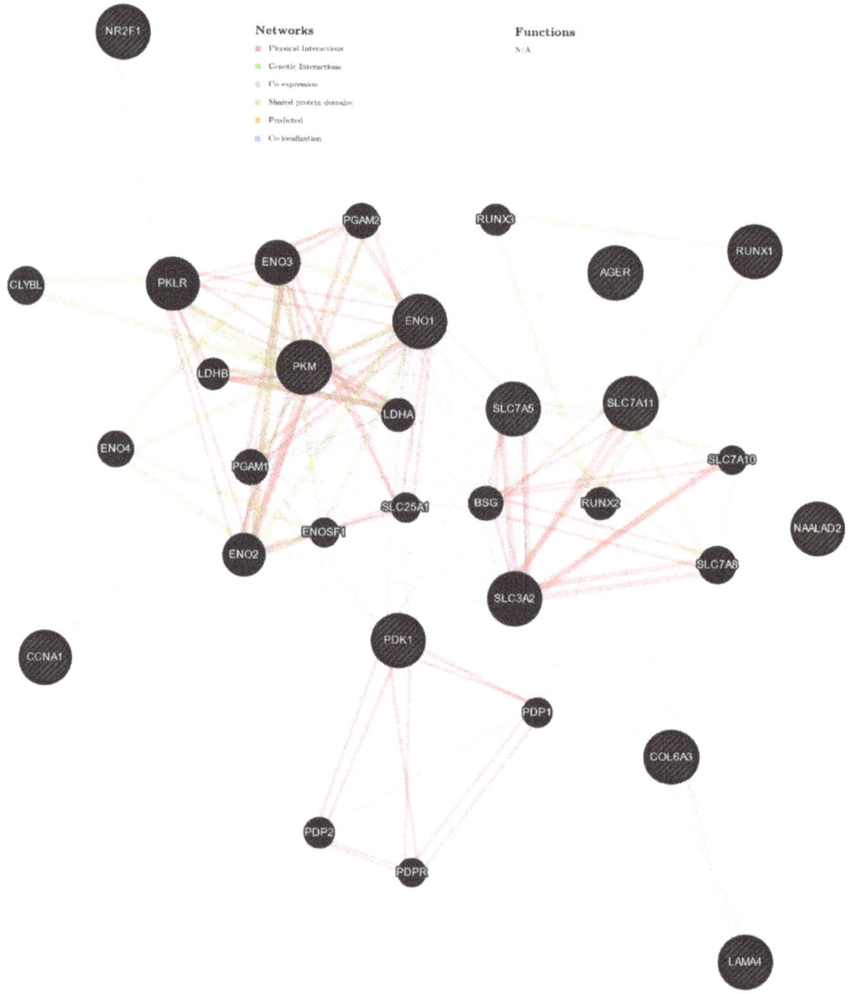

Figure 1. Interaction network constructed for genes involved in central carbon metabolism in cancer (hsa05230) [4] limited to *Homo sapiens* (https://genemania.org/) [24]. The GeneMANIA is a prediction server used for biological network integration for gene prioritization and predicting gene function. The server additionally adds genes based on known interactions. Additional genes are represented by gray, unstriped circles. Selected genes are represented by circles with stripes. The colors of the line suggest the type of interaction, that is, red—physical interactions; purple—co-expression; orange—predicted; blue—co-localization; light blue—pathway; green—genetic interactions; olive—shared protein domains. Interactors are shown with the official gene symbol. *NAALAD2* is the only gene found outside the network. Most studies indicate that *NAALAD2* is involved in prostate cancer. Sidorkiewicz et al. [4] may be the first to have correlated this gene with endometrial cancer (EC). However, the expression of *NAALAD2* was decreased in the endometrium during cancer [4]. Abbreviations: *AGER*—the gene encoding receptor advanced glycation end-products; *ENO2*—enolase 2;

ENO1—enolase 1; *PKM*—pyruvate kinase isozymes M1/M2; *PGAM2*—phosphoglycerate mutase 2; *ENO3*—enolase 3; *CCNA1*—cyclin A1; *ENO4*—enolase 4; *ENOSF1*—enolase superfamily member 1; *CLYBL*—citramalyl-CoA lyase; *NAALAD2*—N-acetylated alpha-linked acidic dipeptidase 2; *LAMA4*—laminin subunit alpha 4; *COL6A3*—collagen type VI alpha 3 chain; *NR2F1*—nuclear receptor subfamily 2 group F member 1; *PDP2*—pyruvate dehydrogenase phosphatase catalytic subunit 2; *PDPR*—pyruvate dehydrogenase phosphatase regulatory subunit; *PDP1*—pyruvate dehydrogenase phosphatase catalytic subunit 1; *PDK1*—pyruvate dehydrogenase kinase 1; *RUNX1*—RUNX family transcription factor 1; *RUNX2*—RUNX family transcription factor 2; *RUNX3*—RUNX family transcription factor 3; *CCNA1*—cyclin A1; *LDHA*—lactate dehydrogenase A; *LDHB*—lactate dehydrogenase B; BSG—basigin; *PKLR*—pyruvate kinase L/R; *PGAM1*—phosphoglycerate mutase 1; *SLC25A1*—solute carrier family 25 member 1; *SLC7A5*—solute carrier family 7 member 5; *SLC7A8*—solute carrier family 7 member 8; *SLC7A11*—solute carrier family 7 member 11. N/A—not applicable. See File S1.

Table 1. In silico analysis revealed that the gene network is involved in multiple metabolic functions.

Function	Official Symbol	Number of Genes
pyruvate metabolic process	*PDK1, PDP1, PDP2, PDPR, LDHA, PKLR, PGAM1, ENO2, ENO1, ENO3*	13
glucose catabolic process to pyruvate	*PKLR, PGAM1, ENO2, PKM, ENO1, ENO3, PGAM2*	7
glycolytic process through fructose-6-phosphate	*PKLR, PGAM1, ENO2, PKM, ENO1, ENO3, PGAM2*	7
glycolytic process through glucose-6-phosphate	*PKLR, PGAM1, ENO2, PKM, ENO1, ENO3, PGAM2*	7
glucose catabolic process	*PKLR, PGAM1, ENO2, PKM, ENO1, ENO3, PGAM2*	7
NADH metabolic process	*PKLR, PGAM1, ENO2, PKM, ENO1, ENO3, PGAM2*	7
ADP metabolic process	*PKLR, PGAM1, ENO2, PKM, ENO1, ENO3, PGAM2, LDHA, ENO4*	9
ATP generation from ADP	*PKLR, PGAM1, ENO2, PKM, ENO1, ENO3, PGAM2, LDHA, ENO4*	9
NAD metabolic process	*PKLR, PGAM1, ENO2, PKM, ENO1, ENO3, PGAM2*	7
purine ribonucleoside diphosphate metabolic process	*PKLR, PGAM1, ENO2, PKM, ENO1, ENO3, PGAM2, LDHA, ENO4*	9
carbohydrate catabolic process	*PKLR, PGAM1, ENO2, PKM, ENO1, ENO3, PGAM2, LDHA, ENO4, ENOSF1*	10
purine nucleoside diphosphate metabolic process	*PKLR, PGAM1, ENO2, PKM, ENO1, ENO3, PGAM2, LDHA, ENO4*	9
ribonucleoside diphosphate metabolic process	*PKLR, PGAM1, ENO2, PKM, ENO1, ENO3, PGAM2, LDHA, ENO4*	9
nucleoside diphosphate metabolic process	*PKLR, PGAM1, ENO2, PKM, ENO1, ENO3, PGAM2, LDHA, ENO4*	9
glucose metabolic process	*PKLR, PGAM1, ENO2, PKM, ENO1, ENO3, PGAM2, PDK1, SLC25A1*	9
hexose catabolic process	*PKLR, PGAM1, ENO2, PKM, ENO1, ENO3, PGAM2*	7

Table 1. *Cont.*

Function	Official Symbol	Number of Genes
monosaccharide catabolic process	*PKLR, PGAM1, ENO2, PKM, ENO1, ENO3, PGAM2*	7
hexose metabolic process	*PKLR, PGAM1, ENO2, PKM, ENO1, ENO3, PGAM2, PDK1, SLC25A1*	9
glycolytic process	*PKLR, PGAM1, ENO2, PKM, ENO1, ENO3, PGAM2*	7
ATP metabolic process	*PKLR, PGAM1, ENO2, PKM, ENO1, ENO3, PGAM2, LDHA, ENO4*	9
monosaccharide metabolic process	*PKLR, PGAM1, ENO2, PKM, ENO1, ENO3, PGAM2, PDK1, SLC25A1*	9
hexose biosynthetic process	*SLC25A1, PGAM1, ENO2, ENO1, ENO3, PGAM2*	6
regulation of sulfur metabolic process	*PDP2, PDPR, PDP1, PDK1*	4
monosaccharide biosynthetic process	*SLC25A1, PGAM1, ENO2, ENO1, ENO3, PGAM2*	6
regulation of purine nucleotide metabolic process	*PGAM1, PDP2, PDPR, PDP1, PDK1, ENO1*	6
regulation of nucleotide metabolic process	*PGAM1, PDP2, PDPR, PDP1, PDK1, ENO1*	6
thioester biosynthetic process	*PDP2, PDPR, PDP1, PDK1, SLC25A1*	5
acyl-CoA biosynthetic process	*PDP2, PDPR, PDP1, PDK1, SLC25A1*	5
acetyl-CoA metabolic process	*PDP2, PDPR, PDP1, PDK1*	4
acyl-CoA metabolic process	*PDP2, PDPR, PDP1, PDK1, SLC25A1*	5
carbohydrate biosynthetic process	*SLC25A1, PGAM1, ENO2, ENO1, ENO3, PGAM2*	6
regulation of fatty acid metabolic process	*PDP2, PDPR, PDP1, PDK1*	4
cellular ketone metabolic process	*PDP2, PDPR, PDP1, PDK1*	4

According to The Cancer Genome Atlas, 20,000 primary cancers have been identified in this novel look at the etiology of cancer. A new classification of EC by The Cancer Genome Atlas revealed that metabolic reprogramming may be one of the causes of cancer progression in women [4,25]. Studies have indicated malfunctions in cell metabolism driven by oncogenes [25]. Therefore, malfunctions in metabolic pathways may be a characteristic feature of cancer [26,27]. However, so far only the Warburg effect has been focused on as a metabolic cause of EC [28–30]. In this review, we would like to demonstrate that RAGE signaling pathways may play a crucial role in the progression of metabolic cancer in the female reproductive tract.

Previous studies have shown that mTOR and PI3K/AKT metabolic signaling pathways are associated with EC progression [4,25,31]. Nevertheless, Ramasubbu and Devi Rajeswari [32] indicated that RAGE may inhibit the mammalian target of rapamycin (mTOR) and phosphatidyl inositol 3-kinase-AKT (PI3K/AKT) signaling pathways during diabetes. Thus, RAGE signaling pathways may play a role in cancer treatments.

Nevertheless, mTOR and PI3K/AKT signaling pathways are involved in cell proliferation and microvessel formation in EC [5]. Moreover, RAGE during metabolic disorders is associated with new microvessel formation [33].

Zheng and co-workers [5] revealed that RAGE may be associated as a potential regulatory factor of microvessel formation in EC. Studies have indicated that a similar phenomenon has been observed in other cancer types [34,35]. Thus, RAGE signaling pathways, as well as mTOR and PI3K/AKT signaling pathways, may be involved in microvessel formation during EC growth [16,34,35]. Studies have indicated that RAGE ligands may also play a key role in the progression of microvessel formation during

EC [17,29]. Overall, RAGE and its ligands are involved in metabolic complications as well as microvessel formation during numerous pathological conditions [8,9,12–15,33–35].

The amount of RAGE protein is elevated in the endometrium during type 1 diabetes, as well as with a high-fat diet [6]. Studies have shown that the amount of RAGE is the highest in EC, particularly in less differentiated tumors [5,36]. Consequently, we may observe the elevated level of advanced glycation end-products (AGEs) in EC [5,36]. Thus, RAGE and its ligands may be associated with progression of EC (https://www.proteinatlas.org/ENSG00000204305-AGER/pathology, accessed on 1 August 2024).

AGEs are formed during the Maillard reaction. The Maillard reaction is a non-enzymatic process in which glucose reacts with protein, i.e., glycation. AGEs are accumulated in our body through high glucose levels or ingestion [37]. The main precursor of AGEs is methylglyoxal (MGO). However, under physiological conditions, glyoxalase 1 (GLO1) is responsible for the detoxification of MGO [8,9,12,38]. Studies have indicated that the amount of AGEs is elevated during pathophysiological conditions such as diabetes, neurological diseases, and cancer [8–15,39,40]. Moreover, reports have shown that AGEs trigger disorders by several mechanisms: (1) AGE intracellular accumulation; (2) disturbances in the proper structure and function of proteins binding to proteins; and (3) activation of the RAGE signaling pathway [8,9,12–15,39]. Previous studies have indicated that the pathological process in the cell is preceded by an increased amount of RAGE-AGEs [41]. Next, the studies revealed the various forms of stress in the cell during disorders [41]. Our studies revealed the pathological process of RAGE-AGEs in the endometrium during the estrous cycle [6]. Therefore, we may speculate that RAGE-AGEs may be involved in the pathophysiological processes of EC [42,43].

3. RAGE and Its Ligands in Endometrial Cancer (EC)

Studies have indicated that patients with diabetes are at high risk of cancer progression [4,5,36]. Our data revealed that the expression of RAGE and its ligands is elevated in diabetic patients [8,9,12–15,40,44]. It can therefore be inferred that endometrial carcinogenesis may be related to increased expression of RAGE and its ligands. RAGE binds with a variety of ligands, especially proinflammatory ones, and is engaged with cytoskeletal dynamics [8,9,13,14]. Studies have shown that the amounts of proinflammatory high-mobility group box 1 (HMGB1) and S 100 calcium-binding protein B (S100B) ligands increase in cancer [42,43,45,46]. GeneMANIA analysis indicated that *HMGB1* and *S100B* interact with *AGER* (the gene encoding RAGE) through physical-, predicted-, and co-localized interactions (Figure 2). These analyses revealed another important interaction between *AGER/RAGE* and *diaphanous-related formin 1* (*Diaph1*; Figure 2), but an exact role of these molecules is unclear in EC (https://www.proteinatlas.org/ENSG00000204305-AGER/pathology, accessed on 1 August 2024; https://www.proteinatlas.org/ENSG00000131504-DIAPH1/pathology, accessed on 1 August 2024).

3.1. *HMGB1*

Our studies have indicated that the expression of HMGB1 is elevated in the diabetic sciatic nerve as well as in the spinal cord harvested from SOD1 G93A mice [8–15]. Moreover, further studies revealed that increased expression of HMGB1 is present in Parkinson's, Alzheimer's, cardiovascular diseases, stroke, retinopathy, neuropathy, as well as amyotrophic lateral sclerosis [12,47–50]. Previous studies revealed that the amount of HMGB1 is elevated in the endometrium harvested from type 1 diabetic mice and mice with a high-fat diet [6]. Our studies have shown that HMGB1 is associated with the inflammation process in the uterus [6]. We may suppose that HMGB1 is related to a chronic pathological process that takes place in the endometrium (https://www.proteinatlas.org/ENSG00000189403-HMGB1/pathology, accessed on 1 August 2024). HMGB1 in hormone-related cancer may be a potential therapeutic target [45]. This phenomenon has not been observed in healthy cells [51].

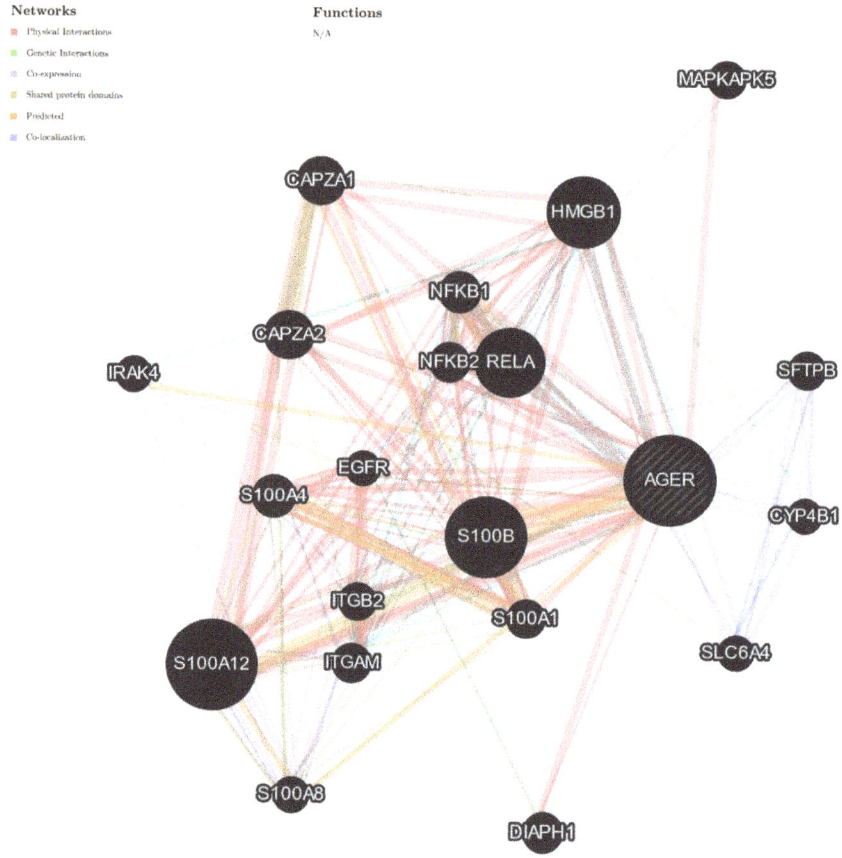

Figure 2. Graph representing the interaction network of *AGER* (the gene encoding RAGE) with genes encoding RAGE ligands. *HMGB1*, *S100B*, and *Diaph1* are the most well-known RAGE ligands. The interaction of *AGER/RAGE* with *HMGB1*, *S100B*, and *Diaph1* may be crucial for EC progression. The interaction network includes the cancer-related factors *NFKB1*, *NFKB2*, and *EGFR*. The colors of the line suggest the type of interaction, that is, red—physical interactions; purple—co-expression; orange—predicted; blue—co-localization; light blue—pathway; green—genetic interactions; olive—shared protein domains. Limited to *Homo sapiens*. Abbreviations: HMGB1—high-mobility group box 1; *S100B*—S100 calcium-binding protein B; *Diaph1*—diaphanous-related formin 1; *MAPKAPK5*—MAPK-activated protein kinase 5; *CAPZA1*—capping actin protein of muscle z-line subunit alpha 1; *CAPZA2*—capping actin protein of muscle z-line subunit alpha 2; *IRAK4*—interleukin 1 receptor-associated kinase 4; *NFKB2*—nuclear factor kappa B subunit 2; *NFKB1*—nuclear factor kappa B subunit 1; *RELA*—RELA proto-oncogene, NFKB subunit; *EGFR*—epidermal growth factor receptor; *S100A4*—S100 calcium-binding protein A4; *ITGB2*—integrin subunit beta 2; *SFTPB*—surfactant protein B; *CYP4B1*—cytochrome P450 family 4 subfamily B member 1; *S100A1*—S100 calcium-binding protein A1; *SLC6A4*—solute carrier family 6 member 4; *ITGAM*—integrin alpha M; *S100A8*—S100 calcium-binding protein A8; *S100A12*—S100 calcium-binding protein A12. See File S2. N/A—not applicable. The interaction network using GeneMANIA was also created in the publication Zglejc-Waszak et al. [8]. These are not the same interaction networks as in the previous publication [8]. The similarity may result from the databases used by the GeneMANIA server.

Histologically, EC may be classified into three grades: grade I—well differentiated, with a better prognosis; grade II—moderately differentiated; and grade III—poorly differentiated, with a worse prognosis. Luan et al. [52] revealed that HMGB1 is negatively correlated with the development of endometrial carcinoma and prevents cancer cell invasion and metastasis by inhibiting the process of epithelial-to-mesenchymal transition. Thus, we may suppose that the role of HMGB1 is not significant in EC type II, as type II ECs are poorly differentiated [52]. It should be stressed that HMGB1 is a RAGE ligand, as the RAGE-HMGB1 interaction may have a strong impact on the progression of endometrial carcinoma [42,52]. Studies have indicated that HMGB1 interacts with RAGE in tumor cells [51].

Extracellular HMGB1 is a proinflammatory ligand that binds to the V domain of RAGE and thereby activates Janus kinase-signal transduction, the transcription activation (JAK/STAT) signaling pathway, and nuclear factor KB-dependent (NFKB) cytokine production (Figure 3) [12,53]. Studies have shown that cancer cells release HMGB1 [54]. Increasing amounts of HMGB1 activate the RAGE signaling pathway. Feedback loops between HMGB1 and RAGE have been observed during the progression of cancer [8,54]. We hypothesize that blocking the cross-talk between RAGE and HMGB1 may inhibit cancer progression. Researchers should consider the RAGE-HMGB1-dependent signaling pathway when searching for therapeutic targets to prevent EC progression.

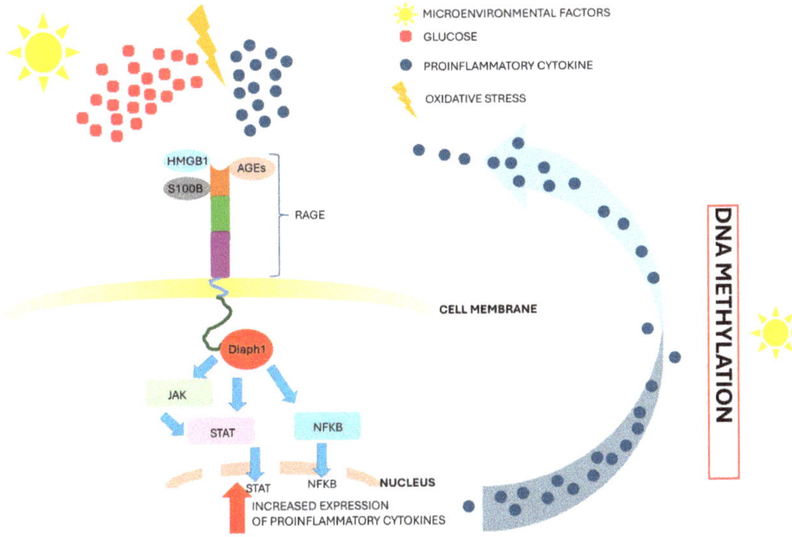

Figure 3. Schematic of the RAGE signaling pathway in EC and potential therapeutic targets. High glucose levels, oxidative stress, and local inflammation activate the RAGE signaling pathway. The V domain (extracellular domain) of RAGE interacts with HMGB1, S100B, and AGEs. HMGB1, S100B, and AGEs are proinflammatory RAGE ligands. Diaph1 interacts with the cytoplasmatic domain. Studies have indicated that Diaph1 may be a crucial player in the downstream RAGE signaling pathway. The signal cascade activates transcription factors (NFKB, STAT) that increase the amount of proinflammatory cytokines. Moreover, inhibiting the RAGE-Diaph1 interaction may contribute to reducing the production of proinflammatory cytokines. However, DNA methylation may have a key impact on RAGE-dependent cell signaling. Local environmental factors, hyperglycemia, oxidative stress, and inflammation may induce malfunctions in DNA methylation and, thus, disturb the epigenetic pattern of RAGE signaling pathways. Abbreviations: AGEs—advanced glycation end-products; RAGE—receptor for advanced glycation end-products; S100B—S100 calcium-binding protein B; HMGB1—high-mobility group box 1; Diaph1—diaphanous related formin 1; NFKB—nuclear factor kappa-light-chain enhancer of activated B cells; STAT—signal transducer and activator of transcription; JAK—Janus-activated kinases.

3.2. *S100B*

The S100B is part of the family of small molecular weight calcium-binding proteins [8,42,55]. Our studies have shown that the amount of S100B is increased in the diabetic endometrium [6]. Most studies implicated S100B in inflammation and cancer progression. That is why this molecule is called a proinflammatory RAGE ligand and a marker of neurodegenerative diseases [12,42,56–58]. Studies confirmed that S100B may be considered a tumor marker [46]. Elevated serum S100B levels have already been proposed as a biomarker for lung cancer and melanoma [59–61]. S100B interacts with cellular tumor antigen p53 [62]. Studies have indicated that S100B may modulate p53 functions in tumor suppression and, thus, stimulate cancer progression [62,63]. Protein p53 prevents genome mutation as well as tumor formation [64]. p53 plays a prominent role in DNA repair, apoptosis control, and the cell cycle [46,64]. The data suggest that S100B may be involved in EC progression (https://www.proteinatlas.org/ENSG00000160307-S100B/pathology, accessed on 1 August 2024). However, high-throughput studies revealed that S100B does not correlate with the estrogen-negative group of cancer [46]. Yen et al. [46] have shown that in breast cancer the amount of S100B was decreased when compared to healthy tissue. This mode of S100B activity may be specific to breast cancer [46]. The interaction of S100B with RAGE deserves attention in the next steps of EC research.

3.3. *Diaph1*

Diaph1 is an intracellular ligand of RAGE. The cytoplasmatic domain of RAGE interacts with the FH1 domain of Diaph1. Diaph1 activity is strictly autoregulated by the DID domain and the terminal DAD domain. However, the FH2 domain is involved in actin polymerization and binds to profilin 1 (PFN1) [8]. The RAGE-Diaph1 signaling pathway was first identified in disorders such as diabetes, inflammation, and neurodegenerative diseases [8,12,14,65,66]. Over the last decade, Diaph1 has gained attention as a significant contributor to the pathogenesis of a few neurodegenerative disorders, such as Alzheimer's, Parkinson's, Huntington's, and Creutzfeldt–Jakob's disease, and various neurodegenerative conditions, such as diabetic neuropathy, amyotrophic lateral sclerosis, amyloid polyneuropathy, Charcot neuropathy, vasculitis neuropathy, and cancer [8,12,14,67]; however, the detailed mechanisms of the Diaph1 contribution to disorders remain unclear (https://www.proteinatlas.org/ENSG00000131504-DIAPH1/pathology, accessed on 1 August 2024).

Recent studies have shown that in animal models of neurodegenerative diseases, the pharmacological or genetic blocking of Diaph1 attenuates inflammation and Diaph1-associated perturbations [8,9,14,68–72]. Studies revealed that Diaph1 deletion may improve sciatic nerve regeneration in diabetic mice [8,14,68–70].

RAGE-Diaph1 signaling pathways trigger the NFKB-dependent signaling cascade and, thus, proinflammatory cytokine production [8]. Nevertheless, Diaph1, as a member of the formin family, is involved in the dynamics of the actin cytoskeleton [67]. Formin, Diaph1, is involved in actin elongation as well as depolymerization through interaction with PFN1 or cofilin 1 (CFL1, Figure 4) [73]. PFN1 and CFL1 are important proteins for proper actin polymerization and elongation [73]. However, studies have indicated that high levels of PFN1 may inhibit actin elongation [74,75]. PFN1 may trigger actin elongation and the RhoA-dependent signaling cascade, and in it is the RAGE signaling pathway [76–79].

These cytoskeletal proteins also play a role in human cancer cells [80–82]. Recent research shows that cytoskeletal proteins play an important role in the development of human diseases [9,14,80–82]. Therefore, they may be a new therapeutic target in cancer treatment.

Cancer cells have a potential for growth, migration, and invasion. The proper functioning of the cytoskeleton is important in these processes [80–82]. Diaph1 and cytoskeletal proteins may regulate cancer cell growth and invasion by the remodeling of the actin cytoskeleton [14,80–82]. We observed that global deletion or silencing of Diaph1 may have an impact on actin cytoskeletal dynamics during human diseases. Data suggest that attenuation of Diaph1 can reduce F-actin polymerization in cells [39]. However, to date, we do not know the effect of Diaph1 deletion on the dynamics of the actin cytoskeleton in EC cells.

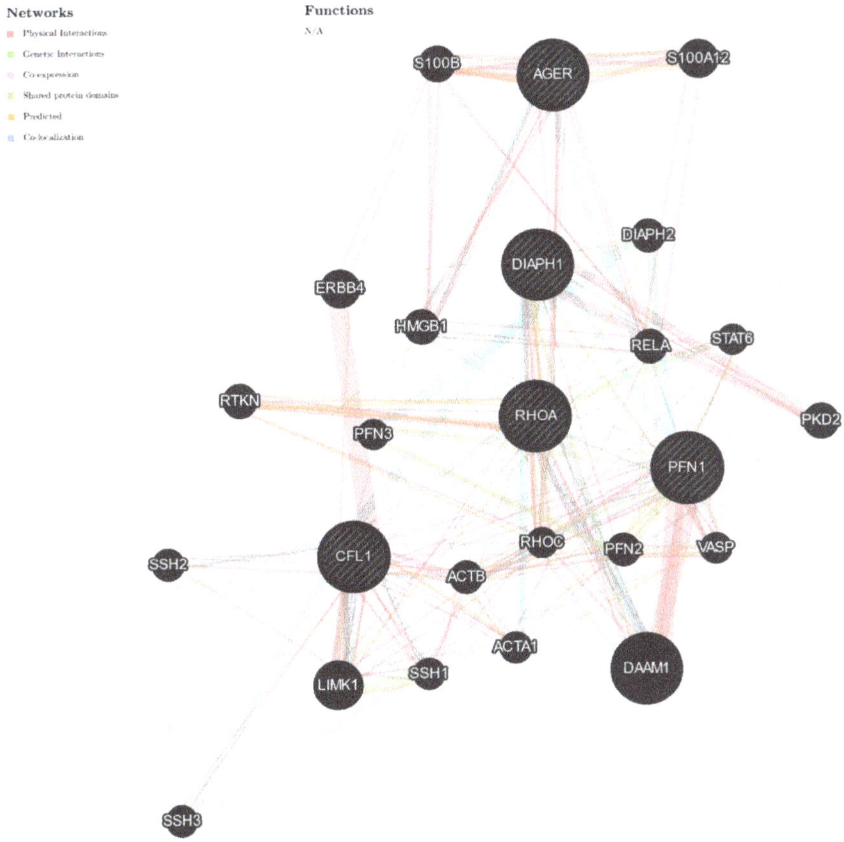

Figure 4. Graph representing the interaction network of *Diaph1* with proteins involved in cytoskeletal dynamics. Formin, Diaph1, is responsible for the polymerization and depolymerization of actin. It interacts with PFN1 and CFL1. Interactions between these molecules engage RhoA to interact with RAGE. Moreover, the cross-talk between RAGE and Diaph1 may play a crucial role in the remodeling of the actin cytoskeleton during the progression of EC. *AGER* (the gene encoding RAGE), *Diaph1*, *PFN1*, *CFL1*, and *RhoA* are connected in one network. The network consists of 25 genes (official symbol). STAT6 belongs to the STAT family. The STAT pathway may be dependent on the proper function of the actin cytoskeleton. The server additionally adds genes based on known interactions. Additional genes are represented by gray, unstriped circles (https://genemania.org/) [24]. The colors of the line suggest the type of interaction, that is, red—physical interactions; purple—co-expression; orange—predicted; blue—co-localization; light blue—pathway; green—genetic interactions; olive—shared protein domains. Limited to *Homo sapiens*. Abbreviations: *S100A12*—S100 calcium-binding protein A12; *AGER*—the gene encoding RAGE; *S100B*—S100 calcium-binding protein B; *Diaph1*—diaphanous-related formin 1; *Diaph2*—diaphanous-related formin 2; *PFN1*—profilin 1; *PFN3*—profilin 3; *PFN2*—profilin 2; *HMGB1*—high-mobility group box 1; *ERBB4*—Erb-b2 receptor tyrosine kinase 4; *RELA*—RELA proto-oncogene, NFKB subunit; *STAT6*—signal transducer and activator of transcription 6; *RTKN*—rhotekin; *RHOA*—ras homolog family member A; *PKD2*—polycystin 2; *SSH2*—slingshot

protein phosphatase 2; *CFL1*—cofilin 1; *ACTB*—actin beta; *SSH1*—slingshot protein phosphatase 1; *RHOC*—ras homolog family member C; *SSH3*—slingshot protein phosphatase 3; *VASP*—vasodilator stimulated phosphoprotein; *LIMK1*—LIM domain kinase 1; *ACTA1*—actin alpha 1; *DAAM1*—dishevelled associated activator of morphogenesis 1. N/A—not applicable. See File S3. The interaction network using GeneMANIA was created in the publication by Zglejc-Waszak et al. [8]. These are not the same interaction networks as in the previous publication [8]. The similarity may result from the databases used by the GeneMANIA server.

Previous studies have shown that RAGE and its proinflammatory ligands are involved in actin polymerization in breast cancer cells [83]. Moreover, the molecular complex of RAGE and its ligands may promote the migration and invasion of human breast cancer cells through actin cytoskeleton modifications [83]. We can suppose that signal transduction in the RAGE pathway occurs as a result of the proper polymerization of actin [39,84,85]. Overall, the RAGE-Diaph1 interaction and, thus, cytoskeletal dynamics may be involved in EC progression. However, further studies are necessary to clarify this mechanism.

4. Cancer and Diabetes

Diabetes mellitus is a set of metabolic diseases accompanied by high glucose and the development of various disorders [8,12,86]. In recent years, many investigations revealed an association between diabetes and cancer progression [86,87]. However, in this review, we do not describe all the similarities between diabetes and cancer; rather, we will focus on the role of RAGE-dependent mechanisms in diabetes and cancer.

RAGE is a protein that increases with chronic inflammation, oxidative stress, and high glucose levels. These pathological conditions are characteristic not only for diabetic complications but also for cancer. Therefore, RAGE may be involved in the process of carcinogenesis in the endometrium [42,86,87]. Contrary to appearances, cancer is a disease with a metabolic disorder. High-throughput studies have demonstrated altered expression of metabolism-related genes in EC [4]. Moreover, a disturbed metabolic mechanism is a common feature of most cancers, regardless of where they occur [88]. Neoplasm consumes very large amounts of glucose compared to healthy tissue; this phenomenon is known as the Warburg effect [4,88,89]. The hyperglycemia milieu causes an increased influx of AGEs, the activation of RAGE and its proinflammatory ligands, as well as formins involved in the dynamics of the actin cytoskeleton [8,9,14]. We observe this pathological mechanism in both diabetes complications and cancer.

Studies have shown that diabetes doubles the risk of developing liver, pancreas, and EC. However, no relationship was found between diabetes and lung cancer, but it was shown that uncontrolled hyperglycemia reduces the likelihood of prostate cancer [86,87]. The reasons for the relationship between cancer and diabetes have been the subject of debate for several decades. We are currently investigating a common signaling pathway, the RAGE-dependent pathway.

Our studies have indicated that diabetes has an impact on female reproductive systems [6]. Diabetes contributes to increased inflammation in the uterus during the estrous cycle [6]. Inflammation is a key to creating an environment for cancer progression [42,86,87]. Chronic local inflammation causes an increase in the amount of S100B and HMGB1 and, consequently, activation of the RAGE-dependent signaling pathway [6,8,90,91]. We assume that RAGE-HMGB1-S100B interactions may contribute to the pathogenesis related to diabetes and cancer [42,52,59–61]. Studies have indicated that silencing S100B and HMGB1 delays diabetic complications and cancer progression [42,92].

Reports have indicated that increasing oxidative stress is characteristic of cancer. Oxidative stress induces RAGE signaling pathways in cancer cells [21]. Activation of the RAGE signaling pathway increases the amount of proinflammatory cytokines [42,52,59–61]. During the development of cancer, there is an accumulation of negative factors: high glucose levels, inflammation, and oxidative stress. Intracorporeal homeostasis is disturbed. A high concentration of AGEs causes mutagenesis, protein misfolding, and, thus, loss of protein functions [8,9,12–15]. All these factors stimulate the proliferation and migration of cancer cells. Moreover, the RAGE pathway leads to the activation of the PI3K/Akt and NFKB-dependent signaling cascades in cancer cells. A large amount of evidence suggests that RAGE signaling pathways are related to cancer as well as diabetic perturbations [31,32].

Evidence indicates that blocking RAGE transduction may slow down cancer progression. One of the molecules that can inhibit the activity of the RAGE pathway is its variant circulating in the plasma [93,94]. It is soluble RAGE (sRAGE). sRAGE can sequester proinflammatory RAGE ligands and, thus, reduce inflammation and oxidative stress during cancer. sRAGE may be a hope for stopping cancer development [95]. Moreover, studies report that sRAGE may be used as a biomarker because low levels of circulating sRAGE may indicate the risk of cancer progression and metastasis [96]. However, further studies are necessary to clarify the role of sRAGE as a therapeutic target against cancer development.

Mangigrasso et al. [69] found a small molecule, RAGE229, that may have the ability to block the RAGE signaling pathway. RAGE229 interacts with the cytoplasmatic domain of the AGE receptor and, thus, inhibits the cross-talk between RAGE and Diaph1 [68]. The cytoplasmic domain is the site of Diaph1 binding to RAGE. Studies in a mouse model showed that the abolition of the RAGE-Diaph1 interaction may diminish inflammation and oxidative stress during perturbations [69]. To date, there is very limited knowledge on the role of Diaph1 in the progression of cancer. However, the most recent evidence indicates that Diaph1 may play a crucial role in cancer with accompanied inflammation and oxidative stress [70].

Moreover, the cross-talk between RAGE-Diaph1 is crucial during micovessel formation [15,20]. Tumor vessels are a non-physiological structure and may complicate cancer treatment [97]. Blood vessels supply cancer cells with nutrients and oxygen. These ingredients are necessary for further progression/invasion of cancer. Hence, RAGE-Diaph1 interaction may be a key factor in cancer treatment. It is well known that cancer cells promote vascularization as well as innervation. Hence, we cannot exclude the role of axonogenesis in the progression of carcinogenesis [98]. Studies have indicated that RAGE and its ligands are present in nervous cells as well as tissue [8–11,44,99]. The role of RAGE signaling during neurodegenerative diseases is well established [8,12]. The cross-talk between RAGE and Diaph1 in the neurological complications of diabetes and cancer should be the subject of further research. In this review, we have assumed that the RAGE cascade is crucial during the progression of cancer. Therefore, in the process of cancer treatment, we should look at the problem holistically. The therapy should cover many aspects key to the development of the cancer, such as inflammation, high glucose levels, oxidative stress, axonogenesis, and vasculogenesis. [8,12,97,98].

Therefore, blocking the RAGE signaling pathway may be a milestone in the treatment of many pathological conditions caused by high glucose levels, oxidative stress, and inflammation. However, the switch that determines whether it will be a diabetes- or cancer-related disorder may depend on epigenetic modifications.

5. DNA Methylation in Endometrial Cancer (EC)

DNA methylation is one of the epigenetic modifications. Numerous studies have indicated that epigenetic modifications may be linked to gynecological malignancies [100,101]. Malfunctions in DNA methylation may play a role in the onset and progression of EC, as abnormal epigenetic patterns may be acquired throughout life. Thus, epigenetic modifications may contribute to an increased risk of gynecological malignancies [100,101].

Methylation remodeling is dependent on DNA methyltransferases, i.e., DNMT1, DNMT3a, and DNMT3b [102]. Our studies indicated that DNA methylation is maintained by the methylation complex in the uterus tissues [102,103]. The main elements of the methylation complex include DNA methyltransferases, the tripartite motif containing 28 (TRIM28), and zinc finger protein 57 (ZFP57) [103].

Briefly, studies have revealed that zinc finger protein 57 (ZFP57) recognizes methylation sites within a DNA sequence. Next, ZFP57 interacts with TRIM28, which triggers and attracts DNA methyltransferases [103]. Therefore, DNA methylation is maintained and determined by methylation complex elements, such as ZFP57, TRIM28, DNMT1, DNMT3a, and DNMT3b [100–103].

Uterine tissues are extremely sensitive to environmental factors [104]. Our studies indicated that periconceptional undernutrition affects in utero methyltransferase expression and steroid hormone concentrations in uterine flushings and blood plasma during the peri-implantation period in domestic pigs. Studies have shown that nutrition may alter the DNA methylation levels in the uterus [104]. DNA methylation regulates gene expression and, thus, the activity of proteins, as well as signaling pathways in cells/tissues. We documented that under-nutrition alters the transcriptomic profile in the endometrium as well as in the myometrium [105,106]. In this review, we would like to demonstrate alterations in DNA methylation that influence the RAGE signaling pathway.

Many serious complications have been found to be the result of RAGE-dependent epigenetic modifications [8,9,12–15]. Kan and co-workers [107] revealed that RAGE gene promoter methylation influences diabetic retinitis. They observed that DNA methylation inhibits the activity of RAGE signaling pathways [107]. Studies showed that if the RAGE pathway is not activated, it results in a reduction in proinflammatory cytokines and, thus, the elimination of inflammation [8,91,107–109]. Moreover, Wu et al. [108] revealed that RAGE is regulated epigenetically by an altered microenvironment.

AGEs may alter the microenvironment in a cell and influence the RAGE signaling pathways [8,19,108]. They interact with RAGE and trigger downstream signaling pathways. Studies have indicated that the molecular interaction between AGEs and RAGE increases the production of proinflammatory cytokines. Cytokines induce inflammation and, thus, change the microenvironment in the cell. Chronic inflammation triggers the RAGE signaling pathways and increases AGE levels. Therefore, we observed feedback loops between inflammation, proinflammatory cytokines, AGEs, and RAGE signaling pathways (Figure 3) [8,19,108]. Overall, if we reduce the inflammatory environment, we inhibit the RAGE signaling pathways. Therefore, we observe epigenetic regulation of the RAGE signaling pathway.

Epigenetic modifications are sensitive to microenvironment alternations [109,110]. We may observe an altered microenvironment during cancer. In the neoplasm, we may observe metabolic alterations, high glucose levels, oxidation stress, and inflammation. All these factors can change the cell microenvironment and influence the epigenetic modifications, especially DNA methylation, which is important in the activity of the RAGE signaling pathway [107–109].

Sidorkiewicz et al. [4] revealed that metabolic status may be involved in EC progression. The GeneMANIA [24] analysis revealed that *SLC7A11, SLC7A5, RUNX1, LAMA4, COL6A3, PDK1, CCNA1, ENO1, PKM, NR2F1, NAALAD2* [4], *DNMT1, DNMT3a, DNMT3b, TRIM28,* and *ZFP57* (methylation complex genes) are involved in two networks (Figure 5). We observed the direct interaction between methylation complex genes and molecules involved in metabolism during the progression of EC (Figure 5). The in silico analysis revealed that *DNMT1* directly interacts with *RUNX1, ENO1, SLC7A5,* and the cross-talk *TRIM28* with *RUNX1, ENO1, PKM,* and *CCNA1* (Figure 5). We suppose that methylation complex molecules may be involved in the regulation of the central carbon metabolism pathway (hsa05230) in EC [4]. Analysis revealed that *DNMT1* is involved in DNA methylation or demethylation, DNA modification, DNA methylation-dependent heterochromatin assembly, regulation of histone H3-K9 methylation, methylation, and the regulation of the DNA methylation-dependent heterochromatin assembly function (Figure 5). Nevertheless, *TRIM28* is engaged in the regulation of DNA methylation-dependent heterochromatin assembly and the DNA methylation-dependent heterochromatin assembly function (Figure 5). Our in silico analysis showed the methylation complex, and, thus, DNA methylation may be involved in EC (Figure 5).

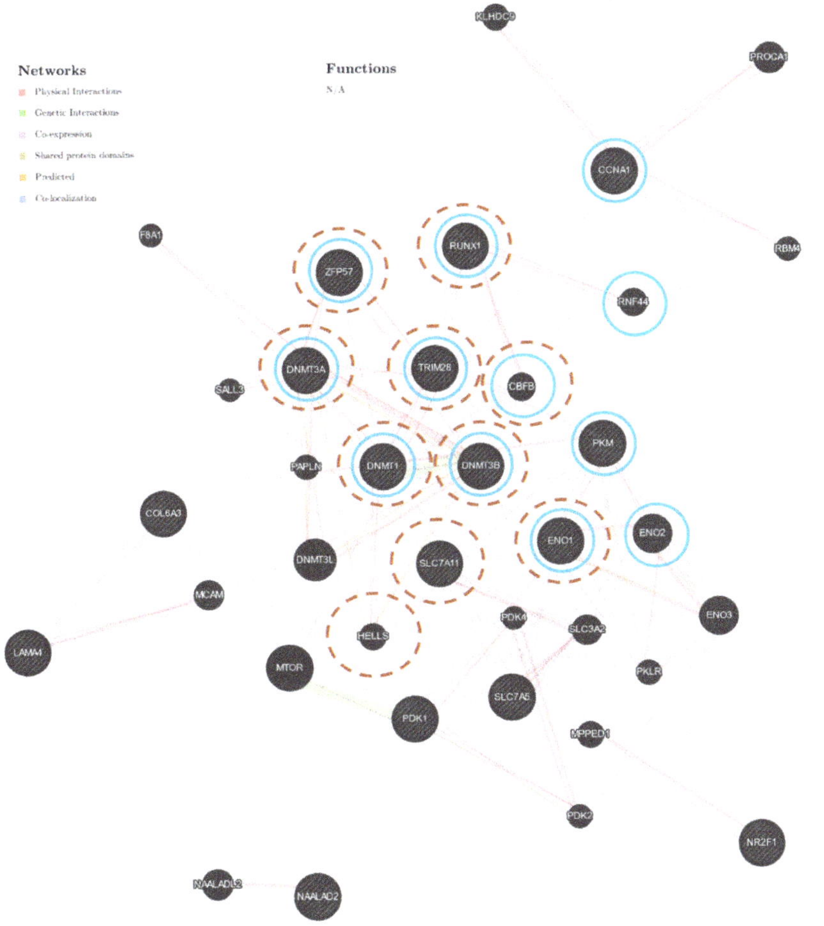

Figure 5. Graph representing the interaction networks of selected genes. The GeneMANIA network indicates the direct interaction between the methylation complex genes and molecules involved in metabolism during the progression of EC [4]. The in silico analysis revealed that *TRIM28* (blue circles) and *DNMT1* (orange, dashed circles) interacted with genes engaged in central carbon metabolism in cancer (hsa05230) [4], limited to *Homo sapiens* (https://genemania.org/) [24]. The colors of the line suggest the type of interaction, that is, red—physical interactions; purple—co-expression; orange—predicted; blue—co-localization; light blue—pathway; green—genetic interactions; olive—shared protein domains. Selected genes are represented by circles with stripes. Abbreviations: *MCAM*—melanoma cell adhesion molecule; *RNF44*—ring finger protein 44; *CBFB*—core-binding factor subunit beta; *HELLS*—helicase, lymphoid specific; *KLHDC9*—kelch domain-containing 9; *MPPED1*—metallophosphoesterase domain-containing 1; *PKLR*—pyruvate kinase L/R; *PAPLN*—papilin, proteoglycan-like sulfated glycoprotein; *RBM4*—RNA-binding motif protein 4; *PDK2*—pyruvate dehydrogenase kinase 2; *PDK4*—pyruvate dehydrogenase kinase 4; *F8A1*—coagulation factor VIII associated 1; *SALL3*—spalt-like transcription factor 3; *SLC3A2*—solute carrier family 3 member 2; *NAALADL2*—N-acetylated alpha-linked acidic dipeptidase-like 2; *PROCA1*—protein interacting with cyclin A1; *ENO2*—enolase 2; *ENO3*—enolase 3; *DNMT3L*—DNA methyltransferase 3-like; *MTOR*—mechanistic target of rapamycin kinase; *TRIM28*—tripartite motif-containing 28;

CCNA1—cyclin A1; PDK1—pyruvate dehydrogenase kinase 1; *PKM*—pyruvate kinase M1/2; *ENO1*—enolase 1; *RUNX1*—RUNX family transcription factor 1; *DNMT1*—DNA methyltransferase 1, *LAMA4*—laminin subunit alpha 4, *DNMT3A*—DNA methyltransferase 3 alpha, *NR2F1*—nuclear receptor subfamily 2 group F member 1; *DNMT3B*—DNA methyltransferase 3 beta; *SLC7A5*—solute carrier family 7 member 5; *COL6A3*—collagen type VI alpha 3 chain; *SLC7A11*—solute carrier family 7 member 11; *ZFP57*—zinc finger protein 57. N/A—not applicable. See File S4.

Future studies on the role of DNA methylation in the activity of RAGE signaling pathways will likely accelerate our understanding of the complex signaling events in EC [111]. In the review, we emphasize the role of a holistic view of the cause of gynecological malignancies (https://www.proteinatlas.org/ENSG00000130816-DNMT1/pathology, accessed on 1 August 2024; https://www.proteinatlas.org/ENSG00000119772-DNMT3A/pathology, accessed on 1 August 2024; https://www.proteinatlas.org/ENSG00000130726-TRIM28/pathology, accessed on 1 August 2024; https://www.proteinatlas.org/ENSG00000204644-ZFP57/pathology, accessed on 1 August 2024; https://www.proteinatlas.org/ENSG00000088305-DNMT3B/pathology, accessed on 1 August 2024).

Promoter methylation cooperates with single nucleotide polymorphisms (SNPs) to modulate RAGE transcription and may alter the perturbation risks. Studies have indicated that alle-374T is associated with non-proliferative retinopathy. Moreover, studies have shown that the rs1800624 and rs1800625 alleles are correlated with ulcerative colitis. Studies have shown that the mentioned polymorphisms in the promoter activate transcription of the *RAGE/AGER* gene. We also propose that the methylation status and *RAGE* promoter genotype could jointly serve as clinical biomarkers to assist in perturbation risk assessments. However, further studies are necessary to decipher the SNPs in EC.

6. Conclusions

The data on the potential role of RAGE signaling pathways in EC are growing. Environmental factors such as hyperglycemia, inflammation, and oxidative stress may have an impact on the progression of EC. It is possible that RAGE signaling pathways are epigenetically controlled, particularly through DNA methylation. DNA methylation may play a crucial role in the progression of EC. These data justify further studies to fully elucidate the role of DNA methylation and RAGE signaling pathways in gynecological malignancies.

Supplementary Materials: The following supporting information can be downloaded at https://www.mdpi.com/article/10.3390/cancers16183192/s1, Table S1: In silico analysis revealed that the gene network is involved in multiple biological functions; File S1: Gene functions in the network. Supplementary data for Figure 1; File S2: Gene functions in the network. Supplementary data for Figure 2; File S3: Gene functions in the network. Supplementary data for Figure 4; File S4: Gene functions in the network. Supplementary data for Figure 5.

Author Contributions: Conceptualization, K.Z.-W.; methodology, K.Z.-W. and M.J.; software, K.Z.-W.; validation, K.Z.-W. and M.J.; formal analysis, K.Z.-W.; investigation, K.Z.-W.; resources, K.Z.-W.; data curation, K.Z.-W., M.J. and J.W.; writing—original draft preparation, K.Z.-W.; writing—review and editing, K.Z.-W., M.T. and M.J.; visualization, K.Z.-W. and M.T.; supervision, M.J. and J.W.; project administration, K.Z.-W. and J.W.; funding acquisition, J.W. All authors have read and agreed to the published version of the manuscript.

Funding: This research received no external funding.

Conflicts of Interest: The authors declare no conflicts of interest.

References

1. Fazeli, A.; Holt, W.V. Cross talk during the periconception period. *Theriogenology* **2016**, *86*, 438–442. [CrossRef] [PubMed]
2. Lee, J.Y.; Lee, M.; Lee, S.K. Role of endometrial immune cells in implantation. *Clin. Exp. Reprod. Med.* **2011**, *38*, 119–125. [CrossRef] [PubMed]
3. Byrne, F.L.; Martin, A.R.; Kosasih, M.; Caruana, B.T.; Farrell, R. The Role of Hyperglycemia in Endometrial Cancer Pathogenesis. *Cancers* **2020**, *12*, 1191. [CrossRef]

4. Sidorkiewicz, I.; Jóźwik, M.; Buczyńska, A.; Erol, A.; Jóźwik, M.; Moniuszko, M.; Jarząbek, K.; Niemira, M.; Krętowski, A. Identification and subsequent validation of transcriptomic signature associated with metabolic status in endometrial cancer. *Sci. Rep.* **2023**, *13*, 13763. [CrossRef] [PubMed]
5. Zheng, L.; Li, D.; Zhou, Y.M.; Yang, H.; Cheng, D.; Ma, X.X. Effects of receptor for advanced glycation endproducts on microvessel formation in endometrial cancer. *BMC Cancer* **2016**, *16*, 93. [CrossRef]
6. Zglejc-Waszak, K.; Korytko, A.; Pomianowski, A.; Wojtkiewicz, J.; Wąsowicz, K.; Juranek, J.K. A mouse model of uterine exposure to long-term hyperglycemia and a high-fat diet. *Anim. Sci. Pap. Rep.* **2024**, *42*, 203–216. [CrossRef]
7. Pintican, R.; Bura, V.; Zerunian, M.; Smith, J.; Addley, H.; Freeman, S.; Caruso, D.; Laghi, A.; Sala, E.; Jimenez-Linan, M. MRI of the endometrium—From normal appearances to rare pathology. *Br. J. Radiol.* **2021**, *94*, 20201347. [CrossRef]
8. Zglejc-Waszak, K.; Mukherjee, K.; Juranek, J.K. The cross-talk between RAGE and DIAPH1 in neurological complications of diabetes: A review. *Eur. J. Neurosci.* **2021**, *54*, 5982–5999. [CrossRef]
9. Zglejc-Waszak, K.; Mukherjee, K.; Korytko, A.; Lewczuk, B.; Pomianowski, A.; Wojtkiewicz, J.; Banach, M.; Załęcki, M.; Nowicka, N.; Jarosławska, J.; et al. Novel insights into the nervous system affected by prolonged hyperglycemia. *J. Mol. Med.* **2023**, *101*, 1015–1028. [CrossRef]
10. Nowicka, N.; Zglejc-Waszak, K.; Juranek, J.; Korytko, A.; Wąsowicz, K.; Chmielewska-Krzesińska, M.; Wojtkiewicz, J. Novel insights into RAGE signaling pathways during the progression of amyotrophic lateral sclerosis in RAGE-deficient SOD1 G93A mice. *PLoS ONE* **2024**, *19*, e0299567. [CrossRef]
11. Nowicka, N.; Szymańska, K.; Juranek, J.; Zglejc-Waszak, K.; Korytko, A.; Załęcki, M.; Chmielewska-Krzesińska, M.; Wąsowicz, K.; Wojtkiewicz, J. The Involvement of RAGE and Its Ligands during Progression of ALS in SOD1 G93A Transgenic Mice. *Int. J. Mol. Sci.* **2022**, *23*, 2184. [CrossRef] [PubMed]
12. Juranek, J.; Mukherjee, K.; Kordas, B.; Załęcki, M.; Korytko, A.; Zglejc-Waszak, K.; Szuszkiewicz, J.; Banach, M. Role of RAGE in the Pathogenesis of Neurological Disorders. *Neurosci. Bull.* **2022**, *38*, 1248–1262. [CrossRef] [PubMed]
13. Zglejc-Waszak, K.; Schmidt, A.M.; Juranek, J.K. The receptor for advanced glycation end products and its ligands' expression in OVE26 diabetic sciatic nerve during the development of length-dependent neuropathy. *Neuropathology* **2023**, *43*, 84–94. [CrossRef]
14. Zglejc-Waszak, K.; Pomianowski, A.; Wojtkiewicz, J.; Banach, M.; Juranek, J.K. New insights into RAGE/Diaph1 interaction as a modulator of actin cytoskeleton dynamics in peripheral nervous system in long-term hyperglycaemia. *Eur. J. Neurosci.* **2023**, *57*, 1642–1656. [CrossRef] [PubMed]
15. Jaroslawska, J.; Korytko, A.; Zglejc-Waszak, K.; Antonowski, T.; Pomianowski, A.S.; Wasowicz, K.; Wojtkiewicz, J.; Juranek, J.K. Peripheral Neuropathy Presents Similar Symptoms and Pathological Changes in Both High-Fat Diet and Pharmacologically Induced Pre- and Diabetic Mouse Models. *Life* **2021**, *11*, 126. [CrossRef]
16. Bao, J.M.; He, M.Y.; Liu, Y.W.; Lu, Y.J.; Hong, Y.Q.; Luo, H.H.; Ren, Z.L.; Zhao, S.C.; Jiang, Y. AGE/RAGE/Akt pathway contributes to prostate cancer cell proliferation by promoting Rb phosphorylation and degradation. *Am. J. Cancer Res.* **2015**, *5*, 1741–1750. [CrossRef]
17. Xu, X.; Zhu, H.; Wang, T.; Sun, Y.; Ni, P.; Liu, Y.; Tian, S.; Amoah Barnie, P.; Shen, H.; Xu, W.; et al. Exogenous high-mobility group box 1 inhibits apoptosis and promotes the proliferation of lewis cells via RAGE/TLR4-dependent signal pathways. *Scand. J. Immunol.* **2014**, *79*, 386–394. [CrossRef]
18. Ishibashi, Y.; Matsui, T.; Takeuchi, M.; Yamagishi, S. Metformin inhibits advanced glycation end products (AGEs)-induced growth and VEGF expression in MCF-7 breast cancer cells by suppressing AGEs receptor expression via AMP-activated protein kinase. *Horm. Metab. Res.* **2013**, *45*, 387–390. [CrossRef]
19. Nowicka, N.; Juranek, J.; Juranek, J.K.; Wojtkiewicz, J. Risk Factors and Emerging Therapies in Amyotrophic Lateral Sclerosis. *Int. J. Mol. Sci.* **2019**, *20*, 2616. [CrossRef]
20. Manigrasso, M.B.; Juranek, J.; Ramasamy, R.; Schmidt, A.M. Unlocking the biology of RAGE in diabetic microvascular complications. *Trends Endocrinol. Metab.* **2014**, *25*, 15–22. [CrossRef]
21. Daffu, G.; del Pozo, C.H.; O'Shea, K.M.; Ananthakrishnan, R.; Ramasamy, R.; Schmidt, A.M. Radical roles for RAGE in the pathogenesis of oxidative stress in cardiovascular diseases and beyond. *Int. J. Mol. Sci.* **2013**, *14*, 19891–19910. [CrossRef] [PubMed]
22. International Agency for Research on Cancer. *World Cancer Report 2014*; World Health Organization: Geneva, Switzerland, 2014; Chapter 5.12; ISBN 978-92-832-0429-9.
23. International Agency for Research on Cancer. *World Cancer Report: Cancer Research for Cancer Prevention 2020*; World Cancer Reports; International Agency for Research on Cancer: Lyon, France, 2020; ISBN 24978-92-832-0447-3.
24. Franz, M.; Rodriguez, H.; Lopes, C.; Zuberi, K.; Montojo, J.; Bader, G.D.; Morris, Q. GeneMANIA update 2018. *Nucleic Acids Res.* **2018**, *W1*, W60–W64. [CrossRef] [PubMed]
25. Nagarajan, A.; Malvi, P.; Wajapeyee, N. Oncogene-directed alterations in cancer cell metabolism. *Trends Cancer* **2016**, *2*, 365–377. [CrossRef] [PubMed]
26. Hanahan, D.; Weinberg, R.A. Hallmarks of cancer: The next generation. *Cell* **2011**, *144*, 646–674. [CrossRef]
27. Hanahan, D.; Weinberg, R.A. The hallmarks of cancer. *Cell* **2000**, *100*, 57–70. [CrossRef] [PubMed]
28. Liberti, M.V.; Locasale, J.W. The Warburg efect: How does it beneft cancer cells? *Trends Biochem. Sci.* **2016**, *41*, 211–218. [CrossRef]
29. Li, W.; Wang, J. Uncovering the underlying mechanisms of cancer metabolism through the landscapes and probability fux quantifcations. *IScience* **2020**, *23*, 101002. [CrossRef]

30. Byrne, F.L.; Poon, I.K.; Modesitt, S.C.; Tomsig, J.L.; Chow, J.D.; Healy, M.E.; Baker, W.D.; Atkins, K.A.; Lancaster, J.M.; Marchion, D.C.; et al. Metabolic vulnerabilities in endometrial cancer. *Cancer Res.* **2014**, *74*, 5832–5845. [CrossRef]
31. Roncolato, F.; Lindemann, K.; Willson, M.L.; Martyn, J.; Mileshkin, L. PI3K/AKT/mTOR inhibitors for advanced or recurrent endometrial cancer. *Cochrane Database Syst. Rev.* **2019**, *10*, CD012160. [CrossRef]
32. Ramasubbu, K.; Devi Rajeswari, V. Impairment of insulin signaling pathway PI3K/Akt/mTOR and insulin resistance induced AGEs on diabetes mellitus and neurodegenerative diseases: A perspective review. *Mol. Cell Biochem.* **2023**, *478*, 1307–1324. [CrossRef]
33. Jarosławska, J.; Kordas, B.; Miłowski, T.; Juranek, J.K. Mammalian Diaphanous1 signalling in neurovascular complications of diabetes. *Eur. J. Neurosci.* **2024**, *59*, 2628–2645. [CrossRef] [PubMed]
34. Guo, Y.; Xia, P.; Zheng, J.J.; Sun, X.B.; Pan, X.D.; Zhang, X.; Wu, C.Z. Receptors for advanced glycation end products (RAGE) is associated with microvessel density and is a prognostic biomarker for clear cell renal cell carcinoma. *Biomed. Pharmacother.* **2015**, *73*, 147–153. [CrossRef] [PubMed]
35. Liang, H.; Zhong, Y.; Zhou, S.; Peng, L. Knockdown of RAGE expression inhibits colorectal cancer cell invasion and suppresses angiogenesis in vitro and in vivo. *Cancer Lett.* **2011**, *313*, 91–98. [CrossRef] [PubMed]
36. Healey, G.D.; Pan-Castillo, B.; Garcia-Parra, J.; Davies, J.; Roberts, S.; Jones, E.; Dhar, K.; Nandanan, S.; Tofazzal, N.; Piggott, L.; et al. Antibody drug conjugates against the receptor for advanced glycation end products (RAGE), a novel therapeutic target in endometrial cancer. *J. Immunother. Cancer* **2019**, *7*, 280. [CrossRef]
37. Goldin, A.; Beckman, J.A.; Schmidt, A.M.; Creager, M.A. Advanced glycation end products: Sparking the development of diabetic vascular injury. *Circulation* **2006**, *114*, 597–605. [CrossRef]
38. Cerami, C.; Founds, H.; Nicholl, I.; Mitsuhashi, T.; Giordano, D.; Vanpatten, S.; Lee, A.; Al-Abed, Y.; Vlassara, H.; Bucala, R.; et al. Tobacco smoke is a source of toxic reactive glycation products. *Proc. Natl. Acad. Sci. USA* **1997**, *94*, 13915–13920. [CrossRef]
39. Senatus, L.; Egaña-Gorroño, L.; López-Díez, R.; Bergaya, S.; Aranda, J.F.; Amengual, J.; Arivazhagan, L.; Manigrasso, M.B.; Yepuri, G.; Nimma, R.; et al. DIAPH1 mediates progression of atherosclerosis and regulates hepatic lipid metabolism in mice. *Commun. Biol.* **2023**, *6*, 280. [CrossRef] [PubMed]
40. Wendt, T.; Tanji, N.; Guo, J.; Hudson, B.I.; Bierhaus, A.; Ramasamy, R.; Arnold, B.; Nawroth, P.P.; Yan, S.F.; D'Agati, V.; et al. Glucose, glycation, and RAGE: Implications for amplification of cellular dysfunction in diabetic nephropathy. *J. Am. Soc. Nephrol.* **2003**, *14*, 1383–1395. [CrossRef]
41. Schmidt, A.M.; Yan, S.D.; Yan, S.F.; Stern, D.M. The multiligand receptor RAGE as a progression factor amplifying immune and inflammatory responses. *J. Clin. Investig.* **2001**, *108*, 949–955. [CrossRef]
42. Palanissami, G.; Paul, S.F.D. RAGE and Its Ligands: Molecular Interplay between Glycation, Inflammation, and Hallmarks of Cancer-a Review. *Horm. Cancer* **2018**, *9*, 295–325. [CrossRef]
43. Dong, H.; Zhang, Y.; Huang, Y.; Deng, H. Pathophysiology of RAGE in inflammatory diseases. *Front. Immunol.* **2022**, *13*, 931473. [CrossRef] [PubMed]
44. Juranek, J.K.; Aleshin, A.; Rattigan, E.M.; Johnson, L.; Qu, W.; Song, F.; Ananthakrishnan, R.; Quadri, N.; Yan, S.D.; Ramasamy, R.; et al. Morphological Changes and Immunohistochemical Expression of RAGE and its Ligands in the Sciatic Nerve of Hyperglycemic Pig (Sus Scrofa). *Biochem. Insights* **2010**, *2010*, 47–59. [CrossRef] [PubMed]
45. Srinivasan, M.; Banerjee, S.; Palmer, A.; Zheng, G.; Chen, A.; Bosland, M.C.; Kajdacsy-Balla, A.; Kalyanasundaram, R.; Munirathinam, G. HMGB1 in hormone-related cancer: A potential therapeutic target. *Horm. Cancer* **2014**, *5*, 127–139. [CrossRef] [PubMed]
46. Yen, M.C.; Huang, Y.C.; Kan, J.Y.; Kuo, P.L.; Hou, M.F.; Hsu, Y.L. S100B expression in breast cancer as a predictive marker for cancer metastasis. *Int. J. Oncol.* **2018**, *52*, 433–440. [CrossRef]
47. Angelopoulou, E.; Piperi, C.; Papavassiliou, A.G. High-mobility group box 1 in Parkinson's disease: From pathogenesis to therapeutic approaches. *J. Neurochem.* **2018**, *146*, 211–218. [CrossRef]
48. Angelopoulou, E.; Paudel, Y.N.; Piperi, C. Emerging role of S100B protein implication in Parkinson's disease pathogenesis. *Cell Mol. Life Sci.* **2021**, *78*, 1445–1453. [CrossRef]
49. Paudel, Y.N.; Angelopoulou, E.; Piperi, C.; Othman, I.; Aamir, K.; Shaikh, M.F. Impact of HMGB1, RAGE, and TLR4 in Alzheimer's Disease (AD): From Risk Factors to Therapeutic Targeting. *Cells* **2020**, *9*, 383. [CrossRef]
50. Scaffidi, P.; Misteli, T.; Bianchi, M.E. Release of chromatin protein HMGB1 by necrotic cells triggers inflammation. *Nature* **2002**, *418*, 191–195, Erratum in *Nature* **2010**, *467*, 622. [CrossRef] [PubMed]
51. Todorova, J.; Pasheva, E. High mobility group B1 protein interacts with its receptor RAGE in tumor cells but not in normal tissues. *Oncol. Lett.* **2012**, *3*, 214–218. [CrossRef]
52. Luan, X.; Ma, C.; Wang, P.; Lou, F. HMGB1 is negatively correlated with the development of endometrial carcinoma and prevents cancer cell invasion and metastasis by inhibiting the process of epithelial-to-mesenchymal transition. *Onco Targets Ther.* **2017**, *10*, 1389–1402. [CrossRef]
53. Hori, O.; Brett, J.; Slattery, T.; Cao, R.; Zhang, J.; Chen, J.X.; Nagashima, M.; Lundh, E.R.; Vijay, S.; Nitecki, D. The receptor for advanced glycation end products (RAGE) is a cellular binding site for amphoterin. Mediation of neurite outgrowth and co-expression of rage and amphoterin in the developing nervous system. *J. Biol. Chem.* **1995**, *270*, 25752–25761. [CrossRef] [PubMed]

54. Kang, R.; Tang, D.; Schapiro, N.E.; Livesey, K.M.; Farkas, A.; Loughran, P.; Bierhaus, A.; Lotze, M.T.; Zeh, H.J. The receptor for advanced glycation end products (RAGE) sustains autophagy and limits apoptosis, promoting pancreatic tumor cell survival. *Cell Death Differ.* **2010**, *17*, 666–676. [CrossRef] [PubMed]
55. Gonzalez, L.L.; Garrie, K.; Turner, M.D. Role of S100 proteins in health and disease. *Biochim. Biophys. Acta Mol. Cell Res.* **2020**, *1867*, 118677. [CrossRef] [PubMed]
56. Leclerc, E.; Vetter, S.W. The role of S100 proteins and their receptor RAGE in pancreatic cancer. *BBA-Mol. Basis Dis.* **2015**, *852*, 2706–2711. [CrossRef]
57. Bresnick, A.R.; Weber, D.J.; Zimmer, D.B. S100 proteins in cancer. *Nat. Rev. Cancer.* **2015**, *15*, 96–109. [CrossRef]
58. Yin, C.; Li, H.; Zhang, B.; Liu, Y.; Lu, G.; Lu, S.; Sun, L.; Qi, Y.; Li, X.; Chen, W. RAGE-binding S100A8/A9 promotes the migration and invasion of human breast cancer cells through actin polymerization and epithelial–mesenchymal transition. *Breast Cancer Res. Treat.* **2013**, *142*, 297–309. [CrossRef]
59. Bonfrer, J.M.; Korse, C.M.; Nieweg, O.E.; Rankin, E.M. The luminescence immunoassay S-100: A sensitive test to measure circulating S-100B: Its prognostic value in malignant melanoma. *Br. J. Cancer* **1998**, *77*, 2210–2214. [CrossRef]
60. Choi, H.; Puvenna, V.; Brennan, C.; Mahmoud, S.; Wang, X.F.; Phillips, M.; Janigro, D.; Mazzone, P. S100B and S100B auto-antibody as biomarkers for early detection of brain metastases in lung cancer. *Transl. Lung Cancer Res.* **2016**, *5*, 413–419. [CrossRef]
61. Heizmann, C.W. S100B protein in clinical diagnostics: Assay specificity. *Clin. Chem.* **2004**, *50*, 249–251. [CrossRef]
62. Lin, J.; Yang, Q.; Wilder, P.T.; Carrier, F.; Weber, D.J. The calcium-binding protein S100B down-regulates p53 and apoptosis in malignant melanoma. *J. Biol. Chem.* **2010**, *285*, 27487–27498. [CrossRef]
63. Yoshimura, C.; Miyafusa, T.; Tsumoto, K. Identification of small-molecule inhibitors of the human S100B-p53 interaction and evaluation of their activity in human melanoma cells. *Bioorg Med. Chem.* **2013**, *21*, 1109–1115. [CrossRef] [PubMed]
64. Surget, S.; Khoury, M.P.; Bourdon, J.C. Uncovering the role of p53 splice variants in human malignancy: A clinical perspective. *Onco Targets Ther.* **2013**, *7*, 57–68. [CrossRef] [PubMed]
65. Shekhtman, A.; Ramasamy, R.; Schmidt, A.M. Glycation & the RAGE axis: Targeting signal trans-duction through DIAPH1. *Expert. Rev. Proteom.* **2017**, *14*, 147–156. [CrossRef]
66. Arivazhagan, L.; Popp, C.J.; Ruiz, H.H.; Wilson, R.A.; Manigrasso, M.B.; Shekhtman, A.; Ramasamy, R.; Sevick, M.A.; Schmidt, A.M. The RAGE/DIAPH1 axis: Mediator of obesity and proposed biomarker of human cardiometabolic disease. *Cardiovasc. Res.* **2024**, *119*, 2813–2824. [CrossRef]
67. Labat-de-Hoz, L.; Alonso, M.A. Formins in Human Disease. *Cells* **2021**, *10*, 2554. [CrossRef]
68. Manigrasso, M.B.; Pan, J.; Rai, V.; Zhang, J.; Reverdatto, S.; Quadri, N.; DeVita, R.J.; Ramasamy, R.; Shekhtman, A.; Schmidt, A.M. Small Molecule Inhibition of Ligand-Stimulated RAGE-DIAPH1 Signal Transduction. *Sci. Rep.* **2016**, *6*, 22450. [CrossRef] [PubMed]
69. Manigrasso, M.B.; Friedman, R.A.; Ramasamy, R.; D'Agati, V.; Schmidt, A.M. Deletion of the formin Diaph1 protects from structural and functional abnormalities in the murine diabetic kidney. *Am. J. Physiol. Renal Physiol.* **2018**, *315*, F1601–F1612. [CrossRef]
70. Manigrasso, M.B.; Rabbani, P.; Egaña-Gorroño, L.; Quadri, N.; Frye, L.; Zhou, B.; Reverdatto, S.; Ramirez, L.S.; Dansereau, S.; Pan, J.; et al. Small-molecule antagonism of the interaction of the RAGE cytoplasmic domain with DIAPH1 reduces diabetic complications in mice. *Sci. Transl. Med.* **2021**, *13*, eabf7084. [CrossRef]
71. Reis, A.H.O.; Figalo, L.B.; Orsini, M.; Lemos, B. The implications of DNA methylation for amyotrophic lateral sclerosis. *An. Acad. Bras. Cienc.* **2023**, *95* (Suppl. S2), e20230277. [CrossRef]
72. Flat, W.; Borowski, S.; Paraschiakos, T.; Blechner, C.; Windhorst, S. DIAPH1 facilitates paclitaxel-mediated cytotoxicity of ovarian cancer cells. *Biochem Pharmacol.* **2022**, *197*, 114898. [CrossRef]
73. Wu, C.H.; Fallini, C.; Ticozzi, N.; Keagle, P.; Sapp, P.C.; Piotrowska, K.; Lowe, P.; Koppers, M.; McKenna-Yasek, D.; Baron, D.M.; et al. Mutations in the profilin 1 gene cause familial amyotrophic lateral sclerosis. *Nature* **2012**, *488*, 499–503. [CrossRef] [PubMed]
74. Lu, Q.; Lu, L.; Chen, W.; Chen, H.; Xu, X.; Zheng, Z. RhoA/mDia-1/profilin-1 signaling targets microvascular endothelial dysfunction in diabetic retinopathy. *Graefes Arch. Clin. Exp. Ophthalmol.* **2015**, *253*, 669–680. [CrossRef] [PubMed]
75. Carlsson, L.; Nyström, L.E.; Sundkvist, I.; Markey, F.; Lindberg, U. Actin polymerizability is influenced by profilin, a low molecular weight protein in non-muscle cells. *J. Mol. Biol.* **1977**, *115*, 465–483. [CrossRef]
76. Da Silva, J.S.; Medina, M.; Zuliani, C.; Di Nardo, A.; Witke, W.; Dotti, C.G. RhoA/ROCK regulation of neuritogenesis via profilin IIa-mediated control of actin stability. *J. Cell Biol.* **2003**, *162*, 1267–1279. [CrossRef]
77. Hirose, A.; Tanikawa, T.; Mori, H.; Okada, Y.; Tanaka, Y. Advanced glycation end products increase endothelial permeability through the RAGE/Rho signaling pathway. *FEBS Lett.* **2010**, *584*, 61–66. [CrossRef]
78. Bros, M.; Haas, K.; Moll, L.; Grabbe, S. RhoA as a Key Regulator of Innate and Adaptive Immunity. *Cells* **2019**, *8*, 733. [CrossRef] [PubMed]
79. Singh, R.; Wang, B.; Shirvaikar, A.; Khan, S.; Kamat, S.; Schelling, J.R.; Konieczkowski, M.; Sedor, J.R. The IL-1 receptor and Rho directly associate to drive cell activation in inflammation. *J. Clin. Investig.* **1999**, *103*, 1561–1570. [CrossRef]
80. Xu, J.; Huang, Y.; Zhao, J.; Wu, L.; Qi, Q.; Liu, Y.; Li, G.; Li, J.; Liu, H.; Wu, H. Cofilin: A Promising Protein Implicated in Cancer Metastasis and Apoptosis. *Front. Cell Dev. Biol.* **2021**, *9*, 599065. [CrossRef]

81. Wang, Y.; Lu, Y.; Wan, R.; Wang, Y.; Zhang, C.; Li, M.; Deng, P.; Cao, L.; Hu, C. Profilin 1 Induces Tumor Metastasis by Promoting Microvesicle Secretion Through the ROCK 1/p-MLC Pathway in Non-Small Cell Lung Cancer. *Front. Pharmacol.* **2022**, *13*, 890891. [CrossRef]
82. Santos, J.C.; Profitós-Pelejà, N.; Sánchez-Vinces, S.; Roué, G. RHOA Therapeutic Targeting in Hema-tological Cancers. *Cells* **2023**, *12*, 433. [CrossRef]
83. Ghavami, S.; Rashedi, I.; Dattilo, B.M.; Eshraghi, M.; Chazin, W.J.; Hashemi, M.; Wesselborg, S.; Kerkhoff, C.; Los, M. S100A8/A9 at low concentration promotes tumor cell growth via RAGE ligation and MAP kinase-dependent pathway. *J. Leucoc. Biol.* **2008**, *83*, 1484–1492. [CrossRef] [PubMed]
84. Young, K.G.; Copeland, J.W. Formins in cell signaling. *Biochim. Biophys. Acta* **2010**, *1803*, 183–190. [CrossRef] [PubMed]
85. Arber, S.; Barbayannis, F.A.; Hanser, H.; Schneider, C.; Stanyon, C.A.; Bernard, O.; Caroni, P. Regulation of actin dynamics through phosphorylation of cofilin by LIM-kinase. *Nature* **1998**, *393*, 805–809. [CrossRef] [PubMed]
86. Giri, B.; Dey, S.; Das, T.; Sarkar, M.; Banerjee, J.; Dash, S.K. Chronic hyperglycemia mediated physiological alteration and metabolic distortion leads to organ dysfunction, infection, cancer progression and other pathophysiological consequences: An update on glucose toxicity. *Biomed. Pharmacother.* **2018**, *107*, 306–328. [CrossRef] [PubMed]
87. Zhu, B.; Qu, S. The Relationship between Diabetes Mellitus and Cancers and Its Underlying Mechanisms. *Front. Endocrinol.* **2022**, *13*, 800995. [CrossRef]
88. Sullivan, L.B.; Gui, D.Y. Vander Heiden MG. Altered metabolite levels in cancer: Implications for tumour biology and cancer therapy. *Nat. Rev. Cancer* **2016**, *16*, 680–693. [CrossRef]
89. Kellenberger, L.D.; Bruin, J.E.; Greenaway, J.; Campbell, N.E.; Moorehead, R.A.; Holloway, A.C.; Petrik, J. The role of dysregulated glucose metabolism in epithelial ovarian cancer. *J. Oncol.* **2010**, *2010*, 514310. [CrossRef]
90. Naka, Y.; Bucciarelli, L.G.; Wendt, T.; Lee, L.K.; Rong, L.L.; Ramasamy, R.; Yan, S.F.; Schmidt, A.M. RAGE axis: Animal models and novel insights into the vascular complications of diabetes. *Arterioscler. Thromb. Vasc. Biol.* **2004**, *24*, 1342–1349. [CrossRef]
91. Juranek, J.; Ray, R.; Banach, M.; Rai, V. Receptor for advanced glycation end-products in neuro-degenerative diseases. *Rev. Neurosci.* **2015**, *26*, 691–698. [CrossRef]
92. Jiang, S.; Chen, X. HMGB1 siRNA can reduce damage to retinal cells induced by high glucose in vitro and in vivo. *Drug Des. Devel Ther.* **2017**, *11*, 783–795. [CrossRef]
93. Juranek, J.K.; Daffu, G.K.; Geddis, M.S.; Li, H.; Rosario, R.; Kaplan, B.J.; Kelly, L.; Schmidt, A.M. Soluble RAGE Treatment Delays Progression of Amyotrophic Lateral Sclerosis in SOD1 Mice. *Front. Cell Neurosci.* **2016**, *10*, 117. [CrossRef] [PubMed]
94. Juranek, J.; Osowski, A.; Wojtkiewicz, J.; Banach, M. Plasma levels of soluble RAGE, AGEs and AOPPs at the early stage of amyotrophic lateral sclerosis: A preliminary study. *Polim. Med.* **2023**, *53*, 105–110. [CrossRef] [PubMed]
95. Aglago, E.K.; Rinaldi, S.; Freisling, H.; Jiao, L.; Hughes, D.J.; Fedirko, V.; Schalkwijk, C.G.; Weiderpass, E.; Dahm, C.C.; Overvad, K.; et al. Soluble Receptor for Advanced Glycation End-products (sRAGE) and Colorectal Cancer Risk: A Case-Control Study Nested within a European Prospective Cohort. *Cancer Epidemiol. Biomark. Prev.* **2021**, *30*, 182–192. [CrossRef] [PubMed]
96. Erusalimsky, J.D. The use of the soluble receptor for advanced glycation-end products (sRAGE) as a potential biomarker of disease risk and adverse outcomes. *Redox Biol.* **2021**, *42*, 101958. [CrossRef]
97. Ganss, R. Tumour vessel remodelling: New opportunities in cancer treatment. *Vasc. Biol.* **2020**, *2*, R35–R43. [CrossRef]
98. Roda, N.; Blandano, G.; Pelicci, P.G. Blood Vessels and Peripheral Nerves as Key Players in Cancer Progression and Therapy Resistance. *Cancers* **2021**, *13*, 4471. [CrossRef] [PubMed]
99. Juranek, J.K.; Geddis, M.S.; Song, F.; Zhang, J.; Garcia, J.; Rosario, R.; Yan, S.F.; Brannagan, T.H.; Schmidt, A.M. RAGE deficiency improves postinjury sciatic nerve regeneration in type 1 diabetic mice. *Diabetes* **2013**, *62*, 931–943. [CrossRef]
100. Inoue, F.; Sone, K.; Toyohara, Y.; Takahashi, Y.; Kukita, A.; Hara, A.; Taguchi, A.; Tanikawa, M.; Tsuruga, T.; Osuga, Y. Targeting Epigenetic Regulators for Endometrial Cancer Therapy: Its Molecular Biology and Potential Clinical Applications. *Int. J. Mol. Sci.* **2021**, *22*, 2305. [CrossRef]
101. Qian, Y.; Shi, L.; Luo, Z. Long Non-coding RNAs in Cancer: Implications for Diagnosis, Prognosis, and Therapy. *Front. Med.* **2020**, *7*, 612393. [CrossRef]
102. Franczak, A.; Zglejc, K.; Waszkiewicz, E.; Wojciechowicz, B.; Martyniak, M.; Sobotka, W.; Okrasa, S.; Kotwica, G. Periconceptional undernutrition affects in utero methyltransferase expression and steroid hormone concentrations in uterine flushings and blood plasma during the peri-implantation period in domestic pigs. *Reprod. Fertil. Dev.* **2017**, *29*, 1499–1508. [CrossRef]
103. Zglejc, K.; Franczak, A. Peri-conceptional under-nutrition alters the expression of TRIM28 and ZFP57 in the endometrium and embryos during peri-implantation period in domestic pigs. *Reprod. Domest. Anim.* **2017**, *52*, 542–550. [CrossRef] [PubMed]
104. Zglejc-Waszak, K.; Waszkiewicz, E.M.; Franczak, A. Periconceptional undernutrition affects the levels of DNA methylation in the peri-implantation pig endometrium and in embryos. *Theriogenology* **2019**, *123*, 185–193. [CrossRef] [PubMed]
105. Drzewiecka, E.M.; Kozlowska, W.; Zmijewska, A.; Franczak, A. Nutritional restriction during the peri-conceptional period alters the myometrial transcriptome during the peri-implantation period. *Sci. Rep.* **2021**, *11*, 21187. [CrossRef] [PubMed]
106. Zglejc, K.; Martyniak, M.; Waszkiewicz, E.; Kotwica, G.; Franczak, A. Peri-conceptional under-nutrition alters transcriptomic profile in the endometrium during the peri-implantation period-The study in domestic pigs. *Reprod. Domest. Anim.* **2018**, *53*, 74–84. [CrossRef]
107. Kan, S.; Wu, J.; Sun, C.; Hao, J.; Wu, Z. Correlation between RAGE gene promoter methylation and diabetic retinal inflammation. *Exp. Ther. Med.* **2018**, *15*, 242–246. [CrossRef]

108. Wu, X.; Shi, X.; Chen, X.; Yin, Z. Advanced glycation end products regulate the receptor of AGEs epigenetically. *Front. Cell Dev. Biol.* **2023**, *11*, 1062229. [CrossRef]
109. Li, P.; Wang, T.; Chen, M.; Chen, J.; Shen, Y.; Chen, L. RAGE-mediated functional DNA methylat-ed modification contributes to cigarette smoke-induced airway inflammation in mice. *Biosci. Rep.* **2021**, *41*, BSR20210308. [CrossRef]
110. Wang, J.; Zhen, Y.; Zhou, Y.; Yan, S.; Jiang, L.; Zhang, L. Promoter methylation cooperates with SNPs to modulate RAGE transcription and alter UC risk. *Biochem. Biophys. Rep.* **2018**, *17*, 17–22. [CrossRef]
111. Peng, Y.; Wang, Y.; Zhou, C.; Mei, W.; Zeng, C. PI3K/Akt/mTOR Pathway and Its Role in Cancer Therapeutics: Are We Making Headway? *Front. Oncol.* **2022**, *12*, 819128. [CrossRef]

cancers

MDPI

Review

Dermatofibrosarcoma Protuberans: An Updated Review of the Literature

Marcin Jozwik [1,*], Katarzyna Bednarczuk [2] and Zofia Osierda [2]

[1] Department of Gynecology and Obstetrics, Collegium Medicum, University of Warmia and Mazury in Olsztyn, 10-045 Olsztyn, Poland

[2] Scientific Circle of the Department of Gynecology and Obstetrics, University of Warmia and Mazury in Olsztyn, 10-045 Olsztyn, Poland; katarzyna.bednarczuk@student.uwm.edu.pl (K.B.); zofia.osierda@student.uwm.edu.pl (Z.O.)

* Correspondence: marcin.jozwik@uwm.edu.pl; Tel.: +48-89-5398742

Simple Summary: Dermatofibrosarcoma protuberans (DFSP) is a rare proliferative condition representing skin sarcomas which is known to locally recur yet very rarely metastasizes. Its genetic background is a reciprocal translocation t(17;22)(q22;q13) that produces *COL1A1-PDGFB* gene fusion. Complete resection is the primary treatment. The aim of this reappraisal is to review various correlates of the condition. Our review underlines that cases of low-to-moderate grade DFSP with excellent prognosis must be distinguished from high grade fibrosarcomatous DFSP with a much worse prognosis.

Abstract: Dermatofibrosarcoma protuberans (DFSP) is a rare proliferative condition representing skin sarcomas which is known to locally recur yet very rarely metastasizes. Its genetic background is a reciprocal translocation t(17;22)(q22;q13) that produces *COL1A1-PDGFB* gene fusion. Complete resection is the primary treatment. The aim of this review is to outline the pathogenesis, diagnosis, and management of DFSP. A clear-cut distinction between low-to-moderate-grade DFSP with excellent prognosis and high-grade fibrosarcomatous DFSP with a much worse prognosis is underlined. Malignant transformation within DFSP (or high histologic grade), older age, being female, large primary tumor size ($\geq$10 cm), narrow surgical margins of excision (<3 cm), surgical margin positivity for tumor cells, short time to recurrence, numerous recurrences, tumor that was recently rapidly enlarging, and presence of pain in the tumor have all been proposed as clinicopathological risk factors for recurrence and metastasis. A tendency for local growth and local relapses of well- and moderately differentiated DFSPs is an argument for their surgical excision, possibly combined with reconstructive surgery, even in patients of advanced age. Another main point of this review is that cases of DFSP with fibrosarcomatous transformation are a challenge and require careful medical attention. Both anatomopathological evaluation of the presence of lymphovascular space invasion and sentinel lymph node biopsy at DFSP surgery merit further study.

Keywords: dermatofibrosarcoma protuberans; soft-tissue tumor; dermal sarcoma

1. Introduction

Dermatofibrosarcoma protuberans (DFSP) is an uncommon skin and/or soft-tissue malignancy. When borne in the skin, it usually stems from the dermis and subcutaneous tissue, but not from the epidermis. As a soft-tissue tumor, it may involve subcutaneous fat or connective tissue [1,2]. Eisen and Tallini state that DFSP originates in the reticular dermis [3]. Fibroblasts or histiocytes are believed to be the cells of its origin, yet the neoplasm has frequently been referred to as a fibrohistiocytic tumor without defining its precise histogenesis [3–9]. Other likely precursors are perineural cells [10,11]. It was first recognized as a separate entity independently by Sherwell and Taylor in 1890 and later described in much detail by Darier and Ferrand in 1924; nonetheless, the full term 'dermatofibrosarcoma protuberans' was proposed by Hoffmann in 1925 [12–15]. The 2012 guideline by the National Comprehensive Cancer Network (NCCN) states that 'typical' DFSP is an uncommon, low- to intermediate-grade sarcoma of fibroblast origin [16].

Information on the incidence patterns of DFSP is still somewhat limited. In a series of 240 patients from the Memorial Sloan-Kettering Cancer Center, New York, NY, there was equal distribution between men and women [17]. Population-based data from the Surveillance, Epidemiology, and End Results (SEER) Program for 1973 to 2002 showed that DFSP's overall annual incidence in the United States was 4.2 per million inhabitants. Women had slightly higher rates of incidence than men (4.4 vs. 4.2 per million per year), the difference being of borderline statistical significance. Interestingly, an ethnic disparity was detected, with annual incidence among African Americans (6.5 per million) being almost double the incidence among Caucasians (3.9 per million) [18]. Data from other SEER Program registries reviewed for the period from 1992 to 2004 demonstrated an overall DFSP incidence of 4.5 per million inhabitants per year and confirmed a higher incidence in women than in men (4.7 vs. 4.4 per million per year, respectively) and in African Americans than in other races [19]. The tumor can occur at any age, yet its incidence peak was observed in patients in their 40s [19]. The largest population-based study of DFSP so far, derived from a cohort of almost 7000 patients observed in the years 2000 to 2010, confirmed its higher incidence among women and African Americans [20]. Somewhat similar trends were shown by data from the Alberta Cancer Registry, Alberta, Canada, where the overall incidence was roughly twice as high as previously reported, 9.3 per million per year. Over the study period (1988 to 2007), this incidence was found to increase by 3.2% per year in women and decrease by 2.7% per year in men [21]. The available European data are as follows: over 3 cases per million inhabitants per year in Eastern France, with men affected 1.2 times more often than women [22], and a more frequent incidence in men than in women (4.4 vs. 4.0 per million per year, respectively) in Sweden [23]. The annual incidence in Denmark for the years 2000–2012 was 5.3 cases per million inhabitants [24]. This relative rarity of DFSP is reflected in the lack of prospective scientific evidence.

Yet, even if infrequent, DFSP represents the most common dermal sarcoma (about 1% of all soft-tissue sarcomas), more than 1% of all head and neck malignant tumors, and 7% of all head and neck sarcomas [25,26].

2. Review of the Literature

2.1. Clinical Presentation

The clinical picture of DFSP varies from plaquelike or small nodular lesions to large uneven masses [27]. Usually, it is a slow-growing, firm, multinodular lesion. The description 'protuberans' in the name of the entity refers to lumps of tissue that form under the surface of the skin [28]. Yet, it has been observed that some cases of DFSP do not protrude above the skin. Consequently, the French Group for Cutaneous Oncology described several variants of the preprotuberant stage of the lesion. These were varied nonprotuberant plaques lasting for a mean of 7 years before the neoplasm became apparently bulging and nodular [29]. We view these preprotuberant variants as precancers.

Typical or low-to-moderate-grade DFSP is generally characterized by slow growth with a tendency to infiltrate surrounding tissues and to persistently recur locally over time, whereas regional and distant metastases are rare. The tumor cells invade subcutaneous tissue in the form of tentacle-like, or villous, projections through the skin septa and fat lobules and surround the skin appendages. These tumor extensions contain few cells and initially look similar to normal fibrous tracts, which makes difficult to determine the true extent of the lesion [3,30]. This infiltration in subcutaneous fat often resembles a honeycomb pattern [31–33]. The longest preoperative duration of DFSP reported in the literature was 60 years [34]; the longest interval from primary excision to local recurrence was 16 years [35]. The pattern of tumor site location is presented in Table 1.

Table 1. Pattern of DFSP tumor site locations in the body.

Number of Patients	Upper Extremity	Lower Extremity	Trunk	Head or Neck	Other Location
n = 240 [17]	29%	23%	31%	14%	2%
n = 368 [26]	34%	29%	37%	-	-
n = 115 [36]	25%	26%	41%	15%	-

A definitive diagnosis is first made by incisional (true-cut) or, less frequently, excisional biopsy in combination with anatomopathological examination, including histologic morphology and immunohistochemistry staining. Fine-needle aspiration biopsies are less frequently performed nowadays, possibly due to the relative inaccuracy of cytologic smears to render the DFSP diagnosis out of a plethora of other spindle cell lesions occurring in the skin and soft tissue [37]. Histologically, DFSP is similar to benign fibrous histiocytoma and deeply infiltrating dermatofibroma. Giant-cell fibroblastoma, occurring predominantly in the first decade of life, is considered a juvenile form of DFSP by some, yet not all, authors [38,39]. Llombart et al. believe that many cases diagnosed in adults actually begin in childhood [30].

2.2. Pathological Findings

Under a microscope, DFSP tumor cells present as uniform spindle cells arranged in a characteristic well-defined storiform or cartwheel-like pattern; they have minimal cytologic atypia, uniform nuclei, absent-to-low mitotic activity, and characteristically stain intensely for CD34 [1,3,36,40–43]. CD34 is a monomeric 115 kDa glycoprotein primarily expressed on normal hematopoietic progenitor cells. A further immunohistochemical profile of DFSP cells includes positive staining for apolipoprotein D and nestin and negative staining for factor XIIIa, stromelysin III, HMGA1, HMGA2, tenascin, D2-40, and CD163 [30]. Possible histologic variants of the neoplasm include pigmented (or Bednář tumor), myxoid, myoid, granular = cell, sclerotic, and atrophic DFSP, giant-cell fibroblastoma, and DFSP with fibrosarcomatous transformation [30,44,45]. However, some authors argue that sclerosis in DFSP may represent an expression of spontaneous tumor regression and discredit the existence of the sclerotic variant of the neoplasm [46]. Composite tumors have also been described [8,47].

Importantly, the above microscopic picture differs in case of fibrosarcomatous transformation. Then, fibrosarcomatous foci look as follows: the cells are mostly fusiform with enlarged atypical nuclei and are often CD34 negative, and cytologic atypia and a high mitotic count are present. In contrast to the storiform pattern in classical DFSP, fibrosarcoma cells grow in a herring-bone arrangement [6,7,34,48]. After Enzinger and Weiss, an important criterion of the diagnosis is that the fibrosarcomatous component must be present in at least 5% of the tumor's volume, whether primary or recurrent [16,34,49,50]. Reports by pathologists indicate that such lesions can be with partial fibrosarcomatous transformation or purely fibrosarcomatous DFSPs encompassing the whole tumor mass [34,45,50]. In the Abbott study of 41 cases, fibrosarcomas arose in 38 (93%) de novo tumors and in 3 (7%) recurrent tumors [50]. In the fibrosarcomatous component of 18 DFSPs from the Goldblum study, 17 resembled fibrosarcoma and 1 malignant fibrous histiocytoma. All these tumors expressed CD34 in the DFSP component but only nine (50%) in the fibrosarcomatous component [42]. In an earlier smaller series, mere focal CD34 immunoreactivity was present in the fibrosarcomatous portion in only one (14%) of seven tumors [41]. In the Mentzel study, only 15 (45%) of 33 fibrosarcomatous lesions demonstrated CD34 positivity [34]. This loss of CD34 expression of varied degree is in line with dedifferentiation in high-grade tumors. Of note, fibrosarcomatous transformation has been linked with the overexpression of p53 protein [6,45,50]. One study suggested the loss of the honeycomb pattern in subcutaneous fat infiltration during fibrosarcomatous change [31]. In another study, necrosis, a high mitotic rate (>10 mitoses per 10 high-power fields), and the presence of pleomorphic areas in fibrosarcomatous DFSPs tended to be related to poor clinical outcomes [34]. Therefore, whether necrosis is a distinctive feature of high-grade DFSP requires confirmation. Table 2 outlines the principal differences between typical DFSPs and cases with fibrosarcomatous transformation. Clearly, fibrosarcomatous transformation heralds a potential for a more aggressive course.

Table 2. Principal clinicopathologic differences between typical dermatofibrosarcoma protuberans (DFSP) and DFSP with fibrosarcomatous change. G1—well differentiated, G2—moderately differentiated, G3—poorly differentiated.

Feature	Typical DFSP	DFSP with Fibrosarcomatous Change
Histologic grade	Low to moderate (G1–G2)	High (G3 present in at least 5% of the mass)
Mitotic activity	Absent to low	High
CD34 positivity	Always present	Often absent
p53 expression	Low-level	Increased
Cellular arrangement	Storiform pattern	Herring-bone pattern
Tumor behavior	Indolent growth of a small mass	Often quick growth of a larger mass
Presence of pain	Rarely present	Often present
Interval to recurrence	Longer	Shorter
Distant metastases	Never or very rarely present	Can be present

Angouridakis et al. stated that approximately 85–90% of all DFSPs are low-grade tumors, whereas the remaining 10–15% contain a high-grade tumor component. This transformation, when presenting in more than 5% of the tumor's volume, leads to a higher incidence of local relapse and distant metastasis [25]. Consequently, the unusual clinical behavior of transformed DFSPs has received special attention from researchers. The most frequent seems to be the above-mentioned fibrosarcomatous change, yet it is not the only one possible. For example, in a Hungarian study of eight lesions with de novo sarcomatous change present, there were five fibrosarcomatous and three malignant fibrous histiocytomatous transformations [51]. Another report described a typical DFSP with several slowly growing recurrences progressing to malignant fibrous histiocytoma over a period of 13 years [4]. Nowadays, malignant fibrous histiocytoma is frequently referred to as pleomorphic dermal sarcoma.

The clinical behavior of the transformed tumor is difficult to predict. Rare studies where histologic comparisons of primary lesions with their consecutive local recurrencies were conducted strongly suggest a gradual replacement of the typical storiform pattern by the fibrosarcomatous herring-bone pattern [52]. Dedifferentiation (that is, the loss of initial differentiation) and increased nuclear atypia and mitoses have been observed in recurrent and metastatic tumors [52].

2.3. Genetic Studies

Of interest, genetic background can be detected in the vast majority of DFSP cases. Early research established that more than 90% of all DFSPs arise from unique unbalanced reciprocal translocations of chromosomes 17 and 22: t(17;22)(q22;q13) and usually demonstrate a supernumerary ring chromosome or chromosomes derived from t(17;22). This genetic alteration can be detected by karyotype, fluorescence in situ hybridization (FISH), or reverse-transcription polymerase chain reaction. The FISH technique is superior and recommended as a routine diagnostic tool, especially in cases with unusual histopathological subtypes and/or immunohistochemical features [53]. The above chromosomal rearrangement results in the chimeric fusion between the collagen type Iα1 gene (*COL1A1*) and the platelet-derived growth factor β-chain gene (*PDGFB*) (specifically, in the fusion of exon 2 of *PDGFB* to various exons of *COL1A1*) [54–56]. The gene product, a COL1A1-PDGFβ fusion protein, binds to the constitutively expressed PDGF receptor and causes a constant activation of PDGF receptor β protein tyrosine kinase, which in turn promotes cell growth in DFSP via autocrine growth stimulation [57–59]. Paracrine growth stimulation is also taken into account [30,60]. Further, in an interesting investigation from Sweden, gene expression profiling of tumors with *COL1A1-PDGFB* fusions identified an array of transcriptionally up-regulated genes in the amplified regions of chromosomes 17 and 22 [61]. Studies using a combination of RNA sequencing and FISH indicated that, apart from the canonical *COL1A1-PDGFB* fusion, a collagen type VI α-3 (*COL6A3*)-platelet-derived growth factor D (*PDGFD*) gene fusion is possible and seems to predispose to DFSP localization in the breast [62]. Moreover, a large-scale Taiwanese study on 188 cases identified additional examples of cryptic *PDGFB*-rearranged and alternative *PDGFD*-rearranged DFSPs, including *COL6A3-PDGFD*-positive cases (again, showing a preference for the female trunk, including the breast) and Elastin Microfibril Interfacer 2 (*EMILIN2*)-*PDGFD*-positive cases (which are male-predominant and mostly fibrosarcomatous) [63]. A recent Chinese work detected a heterozygous germline mutation of *ERCC2* in a 19-year-old man with DFSP [64]; *ERCC2* is a protein involved in transcription-coupled nucleotide excision repair.

2.4. Metastatic Potential and Recurrence

Metastatic DFSP is rare, believed by some to occur in no more than 6% of all cases [65,66]. The rarity of metastatic disease has been linked to DFSP's superficial location, low-to-intermediate histologic grade in the vast majority of cases, and generally small size [65]. Metastasis primarily occurs via the hematogenous route. It typically spreads to the lungs [66,67], yet bones, including the rib cage, the brain, and the heart are other known sites of spread [66]. The detailed postmortem studies published are the most saddening because they testify that such a systemic spread can be virtually to all organs and tissues [3,52,68]. From one study, unusual sites of metastasis were the peritoneum, axillary lymph node, and thoracic vertebrae [49]. The course of the generalized disease can be fulminant [52].

Rare instances of lymphatic spread have been reported as singular case reports. For example, in 1974, Bonnabeau et al. presented a DFSP patient who developed multiple pulmonary and pleural metastases [69]. In a 1975 review of the world literature, Brenner et al. found 17 patients with hematogenous spread and six patients with spread to the lymph nodes, and these authors reported a seventh patient with regional node metastases at that time [70]. Three years later, Kahn et al. published an update of the account, stating as follows: 'More than 400 patients with dermatofibrosarcoma protuberans have been reported in the literature, including the present case, five of these patients had lymph node metastases, 17 patients had hematogenous spread, and three had both lymphatic and blood-borne metastases' [71]. Although infrequent, both hematogenous and lymphatic metastases emphasize the need for a long-term follow-up of the DFSP patient after surgical excision. Unfortunately, distant metastases can arise after adequate surgery and without prior local recurrence of the primary tumor [3,71].

A systematic review comparing oncologic outcomes for DFSP with and without fibrosarcomatous transformation confirmed that the risk of local recurrence, metastasis, and death is significantly elevated in fibrosarcomatous DFSP as compared with DFSP. These are the actual patients who may die from the disease. Therefore, the fibrosarcomatous change in DFSP warrants aggressive treatment and close observation for recurrence and metastasis [48]. Sentinel lymph node biopsy has been advocated in cases with fibrosarcomatous transformation [25]. Unfortunately, this transformation is often not recognized until the final histologic diagnosis [26].

A large retrospective cohort study on 188 patients established that recurrence-free survival is highly significantly shorter in tumors with fibrosarcomatous transformation than in typical tumors. Metastatic disease was seen in no patients with typical lesions, whereas it was confirmed in 17.6% (3 of 17) of patients with fibrosarcomatous transformation ($p < 0.001$) [72]. Other exceptions with a high metastatic rate were the McPeak study, where 5 (5.8%) of 86 patients developed metastases and all of them died of the disease [27], and the Abbott study, where 4 (9.8%) of 41 patients developed metastases and 2 patients died of the disease [50]; however, these were selected populations. A retrospective study on 368 patients from two tertiary sarcoma centers found that, in comparison with patients with typical DFSP, patients with fibrosarcomatous transformation were older by approximately 8 years, female, and with larger, painful tumors that were recently rapidly enlarging [26].

A large analysis of 5249 DFSP cases from the National Cancer Database, USA, for the years 2003–2012 looked not only at clinicopathologic but also socioeconomic corelates. In brief, 3.1% of patients died during an average of 51 months of follow-up, yet this figure did not represent cancer-specific mortality only. Mortality from DFSP was significantly associated with lack of insurance, Medicaid and Medicare insurance, high-grade tumor histology, and positive postoperative margins. Interestingly, specialist treatment at an Integrated Network Cancer Program predicted survival. Higher odds of postoperative radiation therapy were associated with large tumor size, high-grade histology, and positive postoperative margins and inversely associated with treatment at high-volume facilities and non-head and neck tumors. Higher second surgery rates were associated with Hispanic ethnicity, and lower rates were associated with the female sex [73].

In a report combining patient data from three sarcoma treatment centers—the Royal Marsden Hospital, London, UK; The Netherlands Cancer Institute Antoni van Leeuwenhoek, Amsterdam, The Netherlands; and the Erasmus Medical Center-Cancer Institute, Rotterdam, the Netherlands—357 DFSP patients were identified, of whom 41 (11.4%) had a histopathologically confirmed fibrosarcomatous transformation, 4 (1.1%) developed distant metastases at a median time of 68 months, and 2 (0.6%) died of the disease. Patients with transformed lesions had significantly larger tumors and more often received radiotherapy as a treatment modality [67].

In the study by Hayakawa et al., a large size of the primary tumor was found to be a statistically significant risk factor for metastases in DFSP. Moreover, these authors reported on a 37-year-old patient who developed lung metastases from a 5 cm tumor with a histology of typical DFSP without fibrosarcomatous transformation and eventually died of the disease. Consequently, in their series of 67 patients, the metastasis rate was calculated to be 1.7% for typical DFSPs and as high as 57% for fibrosarcomatous cases [49]. We are cautious to accept that typical DFSPs can metastasize. We believe that fibrosarcomatous transformation into the least differentiated high histologic grade (G3) is necessary for the generalized spread of malignant cells. Therefore, we speculate that the sole patient from the Hayakawa study who developed metastases from a typical DFSP could have had a tumor which contained the fibrosarcomatous component at slightly less than 5% of the tumor's volume. Then, anatomopathologic diagnosis with the current criteria would still be typical DFSP, even with some fibrosarcomatous foci present.

Systemic dissemination is strongly associated with previous tumor recurrence and fibrosarcomatous transformation within DFSP [57]. In their review of 115 cases, Taylor and Helwig noted that lymphovascular space invasion is rare in DFSP [36]. Let us underline that lymphovascular space invasion can be focal or substantial and will occur in cases of metastatic potential only, that is, in DFSPs with fibrosarcomatous transformation. Therefore, material from cases with fibrosarcomatous transformation should be examined for the presence of substantial lymphovascular space invasion as a risk factor for and in the early event of generalized disease.

2.5. Differential Diagnosis

Initial errant diagnoses of DFSP may include a wide spectrum of entities: cellular dermatofibroma, cellular leiomyoma, cellular neurofibroma, neurofibroma, fibrosarcoma, low-grade sarcoma, low-grade leiomyosarcoma, low-grade malignant schwannoma, low-grade malignant peripheral nerve tumor, desmoplastic melanoma, spindle cell tumor, and dedifferentiated liposarcoma [1,45]. Llombart et al. added protruding scar, morphea, morpheaform basal cell carcinoma, atrophoderma, and vascular malformations to this list [30]. The cytologic differential diagnosis of DFSP was presented by Domanski and Gustafson [37]. Initial misdiagnosis, prolonged time to accurate diagnosis, and large tumor size at diagnosis are common [16].

2.6. Staging and Grading

To date, there is no definitive staging system for DFSP. Some authors apply the American Joint Committee on Cancer (AJCC) Staging Protocol for Sarcoma of Soft Tissue classification [49]. Others studies use a straightforward distinction: primary tumor vs. local recurrence [17]. The NCCN classification is as follows: stage I is local disease, stage II is regional disease, and stage III is distant disease [16]. Somewhat similarly, the 2018 German dermatologic–oncologic practice guidelines provide the following simplified classification: stage I—primary tumor (localized disease); stage II—lymph node metastasis; stage III—distant metastasis [74].

There is a role for imaging techniques in DFSP. Both ultrasound (7.5–10 MHz) and magnetic resonance imaging can be useful in assessing the extent of the tumor prior to surgery. With suspected local recurrent and/or distant disease, lymph node ultrasound and cross-sectional imaging by computed tomography or magnetic resonance are of value [74].

2.7. Treatment

Complete resection is the primary treatment. The modern options include wide local excision (WLE), Mohs micrographic surgery (MMS), and surgery followed by three-dimensional complete circumferential and peripheral deep margin assessment (or CCPDMA) [66,75,76]. All these techniques rely on the microscopic evaluation of the excised surgical margins, which are possibly narrowest for CCPDMA, medium for MMS, and widest for WLE. After CCPDMA, a Tubingen torte technique on slices from paraffin-embedded tissue taken from the entire circumferential and deep surgical margins with a special staining offers a refinement of final histopathologic assessment. Another variant of Mohs surgery, a slow Mohs surgery (SMS), involves excision of the tumor tissue layer by layer until all the tumor cells are removed, and it has proven to be effective in skin cancer. Some studies note that in some patients with vulvar DFSP, a radical vulvectomy was performed [1,65,77]. A systematic review gave a weak recommendation in favor of MMS over WLE for DFSP excision [76]. In MMS, the excised fresh specimen is frozen and sliced into serial sections for microscopic evaluation of complete margins. There is accumulating evidence that modified MMS with horizontal en face sectioning of formalin-fixed paraffin-embedded blocks, known as slow Mohs surgery, provides better results in terms of complete resection and tissue-sparing capabilities [78–80]. Yet the use of MMS is not indicated for patients with fibrosarcomatous transformation [26,72]. In the Ratner study, as many as 80% of patients required several staged Mohs excisions to achieve complete tumor clearance [81].

An important piece of information came from a recent systematic review with a meta-analysis of eight eligible cohort and case–control studies: the performance of $\geq$3 cm margins in decreasing the local relapse rate was found to be highly significantly better ($p < 0.00001$) than that of <3 cm margins [58]. This is in keeping with a detailed microscopic study with three-dimensional modeling. The likelihood that a given width of excision around the macroscopic DFSP tumor would clear its entire microscopic extent was determined to be as follows: a width of 1 cm around the primary tumor would have left microscopic residual mass in 70.7% of cases; a width of 2 cm in 39.7%; 3 cm, 15.5%; and 5 cm, 5.2% [81]. Goldblum et al. put forth an interesting hypothesis that tumors in which clear margins are achieved may represent a less aggressive subset of DFSPs [42].

Accordingly, there is little doubt that local spread and recurrence are due to inadequate excision, namely, failure to perform complete excision [25,82–84]. Three-dimensional reconstruction of DFSPs has demonstrated tricky tumors with highly irregular shapes and frequent finger-like, or tentacle-like, extensions [81]. These characteristic villous patterns of extension into the subcutaneous fat, fascia, and muscles, and, at the same time, the intention of the surgeon to preserve healthy tissue from resection, represent a surgical challenge [25]. Pathologists indicate that, because of the protuberant, infiltrative growth and low-grade cytologic features of typical DFSP, accurate microscopic assessment of margins can be challenging [45].

The understanding of the role of PDGF receptor β protein tyrosine kinase in DFSP has opened up new possibilities for tailored neoadjuvant therapies. Accordingly, since 2006, imatinib mesylate (Gleevec) has been approved by the Food and Drug Administration in the United States and later by European authorities as a single agent for the treatment of inoperable, primary, locally inoperable, recurrent, and metastatic DFSP [57,66,74]. Imatinib is a tyrosine kinase-inhibitor specifically directed at receptors for Colony Stimulating Factor 1 and PDGFR α and β [60]. The initial results of a pooled analysis of two phase II clinical trials were that the agent induced an objective response rate in approximately 50% of the cases [85]. A later retrospective analysis from a leading Polish oncologic institution on the vicissitudes of 15 patients with advanced DFSP treated with imatinib demonstrated the following results: ten (67%) partial responses, two (13%) stable diseases, and three (20%) progressive diseases [60]. In some patients with advanced disease, imatinib was effective in decreasing the tumor size and making the lesion operable. Seven (47%) out of these fifteen patients underwent resection of residual disease and remained free of disease [60]. In another series, thirteen (47%) patients underwent resection of residual disease following imatinib treatment and nine of them remained free of disease, even though the medication was discontinued [86]. A systematic review on imatinib for locally advanced or metastatic DFSP found that of 152 patients, complete response was observed in 8 (5.2%), partial response in 84 (55.2%), stable disease in 42 (27.6%), and progression in 14 (9.2%). A daily dose of 400 mg imatinib seems more appropriate than that of 800 mg; this is in relation to the adverse and severe adverse effects present in the vast majority of patients [87]. One conclusion of the review was that the medication is useful in inoperable DFSP patients [87]. In a French study from 2021, 27 patients with locally advanced DFSP received the tyrosine kinase inhibitors imatinib or pazopanib for a median duration of 7 months; 24 (89%) of them then underwent surgical excision, and during an over 5-year median follow-up, 23 (85%) patients were disease-free [88].

Because DFSP is relatively sensitive to radiation, radiation therapy may be an important treatment option for inoperable tumors or when postoperative margins are microscopically or macroscopically positive, or for tumors with multiple recurrences. Such a therapy may also be considered a primary treatment option for patients in whom wide excision would result in significant cosmetic or functional impairment. The target volume includes the tumor itself plus any scar(s) from previous surgery plus safety margins of 3–5 cm. With curative intent, a single dose of 2 Gy is usually administered five times a week for a total dose of 60–66 Gy (when microscopic evidence of tumor cells exists) or 66–70 Gy (when there is macroscopic evidence of residual tumor). In a palliative setting, and depending on tumor site and surrounding vital structures, a total dose of 50 Gy may be sufficient [74]. Adjuvant radiation of the tumor bed following the excision of DFSP is not recommended. A systematic review of 12 retrospective clinical trials showed only a weak trend towards lower local recurrence rates after adjuvant postoperative radiotherapy compared to surgery alone [89].

2.8. Prognosis

Let us underline that the existing hard data for the overall prognosis in DFSP are reassuring. Many reported DFSP cohorts noted no presence of metastases nor demise from disease. In an Italian report on 218 patients, the crude cumulative incidence of sarcoma-specific mortality at 5 and 10 years was 1.5% and 2.8%, respectively [83]. The relative 5-year survival in American population-based studies was excellent, at 99.2% (95% confidence intervals: 98.3–100%) [18]. In the Kreicher study, the 10-year relative survival of DFSP patients was 99.1% (95% confidence intervals: 97.6–99.7%) [20]. This generally favorable survival prognosis was confirmed in a recent retrospective analysis where information from the SEER Program for the years 2000–2018 was used. In a cohort of 7567 patients, 89 (1.18%) died of the disease. Significantly higher DFSP-specific mortality was associated with $\geq$10 cm tumor size and high histologic grade (7.07% and 10.08%, respectively) [2].

European guidelines recommend follow-up examinations every 6 months for the first 5 years and at yearly intervals thereafter for up to 10 years. In addition, imaging is reserved for recurrent DFSP or DFSP with fibrosarcomatous transformation, yet without clarification on the interval or type of imaging [57]. The NCCN Guidelines recommend follow-up visits every 6 to 12 months, with regular imaging for patients with high-risk features. Unfortunately, these guidelines do not specify what these high-risk features are, nor do they describe the length of follow-up [12]. In a Dutch study, routine chest X-ray during follow-up did not seem to be useful in patients with typical DFSP, except for those who had fibrosarcomatous changes and thus a relatively high risk for lung metastases [67]. Any suspicious region requires rebiopsy [16]. Patient education about regular self-exams is advised [16].

3. Conclusions

In summary, DFSP is a proliferative condition representing skin sarcomas which are known to locally recur yet very rarely metastasize. It is observed with an incidence of several cases per million inhabitants per year. The vast majority of DFSPs (~90%) harbor unbalanced reciprocal translocations of chromosomes 17 and 22: t(17;22)(q22;q13). Usually, it is a slow-growing, firm, multinodular lesion. Unfortunately, a typical low-or-moderate histologic grade DFSP can undergo sarcomatous transformation to fibrosarcoma or malignant fibrous histiocytoma and such a variant differs both in its histologic composition and clinical behavior. Then, its metastatic spread to all possible organs can be hematogenous and lymphatic and can be the cause of death. Malignant transformation within DFSP (or high histologic grade), older age, being female, large primary tumor size ($\geq$10 cm), narrow surgical margins of excision (<3 cm), surgical margin positivity for tumor cells, short time to recurrence, numerous recurrencies, a tumor that was recently rapidly enlarging, and presence of pain in the tumor have all been proposed as clinicopathologic risk factors for recurrence and metastasis. Wide radial surgical excision with at least 3 cm margins is the gold-standard curative treatment for localized DFSP but may result in functional impairment or cosmetic disfigurement. When needed, skin flap transplantations should be considered, regardless of the patient's age.

4. Future Directions

A repeated surgical excision of low-to-moderate-grade DFSP may offer good local control but may require skin reconstruction with flaps to cover a defect. Such a transplantation should be considered regardless of the patient's age. Cases of typical DFSP with excellent prognosis must be distinguished from fibrosarcomatous DFSP with a much worse prognosis. Adequate staging and grading may be enhanced with modern approaches: anatomopathological evaluation of the presence of lymphovascular space invasion and sentinel lymph node biopsy at DFSP surgery. Both techniques merit further study in fibrosarcomatous DFSP. Possibly, tyrosine kinase inhibitors other than imatinib will offer better disease control in advanced DFSP.

Author Contributions: Conceptualization: M.J.; operative procedure: M.J.; writing—original draft preparation: M.J., K.B. and Z.O.; writing—review and editing: M.J.; funding acquisition: M.J. All authors have contributed substantially to this work. All authors have read and agreed to the published version of the manuscript.

Funding: Funded by the Polish Ministry of Science under the Regional Initiative of Excellence (RID) Program.

Conflicts of Interest: The authors declare no conflicts of interest.

References

1. Edelweiss, M.; Malpica, A. Dermatofibrosarcoma protuberans of the vulva: A clinicopathologic and immunohistochemical study of 13 cases. *Am. J. Surg. Pathol.* **2010**, *34*, 393–400. [CrossRef] [PubMed]

2. Chen, S.; Xiong, L.; Zhao, L.; Li, Y.; Li, L. Survival outcomes and prognostic factors of dermatofibrosarcoma protuberans: A population-based retrospective cohort analysis. *Dermatol. Surg.* **2023**, *49*, 825–831. [CrossRef] [PubMed]
3. Eisen, R.N.; Tallini, G. Metastatic dermatofibrosarcoma protuberans with fibrosarcomatous change in the absence of local recurrence. A case report of simultaneous occurrence with a malignant giant cell tumor of soft parts. *Cancer* **1993**, *72*, 462–468. [CrossRef] [PubMed]
4. O'Dowd, J.; Laidler, P. Progression of dermatofibrosarcoma protuberans to malignant fibrous histiocytoma: Report of a case with implications for tumor histogenesis. *Hum. Pathol.* **1988**, *19*, 368–370. [CrossRef]
5. Aiba, S.; Tabata, N.; Ishii, H.; Ootani, H.; Tagami, H. Dermatofibrosarcoma protuberans is a unique fibrohistiocytic tumour expressing CD34. *Br. J. Dermatol.* **1992**, *127*, 79–84. [CrossRef]
6. Hisaoka, M.; Okamoto, S.; Morimitsu, Y.; Tsuji, S.; Hashimoto, H. Dermatofibrosarcoma protuberans with fibrosarcomatous areas. Molecular abnormalities of the p53 pathway in fibrosarcomatous transformation of dermatofibrosarcoma protuberans. *Virchows Arch.* **1998**, *433*, 323–329. [CrossRef]
7. Sasaki, M.; Ishida, T.; Horiuchi, H.; MacHinami, R. Dermatofibrosarcoma protuberans: An analysis of proliferative activity, DNA flow cytometry and p53 overexpression with emphasis on its progression. *Pathol. Int.* **1999**, *49*, 799–806. [CrossRef]
8. Kholová, I.; Ryška, A.; Dědič, K. Composite tumor consisting of dermatofibrosarcoma protuberans and giant cell fibroblastoma associated with intratumoral endometriosis. Report. of a case. *Pathol. Res. Pract.* **2001**, *197*, 263–267. [CrossRef]
9. Romano, R.C.; Fritchie, K.J. Fibrohistiocytic tumors. *Clin. Lab. Med.* **2017**, *37*, 603–631. [CrossRef]
10. Hashimoto, K.; Brownstein, M.H.; Jakobiec, F.A. Dermatofibrosarcoma protuberans: A tumor with perineural and endoneural cell features. *Arch. Dermatol.* **1974**, *110*, 874–885. [CrossRef]
11. Alguacil-Garcia, A.; Unni, K.K.; Goellner, J.R. Histogenesis of dermatofibrosarcoma protuberans: An ultrastructural study. *Am. J. Clin. Pathol.* **1978**, *69*, 427–434. [CrossRef] [PubMed]
12. Sherwell, S. Morphea. *Arch. Dermatol.* **1890**, *8*, 72–73.
13. Taylor, R.W. Sarcomatous tumors resembling in some respects keloids. *Arch. Dermatol.* **1890**, *8*, 384–387.
14. Darier, J.; Ferrand, M. Dermatofibromes progressifs et récidivants ou fibrosarcomes de la peau. *Ann. Dermatol. Syphiligr.* **1924**, *5*, 545–562.
15. Hoffmann, E. Über das knollentreibende Fibrosarkom der Haut (Dermatofibrosarkoma protuberans). *Dermatol. Z.* **1925**, *43*, 1–28. [CrossRef]
16. Miller, S.J.; Alam, M.; Andersen, J.S.; Berg, D.; Bichakjian, C.K.; Bowen, G.M.; Cheney, R.T.; Glass, L.F.; Grekin, R.C.; Ho, A.L.; et al. Dermatofibrosarcoma protuberans. *J. Natl. Compr. Cancer Netw.* **2012**, *10*, 312–318. [CrossRef]
17. Fields, R.C.; Hameed, M.; Qin, L.-X.; Moraco, N.; Jia, X.; Maki, R.G.; Singer, S.; Brennan, M.F. Dermatofibrosarcoma protuberans (DFSP): Predictors of recurrence and the use of systemic therapy. *Ann. Surg. Oncol.* **2011**, *18*, 328–336. [CrossRef] [PubMed]
18. Criscione, V.D.; Weinstock, M.A. Descriptive epidemiology of dermatofibrosarcoma protuberans in the United States, 1973 to 2002. *J. Am. Acad. Dermatol.* **2007**, *56*, 968–973. [CrossRef]
19. Rouhani, P.; Fletcher, C.D.M.; Devesa, S.S.; Toro, J.R. Cutaneous soft tissue sarcoma incidence patterns in the U.S.: An analysis of 12,114 cases. *Cancer* **2008**, *113*, 616–627. [CrossRef]
20. Kreicher, K.L.; Kurlander, D.E.; Gittleman, H.R.; Barnholtz-Sloan, J.S.; Bordeaux, J.S. Incidence and survival of primary dermatofibrosarcoma protuberans in the United States. *Dermatol. Surg.* **2016**, *42* (Suppl. S1), S24–S31. [CrossRef]
21. Kuzel, P.; Metelitsa, A.I.; Dover, D.C.; Salopek, T.G. Epidemiology of dermatofibrosarcoma protuberans in Alberta, Canada, from 1988 to 2007. *Dermatol. Surg.* **2012**, *38*, 1461–1468. [CrossRef] [PubMed]
22. Monnier, D.; Vidal, C.; Martin, L.; Danzon, A.; Pelletier, F.; Puzenat, E.; Algros, M.P.; Blanc, D.; Laurent, R.; Humbert, P.H.; et al. Dermatofibrosarcoma protuberans: A population-based cancer registry descriptive study of 66 consecutive cases diagnosed between 1982 and 2002. *J. Eur. Acad. Dermatol. Venereol.* **2006**, *20*, 1237–1242. [CrossRef] [PubMed]
23. Hussain, S.K.; Sundquist, J.; Hemminki, K. Incidence trends of squamous cell and rare skin cancers in the Swedish National Cancer Registry point to calendar year and age-dependent increases. *J. Investig. Dermatol.* **2010**, *130*, 1323–1328. [CrossRef] [PubMed]
24. Akram, J.; Wooler, G.; Lock-Andersen, J. Dermatofibrosarcoma protuberans: Clinical series, national Danish incidence data and suggested guidelines. *J. Plast. Surg. Hand Surg.* **2014**, *48*, 67–73. [CrossRef] [PubMed]
25. Angouridakis, N.; Kafas, P.; Jerjes, W.; Triaridis, S.; Upile, T.; Karkavelas, G.; Nikolaou, A. Dermatofibrosarcoma protuberans with fibrosarcomatous transformation of the head and neck. *Head. Neck Oncol.* **2011**, *3*, 5. [CrossRef]
26. Mallett, K.E.; Almubarak, S.; Claxton, R.M.; Ferguson, P.C.; Griffin, A.M.; Rose, P.S.; Wunder, J.S.; Tsoi, K.; Houdek, M.T. Preoperative risk factors for fibrosarcomatous transformation in dermatofibrosarcoma protuberans. *Anticancer Res.* **2022**, *42*, 105–108. [CrossRef]
27. McPeak, C.J.; Cruz, T.; Nicastri, A.D. Dermatofibrosarcoma protuberans: An analysis of 86 cases—Five with metastasis. *Ann. Surg.* **1967**, *166*, 803–816. [CrossRef]
28. Mayo Clinic. Available online: https://www.mayoclinic.org/diseases-conditions/dermatofibrosarcoma-protuberans/cdc-20352949 (accessed on 11 April 2024).
29. Martin, L.; Piette, F.; Blanc, P.; Mortier, L.; Avril, M.-F.; Delaunay, M.; Dreno, B.; Granel, F.; Mantoux, F.; Aubin, F.; et al. Clinical variants of the preprotuberant stage of dermatofibrosarcoma protuberans. *Br. J. Dermatol.* **2005**, *153*, 932–936. [CrossRef]

30. Llombart, B.; Serra-Guillén, C.; Monteagudo, C.; López Guerrero, J.A.; Sanmartín, O. Dermatofibrosarcoma protuberans: A comprehensive review and update on diagnosis and management. *Semin. Diagn. Pathol.* **2013**, *30*, 13–28. [CrossRef]
31. Wrotnowski, U.; Cooper, P.H.; Shmookler, B.M. Fibrosarcomatous change in dermatofibrosarcoma protuberans. *Am. J. Surg. Pathol.* **1988**, *12*, 287–293. [CrossRef]
32. Zizi-Sermpetzoglou, A.; Savvaidou, V.; Fournogerakis, S.; Moustou, E.; Konstantidelli, M.; Vlachakos, N. Dermatofibrosarcoma protuberans of the mons pubis. *Eur. J. Gynaecol. Oncol.* **2012**, *33*, 537–539. [PubMed]
33. Wiszniewska, J.; Roy, A.; Masand, R.P. Myxoid dermatofibrosarcoma protuberans of the vulva: Case report of a rare variant in an unusual location, with unusual morphologic and immunohistochemical features. *Am. J. Dermatopathol.* **2016**, *38*, 226–230. [CrossRef] [PubMed]
34. Mentzel, T.; Beham, A.; Katenkamp, D.; Dei Tos, A.P.; Fletcher, C.D.M. Fibrosarcomatous ("high-grade") dermatofibrosarcoma protuberans: Clinicopathologic and immunohistochemical study of a series of 41 cases with emphasis on prognostic significance. *Am. J. Surg. Pathol.* **1998**, *22*, 576–587. [CrossRef] [PubMed]
35. Orlando, R.; Lumachi, F.; Lirussi, F. Recurrent dermatofibrosarcoma protuberans sixteen years after radical excition. A case report. *Anticancer Res.* **2003**, *23*, 4233–4234. [PubMed]
36. Taylor, H.B.; Helwig, E.B. Dermatofibrosarcoma protuberans: A study of 115 cases. *Cancer* **1962**, *15*, 717–725. [CrossRef]
37. Domanski, H.A.; Gustafson, P. Cytologic features of primary, recurrent, and metastatic dermatofibrosarcoma protuberans. *Cancer* **2002**, *96*, 351–361. [CrossRef]
38. Shmookler, B.M.; Enzinger, F.M.; Weiss, S.W. Giant cell fibroblastoma: A juvenile form of dermatofibrosarcoma protuberans. *Cancer* **1989**, *64*, 2154–2161. [CrossRef]
39. Cin, P.D.; Sciot, R.; de Wever, I.; Brock, P.; Casteels-Van Daele, M.; Van Damme, B.; Van Den Berghe, H. Cytogenetic and immunohistochemical evidence that giant cell fibroblastoma is related to dermatofibrosarcoma protuberans. *Genes. Chromosomes Cancer* **1996**, *15*, 73–75. [CrossRef]
40. Kutzner, H. Expression of the human progenitor cell antigen CD34 (HPCA-1) distinguishes dermatofibrosarcoma protuberans from fibrous histiocytoma in formalin-fixed, paraffin-embedded tissue. *J. Am. Acad. Dermatol.* **1993**, *28*, 613–617. [CrossRef]
41. Goldblum, J.R. CD34 positivity in fibrosarcomas which arise in dermatofibrosarcoma protuberans. *Arch. Pathol. Lab. Med.* **1995**, *119*, 238–241.
42. Goldblum, J.R.; Reith, J.D.; Weiss, S.W. Sarcomas arising in dermatofibrosarcoma protuberans: A reappraisal of biologic behavior in eighteen cases treated by wide local excision with extended clinical follow up. *Am. J. Surg. Pathol.* **2000**, *24*, 1125–1130. [CrossRef] [PubMed]
43. Moodley, M.; Moodley, J. Dermatofibrosarcoma protuberans of the vulva: A case report and review of the literature. *Gynecol. Oncol.* **2000**, *78*, 74–75. [CrossRef] [PubMed]
44. Bednář, B. Storiform neurofibromas of the skin, pigmented and non-pigmented. *Cancer* **1957**, *10*, 368–376. [CrossRef]
45. Jahanseir, K.; Xing, D.; Greipp, P.T.; Sukov, W.R.; Keeney, G.L.; Howitt, B.E.; Schoolmeester, J.K. *PDGFP* rearrangements in dermatomyosarcoma protuberans of the vulva. A study of 11 cases including myxoid and fibrosarcomatous variants. *Int. J. Gynecol. Pathol.* **2018**, *37*, 537–546. [CrossRef] [PubMed]
46. Diaz-Cascajo, C.; Weyers, W.; Borghi, S. Sclerosing dermatofibrosarcoma protuberans. *J. Cutan. Pathol.* **1998**, *25*, 440–444. [CrossRef]
47. de Chadarévian, J.-P.; Coppola, D.; Billmire, D.F. Bednar tumor pattern in recurring giant cell fibroblastoma. *Am. J. Clin. Pathol.* **1993**, *100*, 164–166. [CrossRef]
48. Liang, C.A.; Jambusaria-Pahlajani, A.; Karia, P.S.; Elenitsas, R.; Zhang, P.D.; Schmults, C.D. A systematic review of outcome data for dermatofibrosarcoma protuberans with and without fibrosarcomatous change. *J. Am. Acad. Dermatol.* **2014**, *71*, 781–786. [CrossRef]
49. Hayakawa, K.; Matsumoto, S.; Ae, K.; Tanizawa, T.; Gokita, T.; Funauchi, Y.; Motoi, N. Risk factors for distant metastasis of dermatofibrosarcoma protuberans. *J. Orthop. Traumatol.* **2016**, *17*, 261–266. [CrossRef]
50. Abbott, J.J.; Oliveira, A.M.; Nascimento, A.G. The prognostic significance of fibrosarcomatous transformation in dermatofibrosarcoma protuberance. *Am. J. Surg. Pathol.* **2006**, *30*, 436–443. [CrossRef]
51. Szollosi, Z.; Nemes, Z. Transformed dermatofibrosarcoma protuberans: A clinicopathological study of eight cases. *J. Clin. Pathol.* **2005**, *58*, 751–756. [CrossRef]
52. Onoda, N.; Tsutsumi, Y.; Kakudo, K.; Ozawa, A.; Niizuma, K.; Ohkido, M.; Osamura, R.Y. Pigmented dermatofibrosarcoma protuberans (Bednář tumor). An autopsy case with systemic metastasis. *Acta Pathol. Jpn.* **1990**, *40*, 935–940. [PubMed]
53. Salgado, R.; Llombart, B.; Pujol, R.M.; Fernández-Serra, A.; Sanmartín, O.; Toll, A.; Rubio, L.; Segura, S.; Barranco, C.; Serra-Guillén, C.; et al. Molecular diagnosis of dermatofibrosarcoma protuberans: A comparison between reverse transcriptase-polymerase chain reaction and fluorescence in situ hybridization methodologies. *Genes. Chromosomes Cancer* **2011**, *50*, 510–517. [CrossRef]
54. Simon, M.P.; Pedeutour, F.; Sirvent, N.; Grosgeorge, J.; Minoletti, F.; Coindre, J.M.; Terrier-Lacombe, M.J.; Mandahl, N.; Craver, R.; Blin, N.; et al. Deregulation of the platelet-derived growth factor β-chain gene via fusion with collagen gene *COL1A1* in dermatofibrosarcoma protuberans and giant-cell fibroblastoma. *Nat. Genet.* **1997**, *15*, 95–98. [CrossRef] [PubMed]
55. Vanni, R.; Faa, G.; Dettori, T.; Melis, G.B.; Dumanski, J.P.; O'Brien, K.P. A case of dermatofibrosarcoma protuberans of the vulva with a *COL1A1/PDGFB* fusion identical to a case of giant cell fibroblastoma. *Virchows Arch.* **2000**, *437*, 95–100. [CrossRef] [PubMed]

56. Patel, K.U.; Szabo, S.S.; Hernandez, V.S.; Prieto, V.G.; Abruzzo, L.V.; Lazar, A.J.; López-Terrada, D. Dermatofibrosarcoma protuberans *COL1A1-PDGFB* fusion is identified in virtually all dermatofibrosarcoma protuberans cases when investigated by newly developed multiplex reverse transcription polymerase chain reaction and fluorescence in situ hybridization assays. *Hum. Pathol.* **2008**, *39*, 184–193.
57. Saiag, P.; Grob, J.J.; Lebbe, C.; Malvehy, J.; del Marmol, V.; Pehamberger, H.; Peris, K.; Stratigos, A.; Middelton, M.; Basholt, L.; et al. Diagnosis and treatment of dermatofibrosarcoma protuberans. European consensus-based interdisciplinary guideline. *Eur. J. Cancer* **2015**, *51*, 2604–2608. [CrossRef]
58. Chen, Y.; Jiang, G. Association between surgical excision margins and outcomes in patients with dermatofibrosarcoma protuberans: A metaanalysis. *Dermatol. Ther.* **2021**, *34*, e14954. [CrossRef] [PubMed]
59. Greco, A.; Fusetti, L.; Villa, R.; Sozzi, G.; Minoletti, F.; Mauri, P.; A Pierotti, M. Transforming activity of the chimeric sequence formed by the fusion of collagen gene COL1A1 and the platelet derived growth factor b-chain gene in dermatofibrosarcoma protuberans. *Oncogene* **1998**, *17*, 1313–1319. [CrossRef] [PubMed]
60. Rutkowski, P.; Dębiec-Rychter, M.; Nowecki, Z.; Michej, W.; Symonides, M.; Ptaszynski, K.; Ruka, W. Treatment of advanced dermatofibrosarcoma protuberans with imatinib mesylate with or without surgical resection. *J. Eur. Acad. Dermatol. Venereol.* **2011**, *25*, 264–270. [CrossRef]
61. Köster, J.; Arbajian, E.; Viklund, B.; Isaksson, A.; Hofvander, J.; Haglund, F.; Bauer, H.; Magnusson, L.; Mandahl, N.; Mertens, F. Genomic and transcriptomic features of dermatofibrosarcoma protuberans: Unusual chromosomal origin of the COL1A1-PDGFB fusion gene and synergistic effects of amplified regions in tumor development. *Cancer Genet.* **2020**, *241*, 34–41. [CrossRef]
62. Dickson, B.C.; Hornick, J.L.; Fletcher, C.D.; Demicco, E.G.; Howarth, D.J.; Swanson, D.; Zhang, L.; Sung, Y.S.; Antonescu, C.R. Dermatofibrosarcoma protuberans with a novel COL6A3-PDGFD fusion gene and apparent predilection for breast. *Genes Chromosomes Cancer* **2018**, *57*, 437–445. [CrossRef] [PubMed]
63. Lee, P.-H.; Huang, S.-C.; Wu, P.-S.; Tai, H.-C.; Lee, C.-H.; Lee, J.-C.; Kao, Y.-C.; Tsai, J.-W.; Hsieh, T.-H.; Li, C.-F.; et al. Molecular characterization of dermatofibrosarcoma protuberans. The clinicopathologic significance of uncommon fusion gene rearrangements and their diagnostic importance in the exclusively subcutaneous and circumscribed lesions. *Am. J. Surg. Pathol.* **2022**, *46*, 942–955. [CrossRef] [PubMed]
64. Zhang, Q.; Ju, Y.; You, X.; Sun, T.; Ding, Y. Case report: Identification of a novel heterozygous germline *ERCC2* mutation in a patient with dermatofibrosarcoma protuberans. *Front. Oncol.* **2022**, *12*, 966020. [CrossRef] [PubMed]
65. Soergel, T.M.; Doering, D.L.; O'Connor, D. Metastatic dermatofibrosarcoma protuberans of the vulva. *Gynecol. Oncol.* **1998**, *71*, 320–324. [CrossRef] [PubMed]
66. Jeremic, J.; Stefanovic, A.; Jeremic, K.; Jovic, M.; Pilic, I.; Cvetkovic, A.; Stojanovic, M. Giant dermatofibrosarcoma protuberans vulvae: Rare clinical presentation and literature review. *J. BUON* **2019**, *24*, 1289–1295.
67. Huis in 't Veld, E.A.; van Coevorden, F.; Grünhagen, D.J.; Smith, M.J.; van Akkooi, A.C.; Wouters, M.W.; Hayes, A.J.; Verhoef, C.; Strauss, D.C.; van Houdt, W.J. Outcome after surgical treatment of dermatofibrosarcoma protuberans: Is clinical follow-up always indicated? *Cancer* **2019**, *125*, 735–741. [CrossRef]
68. Ishii, T.; Koide, O. An autopsy case of metastasizing protuberant dermatofibrosarcoma. *Acta Pathol. Jpn.* **1975**, *25*, 503–515. [CrossRef]
69. Bonnabeau, R.C., Jr.; Stoughton, W.B.; Armanious, A.W.; Cuono, C.B.; Mossburg, W.L.; Lancaster, J.R. Dermatofibrosarcoma protuberans. Report of a case with pulmonary metastasis and multiple intrathoracic recurrences. *Oncology* **1974**, *29*, 1–12.
70. Brenner, W.; Schaefler, K.; Chhabra, H.; Postel, A. Dermatofibrosarcoma protuberans metastatic to a regional lymph node. *Cancer* **1975**, *36*, 1897–1902. [CrossRef]
71. Kahn, L.B.; Saxe, N.; Gordon, W.G. Dermatofibrosarcoma protuberans with lymph node and pulmonary metastases. *Arch. Dermatol.* **1978**, *114*, 599–601. [CrossRef]
72. Hoesly, P.M.; Lowe, G.C.; Lohse, C.M.; Brewer, J.D.; Lehman, J.S. Prognostic impact of fibrosarcomatous transformation in dermatofibrosarcoma protuberans: A cohort study. *J. Am. Acad. Dermatol.* **2015**, *72*, 419–425. [CrossRef] [PubMed]
73. Trofymenko, O.; Bordeaux, J.S.; Zeitouni, N.C. Survival in patients with primary dermatofibrosarcoma protuberans: National Cancer Database analysis. *J. Am. Acad. Dermatol.* **2018**, *78*, 1125–1134. [CrossRef] [PubMed]
74. Ugurel, S.; Kortmann, R.-D.; Mohr, P.; Mentzel, T.; Garbe, C.; Breuninger, H.; Bauer, S.; Grabbe, S. S1 guidelines for dermatofibrosarcoma protuberans (DFSP)—Update 2018. *J. Dtsch. Dermatol. Ges.* **2019**, *17*, 663–668. [CrossRef]
75. Mohs, F.E. Chemosurgical treatment of cancer of the extremities and trunk. A microscopically controlled method of excision. *Arch. Surg.* **1948**, *57*, 818–832. [CrossRef]
76. Foroozan, M.; Sei, J.-F.; Amini, M.; Beauchet, A.; Saiag, P. Efficacy of Mohs micrographic surgery for the treatment of dermatofibrosarcoma protuberans. Systematic review. *Arch. Dermatol.* **2012**, *148*, 1055–1063. [CrossRef]
77. Mancari, R.; Cioffi, R.; Magazzino, F.; Attademo, L.; Sant'angelo, M.; Taccagni, G.; Mangili, G.; Pignata, S.; Bergamini, A. Dermatofibrosarcoma protuberans of the vulva: A review of the MITO Rare Cancer Group. *Cancers* **2024**, *16*, 222. [CrossRef] [PubMed]
78. Chaput, B.; Filleron, T.; Le Guellec, S.; Meresse, T.; Courtade-Saïdi, M.; Grolleau, J.-L.; Chevreau, C.; Garrido, I.; Gangloff, D. Dermatofibrosarcoma protuberans: Margins reduction using slow-Mohs micrographic surgery. Experience with 35 patients. *Ann. Chir. Plast. Esthet.* **2014**, *59*, 219–225. [CrossRef]

79. Asilian, A.; Honarjou, N.; Faghihi, G.; Saber, M.; Mozafarpoor, S.; Hafezi, H. An experience of slow-Mohs micrographic surgery for the treatment of Dermatofibrosarcoma protuberans: A long-term cohort study. *J. Cosmet. Dermatol.* **2020**, *19*, 2701–2705. [CrossRef]
80. Algarra-Sahuquillo, J.; Llombart, B.; Serra-Guillen, C.; Sanmartin, O. Slow Mohs micrographic surgery for the treatment of genital dermatofibrosarcoma protuberans: A single-center series of 5 cases. *Dermatol. Surg.* **2024**, *50*, 764–765. [CrossRef]
81. Ratner, D.; Thomas, C.O.; Johnson, T.M.; Sondak, V.K.; Hamilton, T.A.; Nelson, B.R.; Swanson, N.A.; Garcia, C.; Clark, R.E.; Grande, D.J.; et al. Mohs micrographic surgery for the treatment of dermatofibrosarcoma protuberans. Results of a multiinstitutional series with an analysis of the extent of microscopic spread. *J. Am. Acad. Dermatol.* **1997**, *37*, 600–613. [CrossRef]
82. Karlen, R.J.; Johnson, K.; Kashkari, S. Dermatofibrosarcoma protuberans of the vulva. A case report. *J. Reprod. Med.* **1996**, *41*, 267–269.
83. Fiore, M.; Miceli, R.; Mussi, C.; Vullo, S.L.; Mariani, L.; Lozza, L.; Collini, P.; Olmi, P.; Casali, P.G.; Gronchi, A. Dermatofibrosarcoma protuberans treated at a single institution: A surgical disease with a high cure rate. *J. Clin. Oncol.* **2005**, *23*, 7669–7675. [CrossRef] [PubMed]
84. Popov, P.; Böhling, T.; Asko-Seljavaara, S.; Tukiainen, E. Microscopic margins and results of surgery for dermatofibrosarcoma protuberans. *Plast. Reconstr. Surg.* **2007**, *119*, 1779–1784. [CrossRef] [PubMed]
85. Rutkowski, P.; Van Glabbeke, M.; Rankin, C.J.; Ruka, W.; Rubin, B.P.; Debiec-Rychter, M.; Lazar, A.; Gelderblom, H.; Sciot, R.; Lopez-Terrada, D.; et al. Imatinib mesylate in advanced dermatofibrosarcoma protuberans: Pooled analysis of two phase II clinical trials. *J. Clin. Oncol.* **2010**, *28*, 1772–1779. [CrossRef] [PubMed]
86. Rutkowski, P.; Klimczak, A.; Ługowska, I.; Jagielska, B.; Wągrodzki, M.; Dębiec-Rychter, M.; Pieńkowska-Grela, B.; Świtaj, T. Long-term results of treatment of advanced dermatofibrosarcoma protuberans (DFSP) with imatinib mesylate—The impact of fibrosarcomatous transformation. *Eur. J. Surg. Oncol.* **2017**, *43*, 1134–1141. [CrossRef] [PubMed]
87. Navarrete-Dechent, C.; Mori, S.; Barker, C.A.; Dickson, M.A.; Nehal, K.S. Imatinib treatment for locally advanced or metastatic dermatofibrosarcoma protuberans: A systematic review. *JAMA Dermatol.* **2019**, *155*, 361–369. [CrossRef]
88. Beaziz, J.; Battistella, M.; Delyon, J.; Farges, C.; Marco, O.; Pages, C.; Le Maignan, C.; Da Meda, L.; Basset-Seguin, N.; Resche-Rigon, M.; et al. Long-term outcome of neoadjuvant tyrosine kinase inhibitors followed by complete surgery in locally advanced dermatofibrosarcoma protuberans. *Cancers* **2021**, *13*, 2224. [CrossRef]
89. Chen, Y.-T.; Tu, W.-T.; Lee, W.-R.; Huang, Y.-C. The efficacy of adjuvant radiotherapy in dermatofibrosarcoma protuberans: A systemic review and meta-analysis. *J. Eur. Acad. Dermatol. Venereol.* **2016**, *30*, 1107–1114. [CrossRef]

MDPI AG
Grosspeteranlage 5
4052 Basel
Switzerland
Tel.: +41 61 683 77 34

Cancers Editorial Office
E-mail: cancers@mdpi.com
www.mdpi.com/journal/cancers

www.ingramcontent.com/pod-product-compliance
Lightning Source LLC
Chambersburg PA
CBHW062045220926
51850CB00010B/2665